Discourse Analysis and Public Life

T. Ensink, A. van Essen and T. van der Geest (eds.)

DISCOURSE ANALYSIS AND PUBLIC LIFE

Papers of the Groningen Conference on Medical and Political Discourse

1986
FORIS PUBLICATIONS
Dordrecht - Holland/Providence - U.S.A.

Published by:
Foris Publications Holland
P.O. Box 509
3300 AM Dordrecht, The Netherlands

Sole Distributor for the U.S.A. and Canada:
Foris Publications USA, Inc.
P.O. Box 5904
Providence RI 02903
U.S.A.

CIP-DATA

Discourse

Discourse Analysis and Public Life: Papers of the Groningen Conference on Medical and Political Discourse / Titus Ensink, Arthur van Essen, Ton van der Geest (eds.).
- Dordrecht [etc.]: Foris
With index, ref.
ISBN 90-6765-149-4
SISO 499.4 UDC 371.334:[614.253+32-057.1]
Subject headings: medical discourse / political discourse.

ISBN 90 6765 149 4

Printed in the Netherlands by ICG Printing, Dordrecht.

CONTENTS

The relevance of discourse analysis

Titus Ensink, Arthur van Essen and Ton van der Geest

Up to a point a good many social problems may be regarded as communicative problems. Thus in psychiatry the problem of schizophrenia may be viewed as a disorder found in the schizophrenic individual. Alternatively, it may be seen as a communicative problem to be found in the communicative network between the individual who is considered a schizophrenic and people in his environment (Bateson 1972: 201-227).

Similary, the problem of getting opportunities in education may be regarded as a problem of intelligence and abilities of the individual pupil. It may, however, also be understood as a problem occurring in the communication between the school and the pupil. More specifically, the problem may be the result of discrepancies between the communicative system of the school on the one hand, and the communicative system to which the pupil is accustomed, on the other.

However, communication may break down not only as a result of discrepancies between the communicative systems of the participants involved in a conversation. The quality of the communication itself may be another contributory factor, as it may diverge from what may be called adequate, appropriate, or effective standards of specific communication types.

Other areas of social life may be mentioned here as well. In interethnic contacts, in contacts between citizens and the authorities, in contacts between doctors and patients, or in business negotiations, the problems that may arise may be taken either as problems that are peculiar to the situation concerned, or as problems that are caused by discrepancies in the communicative means which are used by those involved in the situation. It is clear, then, that one point of view calls for other solutions to the problems at issue than does the other point of view.

If one adopts the point of view that many of the social

problems mentioned so far are communicative in nature, several questions present themselves. The first is whether communicative problems are the core of the social problem or just a manifestation of other problems, be they psychological, cultural, technological, or whatever. In the former case, a change in communicative habits might offer a solution; in the latter, communicative habits as they interact with other aspects of the social organization have to be the focus of attention.

The second question is which aspects of communication are involved in the problem. The use of different communicative codes (without one party noticing the use of a different code by the other party); discrepancies between the different channels of communication (as between the verbal channel and the paraverbal or behavioural channel); different stores of knowledge or expertise that are drawn upon in communication (again: without one party noticing that the other party has different knowledge at his disposal): all these are communicative if different causes of social problems. And while one cause may be operative in one social area, it may be absent from another.

A third point may concern the question as to whether appropriate or inappropriate means (both in a communicative and in a social sense) are used for a specific communicative situation.

As most communication is organized in forms of verbal interaction, an analysis of the social problems as they occur in communication should be directed towards these forms. Verbal interaction, or discourse, is the specific domain of Sociolinguistics. During the last two decades Sociolinguistics has evolved into an important subfield of both Linguistics and the Social Sciences, and in it, several approaches converge. One trend in Sociolinguistics -the 'macro' trend- is directed towards the establishment of relations between society at large and aspects of language structure, notably those aspects which exhibit stratification across relevant social groups. A fresh and considerable impetus to the growth of Sociolinguistics was given when the stratification of different linguistic behaviours across social classes became a central concern of investigators. Especially when attempts were made to bring the results of these investigations to bear on educational policies, the feasibility to develop a discipline that would have a good deal of social applicability seemed to come in sight. That gave a powerful boost to Sociolinguistics, which from then on began to attract an increasing number of students.

Hymes, admittedly the most eloquent programmatic author in the field of Sociolinguistics, in his paper "The scope of Sociolinguistics" drew a distinction between a 'socially realistic linguistics' on the one hand (under which heading would come the type of macro-sociolinguistics referred to above, as well as the kind of micro-sociolinguistics which is oriented towards the analysis of meaning and speech acts in their dependence upon social context) and a 'socially constituted linguistics' on the other. Hymes himself came down on the side of the latter, in which the social functionality of language use was to occupy a central position. From a realistic point of view such an approach has a decided advantage: the functional perspective enables one to adopt a theoretical position which, at least in principle, is empirically correct. But it also provides a basis on which a socially relevant discipline can be erected:

> "The goals of social relevance and social realism can indeed be accomplished only from the standpoint of the new conception (i.e. socially constituted linguistics), for much of what must be taken into account, much of what is there, organized and used, in actual speech, can only be seen, let alone be understood, when one starts from function and looks for the structure that serves it."
>
> Hymes (1977: 197)

Reviewing the present state of the art, one can only conclude that sociolinguistics has evolved into a branch of a 'socially realistic linguistics': research is being carried out on issues bearing on the relationship between 'sociological' and 'linguistics' facts, be it at a macro- or a micro-level. This development may be viewed as an evolution into what Kuhn has termed a 'normal paradigm'. Seen from this point of view, the development seems sound enough. On the other hand, it would seem that the motive of seeking practical social relevance has receded into the background; that the idea of a 'socially constituted linguistics' has not caught on to the extent that Hymes hoped for, and, in part, predicted. One sector of sociolinguistics, however, might be regarded as an exception.

As a subfield of sociolinguistics Discourse Analysis has grown out of an interest in socially and interactionally accomplished forms of language behaviour. Less so than sociolinguistics, Discourse Analysis has had the pretence of developing practical tools that could be applied in social interaction. The method of Discourse Analysis is reconstructive: the position of those involved in the interaction or discourse at the moment of interaction is reconstructed and used as the basis for explaining the verbal behaviour displayed. Since this basis also contains intersubjective elements, to be documented in the judgement of all members of a community or culture, an analysis will reveal cultural assumptions that are part and parcel of the interaction. A typical representative of this approach is Schegloff (1972): the choice of formulating reference to place is dissected in terms of dependence on the way participants (Schegloff's 'members') in the discourse analyse the location of discourse, the membership of the participants, and the topic of discourse. Although in its method and scope Discourse Analysis keeps close to the moment of interaction, and to the position of those taking part in it, the motive for this approach is provided by realism and much less by the wish to develop tools for use in processes of verbal interaction.

For the very reason that Discourse Analysis keeps close to interaction, the question may well be asked whether the results of Discourse Analysis cannot be brought to bear on it. As it is, many investigations in Discourse Analysis are in fact directed towards verbal interaction in institutional settings, such as classroom interaction (Mehan 1979) interethnic communication in different settings (Gumperz 1982 a and b), medical interviews (special issues of the Journal of Pragmatics 5 (1981), nr. 2/3 and Discourse Processes 7 (1984) nr. 2) interaction in the courtroom (Atkinson & Drew 1979).

It is this combination of close attention to the development of interaction and a keen interest in interaction in institutional settings that suggests the possibility of applying the results of one's analysis. This was the central question put before a conference that was held in Groningen in January 1985, and theme around which the papers presented here revolve. Two types of institutional settings were selected for detailed discussion during the conference. Around one of these, the **medical interview**, a rather extensive body of literature has grown up. The other type of situation, the **political interview**, has been investigated to a lesser extent, at least from the point of view of Discourse Analysis. Both settings play an important part in social life. In medical interviews, in which almost every individual is involved from time to time, decisions are prepared which are vital to the health care of people. In political interviews a good deal of the image-building of politicians takes place and information about politics and policies is presented to the public; hence these interviews play a substantial rôle in the functioning of politics and democracy.

Contributors to the conference were invited to present their views on the possibilities of analysing discourse in either of these two settings, for the purpose of discussing the feasibility of translating the results of the analysis into practical applications. It has not been the organizers' intention to restrict Discourse Analysis to a single approach. To prevent such a thing from happening, scholars from a number of different disciplines were asked to present their views on the central issue of the conference. It will be seen that, even if the subject matter is invariably discourse, not every paper constitutes an example of Discourse Analysis in a narrow sense.

As for the **medical interview**, several forms of doctor-patient conversation are discussed. Thus Bax, Berenst, and Houtkoop report on investigations as to general practitioners; Fehlenberg and Van der Geest analyse conversations in psychosomatic ward rounds. Van der Geest also discusses psychotherapeutic conversations. Fisher & Todd, and Candlin & Lucas, finally, deal with medical conversations with regard to family planning.

Another interesting issue concerns the different topics relating to discourse analysis raised by the participants. Symmetry or asymmetry between GP and patient is discussed not only with respect to its specific contents and linguistic and discourse forms but also with regard to its acceptability in terms of social norms. Fisher & Todd, for example, point to some negative medical effects of asymmetry with respect to the prescription of contraceptives and seem to assume that asymmetry for that reason cannot be accepted. Berenst, Fehlenberg and Van der Geest, on the other hand, adopt a more cautious position in that they accept the view that asymmetry is inherent in institutional contexts and therefore cannot be rejected as such, but should be regarded as an essential or at least unavoidable factor. This fact, however, requires that both GP and patient participate in such a way that the medical as well as the relational aspects of conversation are adequately taken into account.

Another aspect of discourse treated with varying degrees of systematicness and detail by at least some authors concerns the emotional side of conversation in medical contexts as a complicating factor in medication. As the patient introduces at least two problems into the conversation, namely his medical problem and his anxiety about the former, Bax demands from the GP that he also responds appropriately to the latter problem, whenever it is signalled to him by his patients. For this conversational problem Bax offers a theoretical framework to properly deal with the description of emotions.

Other points of interest which, however, are only discussed in passing in this volume, concern 1) the analysis of private topics in conversations with schizophrenic patients by Van Bijsterveld, 2) the analysis of summarizing or formulating techniques in the Rogerian sense as employed by GPs (Houtkoop), and 3) the prescription of contraceptives as a social and micropolitical reflection of society (Fisher & Todd).

The methods of analysis used and/or proposed by the contributors also show remarkable and interesting differences.

Bax, Van Bijsterveld, and Candlin & Lucas, for example, present their data in a pragmatic perspective. The analyses of other contributors, however, (Berenst, Fisher & Todd, Houtkoop) are probably best characterized as discourse-analytic and ethnomethodological. All these studies -both pragmatic and ethnomethodological- are interpretive in character and try to detect some qualitative and inherent aspects of only a small set of data in order to arrive at a more detailed insight into what is going on in the special type of medical conversation under investigation. The question of how much an analysis may contribute to or can be brought to bear on society, however, is less explicitly dealt with. The latter question is central in the studies by Fehlenberg and Van der Geest. In order to cope with this very problem these scholars applied certain statistical procedures to a larger set of data in order to find out which conversational techniques may be more functional and meet more effectively the aims of the medical conversation types they investigated. To this end they extracted from pragmatics, linguistics, and ethnomethodology those variables that they considered to be essential for the purpose.

In sum, it may be said that, as for that part of this volume that deals with the medical interview, and for all the diversity in the topics and the lack of total agreement between the researchers as to theory, norms, and analytic procedures, individual contributions show enough overlap to enable the reader to compare the various studies, to differentiate between them, and to arrive at a carefully considered standpoint, for example, as to the direction research ought to take.

The contributions that are brought together in this volume under the heading of **Political Discourse** show a varied picture. First of all, there is the diversity of forms in which political discourse manifests itself. In contributions by Bormann, Ensink, Van Lint, and Schwitalla, political discourse is conceived of as having the form of a specific genre. Bormann looks at the 1984 American Presidential debates between the candidates Mondale and Reagan; Ensink, Van Lint, and Schwitalla discuss political interviews, i.e. interactional settings specially arranged for the purpose, where some person holding a political office is questioned by a reporter. The contribution by Van Eemeren is also oriented towards a specific genre, namely that of argumentative disputes. Van Eemeren tries to establish a normative basis to which this genre should be oriented. His contribution results in a normative model to be applied to forms of debate; as such, his paper does not confine itself to political discourse. An application of the normative model to a (non-naturalistic) political debate is also presented in the paper. Labov & Labov address themselves to the question of the nature of discourse in formal, public settings, as opposed to discourse in informal, everyday situations. In this respect, their paper is very general in scope, and directed towards a pivotal question of sociolinguistics: what is the relation between forms and styles of speech and situations of speech productions? Their approach is demonstrated in the discourse materials of the public hearings on juvenile delinquency by a U.S. Senate Committee in 1975.

A second aspect in which the contributions on political discourse differ concerns matters of method. The contribution by Labov & Labov is the most strictly sociolinguistic one in character. Their contribution aims at describing the behaviour of a few linguistic categories in public speech, namely quantifiers and attributives. The observed behaviour of these categories, notably some inconsistencies in the use of quantifiers and the specific distribution in the occurrence of non-restrictive attributives, is explained by assuming an orientation of speakers in public discourse towards a set of socially shared moral premises. It appears, then, that the method applied by Labov & Labov, combines descriptive linguistic data with interpretive socio-semantic data within a single analytic framework.

The contributions by Schwitalla and Ensink are closely related to Discourse Analysis. In both papers, examples of political interviews are analysed from the point of view of the organization of the verbal interaction. Rights and duties of the participants, their orientation towards the public in whose behalf the interview occurs, and the 'strategic' aims that participants try to achieve, are introduced into the analysis. Schwitalla pursues a line of research which aims at comparing the behaviour displayed in interviews taken from different periods of recent West-German political history. Ensink aims at showing the peculiarities of political interviews with regard to two central issues in Discourse Analysis, namely cooperation and orientation towards 'face'. In his contribution, Bormann tries to show how, in the discourse of the 1984 Presidental Debates, candidateswere oriented towards so-called 'fantasy themes': socially shared, recognizable schemes which organize experience. In his analysis Bormann shows fantasy themes that are typical of the Democratic, 'New-Deal' tradition, as opposed to those typical of the Republican rhetorical style. Lack of consistency in his orientation towards Democratic fantasy themes on the part of Mondale may be one of the causes of the latter's defeat in the elections.

Van Lint in his paper discusses political interviews from the point of view of a 'purist' typology of texts. His approach concerns a search for principles which would make a 'pure' case of text-type of some kind, and then proceed and confront actually occuring interviews with these principles.

Van Eemeren also shows a normative approach. From the function that should be performed by an argumentative dispute -that is to offer a solution to a difference of opinion between parties- a normative model is derived which should warrant the solution of the conflict. The argumentative model appears as an a **priori** model here: it is not derived from an empirical corpus, but is intended to serve as a guideline for both analysing argumentation and actually arguing.

By and large, two questions pertaining to method appear to be important in the papers on political discourse presented here.

Firstly, there is the question as to whether to start from a descriptive or from a normative standpoint. Descriptive approaches can at best describe things as they occur or as they are done. To derive prescriptions from such an approach is to demand a theoretical surplus which cannot automatically be derived from the descriptive apparatus. Normative approaches start from standards that are to be lived up to. Whether or not it is practically feasible to live up to those standards, whether or not the proposed standards are the best that can be conceived of, whether or not the standard itself is susceptible of evaluation, change, or improvement, are questions that are crucial, even if they are not completely answered here.

The second question bears on the distinction between process and product. Discourse is accomplished as an interactional, ongoing process, evolving in time. What can be recorded, observed, analysed, talked about, however, is the frozen product -in the shape of a text- resulting from this process. This state of affairs is an inevitable one: the process itselfs is less open to recording and observation. A good deal of reflection on methodology in the social sciences is devoted to, or taken up by, this question.

The point at issue here, however, concerns another aspect of the same question: if the results of one's analysis are to be useful in developing tools that can be implemented in interaction, then it would be important to know whether an easy 'fit' is possible between these tools and subsequent interaction. Stappers, in his general commentary on the papers collected here, is rather pessimistic on this point. In fact, none of the authors presented here express themselves clearly on this issue. Those starting from a descriptive standpoint present analyses of discourse, without, however, pursuing their analysis further in the direction of practical applicability. Those starting from a normative point of view do not yet seem prepared to tackle the question of how practicable an orientation towards their norms would turn out to be in actual interaction.

All things considered, the conference was a lot more productive in providing answers to questions which it did not want to ask in the first place than in answering the central question itself -that of the practical applicability of the analysis of discourse. As yet no satisfactory answer to the question seems to be forthcoming.

Acknowledgements

It will be seen that several of the contributions to this volume contain translated excerpts from discourse in languages other than English. Naturally the authors have taken great pains to ensure a faithful rendering of these passages. On our part it would be a gross underestimation of the complexities of translating discourse, however, if we did not recognize that such renderings can be but rough approximations of the original.

The conference received financial support from the Netherlands Organization for the Advancement of Pure Research, Z.W.O., from the University of Groningen, and from the Faculty of Arts of Groningen University.

Contributions that are co-authored were presented at the conference by the author whose name appears in first position.

The contribution by Fisher & Todd is different from the paper which Professor Fisher presented at the conference. For this reason no formal discussion of this paper is included in this volume.

The conference was co-organized by J. Berenst. M. Achterhof was extremely helpful in compiling the bibliography. We greatfully acknowledge their valuable and indispensable contributions.

Titus Ensink
Arthur van Essen
Ton van der Geest

1

Interpretations and explanations in discourse

Modes of 'advising' in family planning

C.N. Candlin and J. Lucas

0.1 Purposes

The particular purpose of this study is to offer an account of the interaction between professional and client in the Family Planning Counselling interview. More specifically, to examine critically the roles and frames of reference of the counsellor as she seeks to offer information and counsel to her client. Central to this activity is the concept of "advising", and the study seeks to elucidate what its modes are and how they are realised in terms of pragmatic principle, discoursal structure and linguistic feature. Within this account, it will be argued that "advising" is a complex discoursal activity and one which gives rise to conflicting ideological interpretation. In the course of exploring this activity the study will suggest a number of hypotheses concerning the interpretation of these and other data from similar encounters, wich may, in addition, have more general relevance to discourse analysis. Finally, the study suggests how its results might form part of counsellor and, conceivably, client training, in order thereby, incidentally, to verify its own argument.

0.2 Setting and Participants

Hale Ho'ola Hou (House of New Life) was founded in April 1975, in Kaumakapili Church "out of concern for the lack of affordable medical care for the urban poor of the Kalihi-Palama (Honolulu, Hawaii) area" (see Hale Ho'ola Hou Kalihi-Palama Health Clinic Annual Report 1983). Three criteria guide its action according to the Annual Report, viz. service must be provided (i) at low cost; (ii) in a non-institutional setting, and (iii) by a multi-lingual staff. The clinic is incorporated in the State of Hawaii as a private non-profit corporation and, in 1983, had 17 full-time employees and 4 part-time employees providing family planning, dental and nutrition services in addition to primary medical care. (see Annual Report op.cit.)

The above constitute the four main service components of Hale Ho'ola Hou, viz. Primary Medical Care, Family Planning, Dental Care, and the Special Supplemental Food Program for Women, Infants, and Children (WIC).

0.3 Preliminaries

In the context of FPC it seemed to us that the non-authoritarian relationship between professional and client (as opposed to that, for example, holding between doctor and patient) within a context in which knowledge was being drawn upon to offer information as well as education, might produce discourse which fluctuated along a continuum, the poles of which were information-giving and seeking on the one hand, and the specifying of contra-indicated behavior on the other. If this were so, then to be a cousellor was pragmatically and discoursally difficult, since neither the authoritarian nor the libertarian role would capture what counselling might turn out to be. This "hunch" was one which initial and subsequent discussions both within and outside the clinic confirmed as warranted, as indeed did the available background literature on the practice of Family Planning Counselling.

1.0 The ideology of Family Planning counselling

Why ideology, and what is its relevance to the analysis of discourse? In offering some answer, we take the position that any analysis of language in use has to see such language as the skilled accomplishment of participants in the service of some social goal and not merely in terms of a text-as-object. Such an approach is interpretive, therefore, not merely descriptive, and implies an assessment by the analyst of the degree to which participants feel that they have achieved these particular goals. For some exemplification from the world of psychiatric counselling we may look to Labov and Fanshel (1977). Nonetheless, such an interpretive account will remain inadequate if we cannot, through what is said and meant, infer and explore the social conditions which imbue both particular performances and particular interpretations. To pursue this any study will need to accommodate not only the distinct perceptions of the participants of the nature, purpose and proceedings of the encounters in which they engage, but, we contend, will also have to understand that discourse regularly naturalises participants' values and beliefs in an unconscious manner.

This constitutes our warrant for taking ideology into account and motivates our interest in explanation. In sum, we take the view that participants use language, employ communication strategies and infer particular meanings without often any conscious awareness of how such usages, in given social conditions, act to betray personal, professional and sectional beliefs and values. Ideology in discourse, following Berger & Luckmann (1966) and, especially, de Souza (1983), reflects a view that talk maintains the reality of its participants through the taken-for-grantedness of its realisations and their value. The routines of conversation, in Berger and Luckmann's terms, reinforce the routines and relationships of everyday life, and confirm participants in roles, behaviours and beliefs. Language, in de Souza's (1983) sense, guides action and commits participants to particular values and intentions. Ideology in discourse analysis, following Candlin (1983c) begins from the point that it is crucial, in such analysis, to display and explain how language can work indirectly and under what conditions it can take effect. What this view of discourse does is to capitalise on the suggestion of Berger & Luckmann (1966) and of Habermas (1972) that the presence of an underlying ideology in talk is revealed at moments of communicative crux where participants' subjective realities are questioned, and turns that into a principled procedure. Ideology in this sense implies critique, that is to expose values and beliefs, make explicit role and function, and attempt to explore the degree of speaker's control over presuppositions and implicatures. In short, this approach seeks to demystify hidden yardsticks against which meanings are constructed. It does so by subjecting the use of particular terms, the choice of phonological and lexico-syntactic realisations, the selection of certain conversational strategies and routines, the uptake of force, the awareness by participants of the norms of interaction and interpretation in encounters, to analysis and to critique. Contradictions within FPC are referrable to the relationship of FPC to forces/factors in the social formation. These contradictions, as we shall see,

A
(i) LINGUISTIC
Linguistic/Discoursal/Pragmatic features
(ii) ETHNOGRAPHIC
Activity types, their macro-structure and participants' expected roles
(iii) SOCIOLOGICAL & SOCIAL PSYCHO LOGICAL

Participants' frames within the activity type, their appraisal of the significance and 'fit' of the linguistic features used

LINKED TO

B
(i) DESCRIPTION
Text as object
(ii) INTERPRETATION
Text as skilled accomplishment of participants
(iii) EXPLANATION
Text as socially shaped and socially shaping

Set against a background of IDEOLOGY (i.e. a set of systems/concepts/ values involved in explaining things, connecting events, placing events and objects in the context of patterns structures and causes) and viewed critically not only descriptively

Involving particular RESEARCH SITES, HYPOTHESES, METHODOLOGY, where moments of communicative crux allow us to display the interrelationship with and between A and B and present our results reflexively to those who are involved.

Figure 1

at the macro level work down the line to particular textual choices at the micro level (cf. Fairclough 1985). In one sense, the purpose of FPC is straightforward; in terms of (HHH)

> "The primary purpose of the FPC session is to assist the client (and partner if included) in making informed decisions regarding fertility management" (p.1)

Yet, as Haselkorn (1968) points out,

> "It becomes quickly evident ... that the legimitation of family planning by no means lessens the fact that this is a highly value-laden arena for social work, perhaps as much as it is for those we seek to serve ..."

and Manisoff (1970) reminds us,

> "Since the welfare and health of many families can be significantly improved by family planning, the subject holds unusual significance. Family Planning concepts and accurate information about family planning size, birth control and fertility are not, generally speaking, clearly understood by those with limited education. Public welfare agencies face a distinct challenge and a unique opportunity in dissipating misinformation and confusion"

We have then, a socially significant educational and informational activity, which by virtue of its intimacy and personal relevance cannot but be imbued by an awareness of the need for self-realization and self-determination, yet which is also subject to pressures of broader social policy. As Haselkorn (1968) keenly indentifies,

> "... the rub comes, as it always does, when one attempts to apply abstract values which collide with subsidiary, competing, or conflicting instrumental values."

This conflict is one characteristic of social work in general, not merely in FPC. What makes FPC particulary problematic, in the views of commentators, is that the issue of "individual freedom versus social responsibility" is exacerbated by what Haselkorn (1968) refers to as "the troublesome value dilemmas" surrounding the public's and the counsellor's views about sex, in short, their ideologies.

These views do not only centre around what individuals regard as "acceptable" sexual behaviour, but also touch on individuals' capacities to discuss such intimacies. Less often acknowledged, perhaps, is the pressure upon workers in FPC to take account of current views on the social order, which directs FPC frequently (and explicitly as we have seen, in the case of Hale Ho'ola Hou) to the poor, the immigrant, the indigent, and the medically high-risk. Notwithstanding the protection of the right of the client to decide, enshrined as Manisoff (1970) points out, in US constitutional law, it would be naive to deny that certain groups experience the FPC event as coercive, and, indeed, that certain FPC workers are engaged in debate on the need, for such high risk groups, to prescribe in any case. These issues constitute, for Manisoff (1970) at least, "the opportunity and the danger" for FPC, and point up the more general dilemma in social work of being, in Haselkorn's (1968) phrase: "and agent of change yet (allowing) people the freedom to resist change".

There is,therefore, a continuum to be negotiated between intervention and the preservation of freedom of choice. It is this ideological dilemma which, in our view in this study, characterises the discourse of FPC, and highlights the ambivalence of frame of reference which we have noted in the literature, our interviews, and in our counselling data. To say this, of course, is in no way to deny what our informants consistently stressed, namely, that their relationship was between professional and client, that clients were to be treated as individuals, that they were responsible for themselves, that counsellors as knowledgeable persons were there to present facts and be non-judgemental. What has to be acknowledged is that avoiding being judgemental in the sense of "advocating a unitary value system" (Haselkorn 1968) does not imply that FPC workers, or FPC in general, are without values. What we hope to show also, is that in the world of FPC, "facts" and "information", like language, are not value-free. They exist on a continuum (in this case between presentation and special advocacy) and critiquing that in context is the function of the approach to discourse analysis we are taking, and, we would argue, the approach to FPC training which we would advocate.

Roles of Counsellors and Client

> "We are client and professional - we're giving information that clients don't have. We are informed. We recognize our limitations, we provide services. They're really clients not patients - they're not sick they're paying for a service" (DB personal communication)

It would be wrong, however, to see the counsellor only as a provider of information; as Deeds (1973) puts it, "if information alone led to action, we would not have smoking problems". Some like Deeds, seek to separate information from education, seeing the latter as "going beyond the facts to developing sound family planning practices". In this view, communication with patients inevitably implies conscious intent to influence behaviour but takes two forms, one (which Deeds (1973) calls "counselling") aimed at "providing the patient emotional support and helping him adjust to his condition and reach his potential", the other ("interviewing") which is designed to "facilitate receiving the most pertinent information needed to make medical and educational diagnoses". The essential characteristic remains, however, the freedom of the client to accept or reject advice. Others, like Manisoff (1970) for example, while separating information offering from counselling, elevate the protection of freedom of choice to a role equivalent to both these:

> "Any attempt to issue a flat directive in this imitate province (apart from legal considerations) not only may fail to convince the client to accept family planning but may reinforce suspicion that society, its institutions and especially its Department of Public Welfare seeks to impose denial of parenthood with the many other penalties of poverty" (Manisoff op.cit p.37)

Moreover, the dilemma is highlighted where the client perceives the FPC as "a person with authority and the power to give or withhold financial assistance" and this is set against the injunction on the FPC, again in Manisoff's words, "to fully perceive, understand and accept her role as a provider of social and educational services in the family planning area, (adopting) a positive attitude towards this role if she is to be helpful to clients" (Manisoff op. cit. p. 50)

In sum, the FPC is required to enact the three roles: the giving and getting of information, the providing of support and the clarifying of problems, in an atmosphere of privacy, positiveness, lack of coercion and "non-judgementalism".

In practice, of course, the dilemma of conflicting perceptions of FPC role between FPC and client indicated above, the existence of external pressures from society captured by Manisoff, make the enactment of the ideal roles fraught with difficulty. It seems, for example, that Deeds' distinction between information and education is hard to make in practice, and, for CR in her work, so is the distinction between education and counselling:

> "You usually don't separate the two, it's really difficult to separate, they go hand in hand" (CR personal communication)

What is more, the variation of perspective between client (interestingly, "patient" in CR's account) and FPC is one which, for her, stems from the counselling interview being a "psycho-social, and not just an educational assessment" that is, "there's a reason for the way that the education is being provided" (CR personal communication). A truer picture is probably that of a continuum between information giving and getting appropriate to an interview, counselling with its involvement in preparation for choice, and, beyond the counsellor unless she is medically qualified, the issuing of directives. In short, the lack of sharp distinction between roles is a FPC characteristic, not easily separatable from some territorial imprecision between the spheres of the "educator", the "social worker" and the "counsellor". There will always be some conflict in practice between a non-judgemental stance which advocates clients making their own decisions on their needs, and one which puts a requirement on the FPC to advocate in particular cases some form of birth control. At such moments, the FPC sustains a conflict between a pressure to dispense and the counsellor's general role of providing the options. Haselkorn (1968) indentifies this conflict as a key issue in the profession's search for role-definition:

> "On balance, it is to social work's credit that in its efforts to establish priorities in the hierarchy of values it is struggling to avoid the dangers on the hand of 'heavy-handed invasiveness' and, on the other, 'let-alonism'. In family planning, as in all social planning, finding the raprochement between either stark alternative that is consistent with its democratic value base is the challenge social work increasingly confronts" (Haselkorn op.cit. p.14)

It is the contention of this paper that the negotiation by the FPC of an appropriate place on the continuum, at different points within her encounter with her client, makes extensive demands on her powers of discourse, and, conversely, it is through her discourse that these conflicts and this negotiation become apparent. From this then follows the reflexive issue of the extent to which participants in this process, client and FPC, are aware of the significance in these terms of the transaction in which they are engaged, and the degree to which they see them as a possible source of anomaly and communicative breakdown. On the face of it this is more subtle an approach to the problems of FPC-client interaction than those our informants commonly identified, viz. insufficient language, lack of client feedback and the disturbing presence of partners.

2. Objects of Focus and interpretive procedures

The foregoing has provided a basis upon which to focus on modes of counselling in FPC, and, in particular, to identify some interpretive procedures, appropriate in our view, to the understanding of counselling discourse.

The interpretive procedures we propose have the status of experimental hypotheses which need validation. Such validation may derive from the triangulated evaluation of interested parties, counsellors and clients, and from laboratory experiment. The procedures themselves have a general cause in a conviction that discourse analysis and pragmatics needs to move beyond botanising to the making of more powerful generalisations about the interpretability of naturally-occurring talk. In that sense, such procedures may have more general relevance beyond FPC; they may offer us a way of comparing the value of utterances across activity types. If so, then this paper will have made a modest contribution to a theory of social action. The immediate cause for the procedures is the work of Labov & Fanshel (1977) but the impulse to more generalisable statements in pragmatics and discourse is to be found in the work of Grice (1976), Leech (1983) and Levinson (1983) on conversational maxims and pragmatic principles, Searle's (1969, 1975) work on the conditions on speech acts, the formulations by ethno-methodologists of interpretive procedures in the manner of Cicourel (1972, 1980), and the applications of the above in the applied linguistic studies of Candlin et al (1980, 1981, 1983).

2.0 The Counsellor as Educator versus the Counsellor as Advisor

In Section 1.2 above we have already proposed that the value of the Counsellor's discourse can most appropriately be understood as fluctuating along a continuum as in the following Figure, where at the extreme left we have Pole A "information-giving and -seeking", and at the extreme right, Pole B "specifying contra-indications".

THE COUNSELLING CONTINUUM

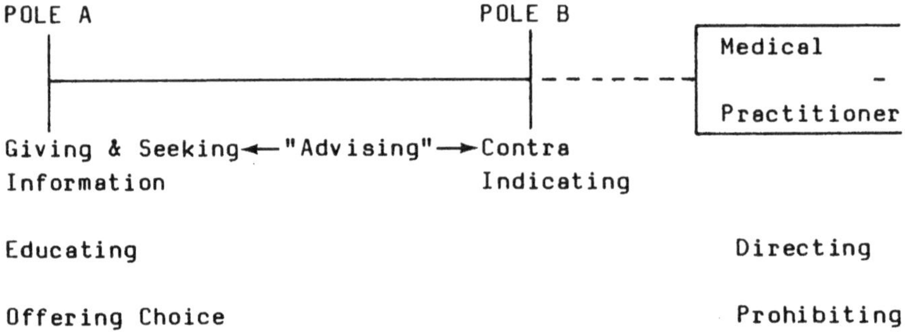

Figure 2

At Pole A, the Counsellor exercises her role as educator, eliciting from the client information of, say, a demographic or medical kind, assessing her knowledge of birth-control procedures and circumstances, and then providing the appropriate information to "fill in gaps". At this pole of the continuum, then, the client is faced with making a decision or a choice (for example of birth-control method, or whether to continue or terminate a pregnancy) and is, ideally, given complete freedom of choice on the basis of this information.

At Pole B, in contrast, the Counsellor is concerned to detect, and thence required the specify those behaviours or conditions of the client which may be medically contraindicated for the decision the client wishes to make. Given, however, that it is the Phsyician's Assistant, or the medical practitioner, who has the authority to issue directives on medical grounds, for example, the refusal to dispense the birthcontrol pill to a heavy smoker, it becomes the responsibility of the Counsellor in her counselling role to "prepare" the client for the possibly prohibitive decision of the medical staff.

> "...if I don't think that she's really not going to be a suitable candidate for the pill ... I have to prepare her for the possibility that the physician's assistant will say 'no, we will not dispense the pill to you' " (CR personal communication)

These two poles capture, however, only part of the interaction between Counsellor and client in FPC. The question arises of what transpires between the two poles? As the Counsellor moves between the two poles, at time drawn towards one or the other, how does her role change and how are these role changes reflected pragmatically and discoursally? It is at this point that we wish to introduce the concept of "advising" as a means of casting light on the nature of this shifting frame of reference. We suggest that as the Counsellor moves along the continuum from Pole A in the direction of Pole B, her discourse takes on the characteristics of advice. In making this assertion, we are, of course, aware that we may be in conflict with the accepted ideology of FPC, as discussed in Section I of this paper. We shall look at one example from our data: Client 3 "JA" has come to the Clinic for a refill of birth-control pills. From her medical chart, the Counsellor sees that not only is JA a heavy smoker, but she is 29 years old, has a family history of diabetes and cancer, and her blood pressure reading has come out slightly above normal - all of which are contraindication of use of the pill. In such a case, information such as:

CR: ... smoking what it does is it changes your circulations and it might be more chance, especially as you get older of strokes

would, we argue, be considered as being offered within the "counselling" frame, and may have been intended by the Counsellor as advice, either to cut down on smoking or to consider another form of birth control. The client, however, who wants both the pill and to continue smoking, prefers to hear the information as "education".

To summarize, what constitutes advice is both complex to determine and discoursally difficult to perform unequivocally. It would seem to involve the following factors, in the context of FPC:

(i) The Counsellor attempts in principle to avoid overt advice, but in the case of contraindicated behaviour must give advice in some form, since she is not empowered to direct

(ii) The client expects to receive advice from the Counsellor but may or may not want to accept such advice in a given case.

As the Counsellor negotiates her place on the continuum between Poles A and B, fluctuating from frame to frame, the client interprets her utterances depending on the frame she perceives the Counsellor to be operating in.

On the basis of this argument, we propose below a set of interpretive procedures for both Counsellor and client, relating in particular to the concept of advice within FPC.

Interpretive Procedure #1

If information given by the Counsellor is directly related to a decision to be made by the client, and to her benefit, such information will be perceived by the client to be advice.

Interpretive Procedure #2

If information which is medically contraindicative is given

by the Counsellor in response to a behaviour or to a request of the client, such information will be perceived by the client to be either advice (or, in its strongest form, prohibition) and will constitute a denial of the request.

Interpretive Procedure #3

If the Counsellor experiences the need to offer advice, she will do so covertly, formulating it as information.

Interpretive Procedure #4

If the client rejects such covert advice, regarding it, for example, as information, the Counsellor must employ other modes of advising.

2. 2. Modes of advising + modes of control

We referred briefly to the question of the giving of advice in relation to the roles and frames of reference of the Family Planning Counsellor. In this context we will address the discoursal modes and strategies employed by the Counsellor in the context of giving advice in FPC, recalling that at the microlevel, FPC as a social institution acts as the "social pivot" between the highest level of the social function and (inter)action. (cf Fairclough 1985 op.cit.)

In particular, we consider these modes of advising in the light of the authority possessed by the Counsellor, both as she perceives it and as it is perceived by her clients. The issue, then, is the negotiation of place on the counselling continuum as the Counsellor goes about the process of advising within the boundaries of her authority.

Much of the authority of the Counsellor arises by virtue of her knowledge and experience in FPC. Within HHH, it is the Counsellor, in this case (CR), a trained social worker, who has expertise in matters which relate to FPC. Her authority has certain limits, however, in that she cannot make medically-related decisions. As we have noted above, such decisions must be referred to the Physician's Assistant.

In her relationship with her clients, the Counsellor in our study stresses that she makes special efforts to de-emphasise her authority, and, in fact, claims to see the concept of authority as detrimental in the establishing and maintaining of an atmosphere conducive to free and open talk between herself and her clients.

> " ... the only way you can have any kind of a good relationship in counselling .. is for the patient to feel she can trust you .. and if you come across as if you're really on a totally different level from what they are, it'll be really difficult for them to open up and let you know what their fears are or what questions they have." (CR: personal communication)

Nonetheless, the role of the Counsellor within her institutional context, and the recourse made to her by her clients, inevitably accord her that ascribed authority. Perceptions of its intensity will, of course, vary from client to client, in part dependent upon the client's background, her experience and her pre-conceived notions of what a Family Planning Counsellor is "like", all in relation to the purposes of the client's visit. A young woman confronted with a very difficult decision, for example, may perceive the counsellor as a caring figure, whereas the client simply intending to obtain birth-control supplies may perceive her as a provider of a service or as a gatekeeper.

Our Counsellor, then, has at least two constraints on her authority:

(i) She lacks the authority to make medically-related decisions
and

(ii) Her awareness of the client's possible perception of her as an authority, constrains her to minimize the authority she does have in order to maintain a relationship with her client of solidarity and trust.

It is our contention that these constraints, taken with earlier comment on the continuum of advice-giving, act to influence the discourse of both Counsellor and client, in particular in the case of the former towards greater indirectness of utterance. An obvious area of application of pragmatics to an understanding of the Counsellor's role, as we have defined it, is that of speech act theory. Indeed, we have already referred explicitly to the work of Searle (1969, 1975) and in stressing the centrality of the concept of "benefit to hearer" and "in the hearer's best interests" to the act of advising, we have already informally drawn on Searlian conditions. We have, however, been at pains to indicate that this concept of "advising", at least as its applies to FPC, is not something that can be identified unerringly. This is not only the case from the viewpoint of the analyst, it is also the case from the viewpoint of the Counsellor, to whom such indeterminacy of performative value is of ideological significance. We find ourselves, then, much in the position of Leech (1977, 1983), concerned that (in his words)

> "...the yes/no conditions imposed by a Searlesque speech-act typology do not justly represent the shifting, continuously variable nature of pragmatic illocutionary force." (Leech 1977 p.3)

Indeed, Leech selects as an example of such speech-actin determinancy the "uncertain boundary", in his words between a directive and a piece of advice. Our data support his contention that this indeterminacy is intentional; necessarily so, we might argue, if the Counsellor is to accommodate the second of the constraints we identify above. FPC, in fact, is an excellent locus for the warranting of Leech's position that it is false to assume that "corresponding to every performative verb there is an illocution in social reality" (Leech op.cit. p.4).

We follow his line, then, that acts are best placed on continua rather than seen as discrete and unproblematically identifiable phenomena. On this argument, then, "advising" would be placed on just such a continuum as we have already placed it (see figure 2), that is, occupying some pragmatic space between "informing" at one Pole and "directing" at the other, on occasion closer to the one and on occasion to the other. (Note here that constraint (i) above compels our Counsellor (CR) to regard "Requesting" as the limit of her pragmatic space, though this would not be true of Counsellors who were RN's (DB personal communication)).

Leech's genial proposal of pragmatic scales offers us the possibility of placing some bounds on these continuous phenomena. In brief, the **cost-benefit scale** specifies how much the act referred to in the propositional content of the speech act is judged to cost or benefit the speaker or the hearer; the **optionality scale** specifies to what degree the performance of the content of this speech act is at the choice of the speaker or hearer, while the third scale, that of **politeness**, is a function of the first two scales; that is, if the cost-benefit factor is held constant, for example, and the optionality factor is increased, the degree of politeness will be increased. If, on the other hand, the optionality factor is held constant and the cost-benefit factor increased, the degree of politeness will also be increased. (For examples of the interplay of these scales, see Leech op. cit.).

In addition to these scales of Leech, we can also have recourse to the proposals of Brown and Levinson (1978) concerning the definition of **politeness**, and its realisation in text. As Leech acknowledges, they augment his analytical proposals. In particular, Brown and Levinson propose a dimension of **power** and a dimension of **solidarity**. **Power** refers to the mutual recognition by both participants that one is in a position of superiority (authority) over another, while **solidarity** refers to the strength of the mutual bond of intimacy between the participants. As a third dimension, they offer that of **imposition**, that is the degree of burden placed or implied by the utterance of one participant upon the other. As with Leech, these axes interact in discourse. The amount of power exercised by one participant over another is calibrated with degree of intimacy between them in the light of the weight of imposition of the propositional content of the proposed message. From the exercise of these variable dimensions derives the degree of indirectness of the utterance, and consequent upon that, the estimation of its degree of politeness.

Leech (1983: p.127) sets out this point as follows:

"(i) the greater the cost of A to h
(ii) the greater the horizontal social distance of h from s
(iii) the greater the authoritative status of h with respect to s
(iv) the greater will be the need for optionality, and correspondingly for indirectness, in the expression of an impositive ..."

FPC consultations provide relevant examples of all these factors, the degree of cost of an action to a client, the amount of optionality that is involved, the degree of power and solidarity between counsellors and client, the act of advising itself. Their interplay affects the quantity and nature of indirectness and the types of politeness strategies used in particular by the Counsellor.

As illustration, we draw upon data from the client #3 "JA". "JA" has presented herself at the Clinic for the primary purpose of obtaining a new supply of birth-control pills. As CR reviews her medical chart, she notices, among several other possible contraindications, that "JA" is 29 years old and smoke cigarettes, both signals that her client is not likely to be a good candidate for the pill, as long as she continues to smoke.

In terms of her authority, CR cannot herself deny "JA" the pills. As we have seen, CR sees her role as preparing the client for the possible subsequent denial of the pill by the medical staff. Whether or not the pill is eventually denied, CR believes that smoking and use of the pill are potentially dangerous to the client. As such, CR sees either a change to an alternative form of birth-control, or abandoning smoking, as preferable courses of action to their concurrent use. The client, on the other hand, sees both changing birth-control method and quitting smoking as being costly to her. The pill is more convenient than other methods, and smoking a pleasurable and too difficult a habit to break.

In terms of the cost-benefit scale, then, the Counsellor perceives a high benefit to "JA's" either changing methods or quitting smoking, whereas "JA" sees both alternatives as very costly. There is no reason why both participants should view the distribution of cost and benefit in the same way. In terms of optionality scale, the degree of optionality from CR's point of view at least, depends on how likely she believes it to be that the Physician's Assistant will refuse to dispense the pill. In terms of power, CR lacks the power to refuse the pill, and in any case, as we have seen, eschews the exercises of overt authority, preferring a relationship of solidarity in which social distance between her and her client is minimized.

How then does the Counsellor exercise the face-threatening act (FTA) (see Brown & Levinson 1978 passim) of advising her client that she should either quit smoking or change her method of birth-control? The data demonstrate a variety of strategies, all of which, in our view, constitute attempts by CR to lead the client towards the realization that the long-term cost not accepting her advice might well outweigh the more immediate cost of abandoning smoking or changing a convenient method of birth-control. In essence,

CR employs a range of strategy: overall she uses negative politeness where she performs the FTA "plus redress to h's want to be unimpinged upon" (Brown & Levinson op.cit.), positive politeness where she performs the FTA plus "redress to h's wants" (Brown & Levinson op.cit.), or going off record and doing the FTA indirectly. What follows is a list of those particular strategies employed by CR in terms of this especially significant encounter. Although it appears from the data to be significant that the strategies are employed in the order that they are, and that the first strategy will typically take precedence in encounters of the type evidenced by "JA's" particular condition, it is likely that other orders of strategy use are both possible and likely, influenced by key variables. Such variables will include: topic of discussion, client type, nature of client's purpose, quality of client's response to the Counsellor on the topic at issue. What we propose here, then, constitutes at best an invitation to further study.

Strategy 1:	Provide relevant information
Strategy 2:	Ascertain h's awareness of this information
Strategy 3:	Shift responsibility for overt FTA to higher authority
Strategy 4:	Focus on A_1 (i.e. giving up smoking) of h but indirectly, with mitigation
Strategy 5:	Abandon focus on A_1 of h, focus on A_2, (i.e issue birthcontrol by contraceptive pills), then resume focus on A_1
Strategy 6:	Claim common ground, empathise
Strategy 7:	Place responsibility on h, be indirect
Strategy 8:	Allocate disproportionate consultation time to A_1 & A_2

(Note: By A_1 here we refer to the issue of giving up smoking, and by A_2 we refer to the issue of birth-control by contraceptive pill)

Soon after the beginning of the consultation, CR employs Strategy #1, that of supplying the information relevant to the issue of smoking and the pill. She explains how the client's family history of both cancer and heart disease could make her a candidate for similar problems, if she takes the pill. She explains how the client's slightly abnormal blood pressure reading might contraindicate her use of the pill. Insofar as this information is known already to the client, we have an instance here of a violation of Grice's (1967) maxim of Quantity. Even the giving of this information is mitigated, however:

> CR: The reason I'm asking you these questions is because sometimes the birth control method you choose can affect your body in different ways and lets say circulation for the pill or hormonal for the pill. which if its family related. you could be more of a likely candidate for that problem .. so we like to know what your family history is .. we like you to be aware of that too.

> CR: It looks like the left side is OK and. like I said. the bottom. this is not to alarm you its just to make you aware.. if its ninety or above there might be some contraindication to the use of the pill or if next time you come back. and its like ten millimetres well want to discuss that since you're using the pill.

Immediately following, CR refers to her client's smoking habit. Here, rather than explaining on-the-record the dangers of smoking and the pill, CR attempts to determine, via Strategy # 2, how much "JA" already knows about the attendant risks. She then fills in the appropriate information.

CR: Ok the other thing that I see from your chart is that you do smoke cigarettes.. do you know about that and how it affects how its affected. with the use of the pill?
JA: Yes I do.
CR: Can you tell me what you know?
JA: Huh
CR: can you tell me what you know?
JA: about smoking and taking the pill?
CR: uh huh
JA: mm ... the risk of getting cancer is higher.
CR: Ok, the risk of cancer with the pill might just be from a hormonal level like if you had cancer in your family, breast

cancer for instance, but smoking what it does is it changes your circulation and it might be more chance especially as you get older of strokes.
JA: Oh

Strategy #3 involves CR telling "JA" that the Physician's Assistant will be talking to her about the problem. In this way, CR escapes the need to accept responsibility for the FTA by placing it on the higher authority.

CR: Uh huh. so thats and you smoke quite a bit and youre twenty nine. so you're in a high risk group so she's definitely gonna talk to you about that today..um, its up. to the physicians assistant if the birth control method is dispensed or not. if its a prescribe method.

Following this, CR begins a line of questioning focussing on the possibility of "JA" quitting smoking (A_1), her reason for smoking, and possible alternatives to this "problem". Once again, CR's questions are heavily mitigated.

CR: have you ever thought about discontinuing smoking?
JA: uh. I thought about it (laughs)
CR: do you think you'd be able to do it?
JA: I don't know (laughs) I guess if I really wanted to.. I've been smoking for a long time.
CR: are you under more stress now?
JA: um. I guess you could say so. yeah cause it was last year that I started smoking more.
CR: do you think if you worked on those things you might be able to cut down?
JA: on the stress you mean?
CR: well. I don't know what the stress is and I don't know if you're open to talking about that but.. from the facial expressions. it seems like you're really hesitant to make a decision to discontinuing smoke. I mean smoking, that gonna have to be something up to you.. do you think if the stress was eliminated that maybe..
JA: I could cut down.

CR: or quit.. for your age its probably better for you to just quit altogether.

CR mitigates even further, saying:

CR: Thats not necessarily a decision you have to make right this minute

and once again refers to the Physician's Assistant, perhaps to justify her persistence in discussing the matter:

CR: I know that B will be talking to you about that. and what we can do is maybe talk about some alternate birth control methods in case she really feels strongly that it wouldn't be real healthy for you to continue using the pill.

With this, CR provides "JA" with a pamphlet on smoking and the pill, and then leaves the topic of smoking (A_1), steering towards the topic of alternative methods of birth-control (A_2). In so doing she effectively approaches A_1 again, but by an indirect route. When "JA" mentions that she has heard about the IUD method, CR takes the opportunity not only to explain the method, but to suggest its particular appropriateness for "JA".

CR: um. the iud might be an appropriate method for you to use since you've had two children.. two full term pregnancies..

After explaining other available methods, CR appears to be moving toward ending the consultation by explaining the examination which is to follow, the hours of the Clinic etc. But before closing the consultation, she hedges, and using Strategy #5, returns to the topic of smoking (A_1) this time referring "JA" to the American Cancer Society for help in assisting her to quit smoking:

CR: I know this is kind of backtracking. um. as far as the cigarettes go. if you feel like you need help with that. theres the American Cancer Society. they have programs to help you with that.
JA: to quit smoking.

CR: yeah..

At this point CR introduces the possibility of her visiting the local mental health clinic, but immediately on performing this more on-record FTA, redresses with negative politeness:

CR: n. if you need a support group or if it gets down to that. and you're going to choose that over the pill or vice versa. or if you felt like whatever stress. you're having is out of control and you don't have insurance at your job. we don't offer that kind of counselling here. all our work is short term but there is a local mental health clinic.
JA: mm mm
CR: according to where you live ... from what I'm getting from you. you seem to be reasonably. a. everythings ok unless I'm not picking up.

The consultation continues, and CR makes use of Strategy #6, claiming common ground as an example of positive politeness, sharing her own experience with smoking and how she (CR) was able to quit:

CR: well. you know it's not easy. cause everybody. well I've got my bad habits too. and its not easy..I smoked for eight years too so I know its not easy.
JA: did you quit?
CR: yeah.

CR's final strategy within the consultation proper is one which returns to the characteristic open-endedness of counselling. Strategy #7 places responsibility for the decision on the client. CR reminds her that now that she is informed of the dangers it is for the client to decide what is best for her. CR also mitigates again here, using phrases such as: "You can't maybe see... but" and "that might make it easier."

CR: I got allergic to the smoke. so that made it easier I think. if there's some reason sometimes that you know it's not good for you. I mean. I knew I could feel the allergy. the bumps on my tongue. for you its the same way. its a little bit different you can't maybe see whats going on with the pill when you're smoking. but if you know from your knowledge has increased now. that might make it easier for you to make a decision about it.

CR: if you feel like you want to come back and talk to me again about alternate birth control. we can do that.. Of course you can always go to another doctor and get pills. but it's just a matter of deciding what's best for you. ok. cause that's kind of how we like to operate.. we like to be concerned with your total health care. ok..

Nonetheless, the references to unseen processes, the possibility of exploring further alternate birth-control methods and the suggestion that non-Clinic doctors might prescribe where the Clinic would not, seem in our view to shift CR towards advising in the negotiation of the pragmatic space between informing and directing action.

We suggest as a final Strategy #8 one which, strictly speaking, is not linked to any particular point within the consultation, nor to any specific utterances. We refer to the proportion of overall consultation time devoted to the twin topics of smoking and the pill. More than two-thirds of the total talking time was so devoted, which indicates its significance to CR (and, presumably to "JA") especially in view of CR's acknowledged complaint that insufficient time was available for client counselling.

In the foregoing we have illustrated how throughout this consultation the Counsellor employs strategies which quite typically shift within the counselling frame along this "advising" continuum. Characteristic in CR's indirectness, evidenced by much mitigation and redressive action, with the client left free to be cooperative or uncooperative. In the remainder of this Section, we wish to examine further this question of cooperativeness, and through more detailed examination to evaluate to complexity of the Counsellor's role and the demands on her pragmatic and discoursal competence.

Central to the concept of FPC, as we have seen, is that the Counsellor and client should interact in an atmosphere of trust and cooperation. Counsellors are there to help and empathise with the concerns and questions of their clients. Indeed, one guarantee of success in FPC is the strength of the relationship that can be established between both parties. To the extent that an atmosphere of cooperativeness and common goal can be created, the more likely that the course of action most conducive to the benefit and lifestyle of the client will be followed. Despite time-pressures, wich in the view of CR "inhibit in-depth counselling", Counsellors should resist decision-making on behalf of their clients. Nonetheless, it would be naive and untrue to surmise that clients and Counsellors will always share the basis of that cooperation, central to the effectiveness of the FPC process. Such a circumstance is provided by the consultation we have been drawing upon in this sub-Section.

To understand the demands made upon CR in this case, we need first to make a distinction within the Gricean concept of "cooperativeness" between that cooperativeness which refers to maintaining the conventions of conversational exchange, for example, responding to questions making such responses relevant to the topic of talk etc., and that deeper cooperativeness which refers to the degree to which the participants share real-world goals. In short, it is routinely possible for co-participants in a discourse to carry out the demands of conversing (cooperating at the level of discourse, if you like) without sharing a common objective for that discourse in terms of the world to which that discourse pragmatically refers. Such a circumstance may regularly be expected in any gate-keeping encounter, one type of which, in part, as we have seen, is the FPC event. In the specific circumstances we outline in this Section, viz. smoking and the birth-control pill, this is characteristically the case. Goals are not shared, since the client wishes the pill (as a convenient mode of birth-control) yet her smoking contraindicates its use, while the Counsellor, as we have seen, has either to suggest abandoning the habit or else advising an alternative mode. Notwithstanding that lack of congruence of real-world goal, the general maxims imposed by FPC on the Counsellor to strive for empathy with her client so as to be able to provide both education and counsel compel her to maintain that discoursal cooperativeness to which we refer. The client, for her part, has her own vested interest in maintaining the discoursal cooperativeness, if only to continue to seek the achievement of her pragmatic goal, viz. that of obtaining both pill and a dispensation to continue smoking. Furthermore, it is the counselling and educative responsibility of the Counsellor to try to bring the client to the point at which she sees the incompatibility.

It is this latter task which constitutes the crux for the discoursal competence of the Counsellor. She specifies contraindicated behaviour, and clearly believes it to be of great benefit to the client if the latter were to change these behaviours. However, because she lacks the authority to be directive, baldly, and in any case does not wish to damage solidarity with her client by being authoritarian, she must find ways to offer advice indirectly. However, in being thus indirect, she also presents the client with the option of rejecting her advice. Furthermore, given the time constraints she is admittedly under, the Counsellor cannot allow the client, in such a crucial circumstances, to move off topic. She needs to maintain client relevance, semantically, discoursally and pragmatically. To do so, she is compelled, we have been arguing, to draw upon a battery of discoursal strategies which in other more canonical cases (such as in police-witness interviews, see Candlin (1983a)) demonstrate the exercise of control, and offer instances of asymmetry. The "powerless" participant (in this case, the client) responds by using particular discoursal strategies, designed to maintain discoursal cooperativeness, and thus to avoid being drawn into a situation where the lack of cooperativeness of pragmatic goal would become obvious and might truncate the encounter. It is precisely to obviate that, and in order to sustain her superordinate goal of maintaining an empathetic relationship with her client that the Counsellor shifts the decision to another authority.

From this assessment we may derive some further interpretive procedures, with which to close this account.

Interpretive Procedure #5

The higher the Counsellor perceives the cost of a medically or socially contraindicated behaviour to a client to be, the more varied strategies of advising she will employ, and the greater time she will devote to discussion with the client of such behaviour.

Interpretive Procedure #6

The greater the degree of mitigation and the greater the indirectness of the Counsellor's advice, the greater will be the optionality on the part of the client to accept or reject the advice.

Interpretive Procedure #7

In order to attain their at times incompatible pragmatic goals, both client and Counsellor will maintain a discoursal cooperativeness in order to sustain the conversation. In the case of the Counsellor, this discourse will, however, be marked by mitigated strategies of discoursal control, in an attempt to keep the client relevant and "on topic". In the case of the client, her discourse will be marked by a high degree of surface cooperativeness, designed to offset her pragmatic uncooperativeness and leave space for its later (possible) attainment.

ACKNOWLEDGEMENTS

Grateful thanks are due to the Executive Director of Hale Ho'ola Hou, Ms Elizabeth Geisting, the Program Coordinator, Ms Margaret Nielsen, and all the Clinic staff for allowing us access on many occasion to the work of the Clinic and for talking time to introduce us to their work and to answer our queries.

We are especially grateful to Ms Candy Radner, the Family Planning Counsellor, on whose work and discourse we came to focus in this study. She allowed us to sit in on her counselling sessions and to audio-record a number of them, and helped us with her comments to understand more fully the delicate relationship between professional and client in her work.

Through the agency of Ms Ceci Ogden of Hawaii Planned Parenthood Inc., we were able to discuss with Ms Diane Baker RN the nature of counselling in an organisation with a different structure and clientele to that of Hale Ho'ola Hou, thus providing a complementary perspective on our study.

Finally, we should like to acknowledge, with considerable gratitude, those clients of the Family Planning Service of the Clinic who gave us access to their counselling sessions and permitted us to make our audio-recordings.

COMMENTS ON C.N. CANDLIN AND J.L. LUCAS

Paul ten Have

The paper by Candlin and Lucas raises a number of important issues concerning a specific type of 'unequal encounter': Family Planning Counselling (FPC). The situation of FPC, as studied by the authors, turns out to be rather complex and FPC discourse may be analyzed in strategic terms as the outcome of ways of dealing with this complexity. On the one hand, counsellors define their work in terms of a general 'ideology of social work'. In this conception clients should be assisted in making their own choices by providing them with relevant information and emotional support. It stresses that counsellors should be non-judgemental and that they should strive for egalitarian and trustful relations with clients. But, on the other hand, in their actual practice counsellors have only a limited amount of time available per client, they work within a larger organization which has the authority to dispense or withhold birth control means, and they have to deal systematically with a rather complicated problem area. This situation makes it hard for counsellors to live up to the ideals of their professional ideology. The paper argues that counsellors are continously making choices from a range of alternatives varying in 'directiveness' and that they put quite an effort in softening and hiding the directive actions that they cannot avoid taking.

More concretely, the authors discuss three kinds of 'frame' that are used by counsellors to structure their encounters with clients. The dominant one is the 'interview', when the Medical Chart gives the agenda for a systematic gathering of information. Gaps in client knowledge, that may show up during this process, may lead to the use of an alternative frame: 'education'. The third frame is that of 'counselling' proper, which is said to include counsellors' "dealing with the present situation of the client, her decisions, her emotional state, her specific needs". The counsellors' intent and the clients' perception as to which frame is relevant at a specific moment may not always coincide. This may specifically be the case when a piece of information may be either seen as 'just information' or as 'advice'. In general the authors note tendencies for advice to be indirect, mitigate, and accompanied by efforts at positive and negative politeness. A parallel set of phenomena is seen to go with the inevitable 'questioning'. Both 'advising' and 'questioning' are suggestive asymmetrical and authoritarian relationships and so run counter to the professed ideology. The authors also note the frequent use of 'formulations' when the counsellors summarize what the client has just said or implied. Although this device is widely used in social work, its 'directive' effects seem to be quite clear. One could also argue that by formulating 'for' the client one suggests that the client's own abilities in this field are somehow defective. To sum up, the authors make it clear that a large proportion of the counsellor's discoursal activities in FPC may be seen as covert forms of asymmetrical, authoritarian and directing behaviour, which are not at all in line with the professed ideology of social work.

As this summary suggests - and as the full text of the paper demonstrates much more clearly - Candlin and Lucas raise many interesting problems for a discourse-analytic treatment of FPC-material. Their discussion uses quite an array of theoretical concepts, including 'ideology', 'strategy', 'frame', 'speech act', 'politeness', and 'interpretive procedures'. They are, I think, successful in evocating the complexities of FPC, but the theoretical articulation of their concepts is not altogether convincing. Neither is it clear to me what precisely their basic analytic framework is.

What I will do in the rest of this brief discussion is to roughly apply some of the general ideas from my own work on doctor-patient interaction to the observations on FPC available in the Candlin-Lucas paper. These ideas are largely drawn from the growing corpus of writings in Conversational Analysis, and specifically from the work of people like Atkinson, Fisher, Frankel, Heritage and Todd. Given the limitations of space and available data my sketch can only be tentative. Although formulated as an analytic alternative, it is at the same time heavily parasitic on the paper that occasioned its formulation here.

The basic idea of such an alternative framework is that participants in a conversation demonstrate, in the situated practices of their utterance construction, how their speech fits into that particular sequential environment, while, at the same time, contributing to the sequential environment for subsequent speakers' utterances. In other words, they 'place' their utterances in their context, which prominently includes preceding utterances, and they 'project' what kinds of utterances can coherently follow theirs. This 'placing' and 'projecting' is done by applying a number of devices for connecting the local instances of speaking with members' typifications of utterances, utterance sequences, interactional formats, and speech exchange systems.

Applying this framework to FPC, we may begin by noting that FPC may be considered a subtype within a much larger class of 'service encounters'. This class of encounters involves two parties, providers and clients, with clear 'rights' and 'duties' for each. These encounters are organized to have one party, the client, give a 'display' of his or her troubles, under the direction of the other, the provider, who is expected to 'do' something with the information given. In this characterization we can already recognize the three types of utterances that together constitute the basic sequence for those encounters. In the first position in this sequence we find utterances by the provider that in some way 'direct' the conversation, i.e. questions. The second position is reserved for trouble-displays and other relevant information given by the client. And in the third position the provider may in some way acknowledge the receipt of the display or show some 'processing' of it. The fact that the provider party has a right to both the first and the last part of this three-part sequence guarantees that this party may - but need not - exercise a tight control over the proceedings. Utterances by providers tend to contain two parts - an acknowledgement and a question - or to be 'double-edged', serving for both third and first position. When this is done, the only way for a client to gain some control over the conversation is by initiating some kind of 'repair' in second position, by giving a 'double-edged' answer, or by adding an initiative to an answer.

Within this large class of service encounters one can observe an extended variety of interactional styles. I should like to suggest four different types as a preliminary of this variety. The first two of these four refer to the style of questioning. In type I the provider controls the exchange strongly by narrow and precise questions which leave the client with only restricted choices, like yes or no, or concrete factual answers. At the other extreme in type II provider questions are little more than general invitations to speak, possibly suggesting an area of discussion and encouraging the client to say what she wants. Corresponding with this type are long, self-directed and story-like evocations of troubles and circumstances. The other two types refer to the variety of options for the third position. In type III acknowledgements are short, neutral or simply deleted, that is, the provider does not show how he or she processes the information given by the client but just goes on to the next question. In contrast, in type IV providers give some elaboration of the preceding displays, a repeat, a summary, formulations of 'gist' or 'upshot'. In this way the information given by the client is, so to speak, preserved for the conversation, for drawing out implications and further discussion 'within' the conversation. These styles seem to imply different 'roles' for the participants and may be combined in various ways. 'Interrogation', for example often seems to combine I and IV, while psychoanalysis may combine II and III. The classical interview style combines I and III, while social work counselling often combines II and IV. As to control of the interaction by the provider, this will be most obvious and direct in type I, but there are also important possibilities for provider control in type IV, by selectively stressing certain aspects or suggesting certain interpretations in a way that established a strong 'preference' for agreement. This type seems specifically efficient for provider-controlled 'conversational mind-work', a kind of interaction that may find the client entrapped in a construction of her 'mind' built up from her own sayings and hard to deny.

Returnings to the FPC material collected by Candlin and Lucas we may say that the counsellors seem to find it hard, given their practical circumstances, to restrict their controlling moves to the third position, although this would be a major recommendation from their ideology. The Medical Chart provides them with a systematic basis for at least touching on all the important aspects of FP problems. This basic 'interview' format can be 'interrupted' at those points when gaps in client-knowledge make themselves felt. At those moments a shift to an 'education' format can be initiated by the client - by a Next Turn Repair Initiator in position 2 - or by the provider - self-initiating in either 1 or 3. In one interesting example, quoted in the paper, the counsellor asked the client for her knowledge - a kind of examination question - as a way to let the client produce a warrant for further 'education' on her part. Such a strategy already takes us in the direction of what I have called 'mind work', where questions are designed to elicit displays that can be 'worked on' in a specific manner in position 3. A practical difficulty in the FPC's studied seems to be that the counsellors do not have the time available that would be needed for a 'complete' social work strategy, combining type II questioning with type IV elaboration. So both the time pressure and the kind of problems she has to deal with - requiring a huge amount of factual information - forces her to use an uneasy mixture of formats and stategies that is only partly compatible with her treatment ideology. So what we can see in the quoted fragments are many signs of 'dispreference', for instance hesitation markers and accounts at the moment of format-switching, and extensive mitigation and other ways of circumlocution when she cannot avoid being 'directive'. On relational and ideological grounds she would prefer to be less imposing, but practical circumstances - time pressure, the necessary 'preparation' for the medical assistant - force her to act differently. The many signs of 'dispreference' attached to what she does do show clients as well as analysts what she would really prefer.

Space forbids that I demonstrate the claims I have made in the above summary treatment. Such a demonstration would also require a more extensive data set. Further research could profitably compare social worker FPC with the ways medical personnel deals with FP problems (see Todd, 1983). Detailed research could throw some lights on both ideological preferences and practical effectiveness of various sequential options open for providers of FPC.

NOTE

Due to space limitations I could not explain the meaning of the various analytic concepts drawn from Conversational Analysis. Accessible overviews can be found in Heritage, 1984, chapter 8, and Levinson, 1983, chapter 6.

2

Friendly persuasions

The negotiation of decisions to use oral contraceptives

S. Fisher and A.D. Todd

Recently Semantha, an 18 year old, middle class, female student told the following tale. She had just become sexually active, and not wanting to get pregnant, she decided to find out more about birth control. She made an appointment at the student health center on campus to attend a twenty minute presentation about the available birth control methods. After carefully considering her options, she decided the diaphragm best met her needs. Her sexual activity was infrequent; therefore, she felt that the risks inherent in the other methods of birth control were not justified. With this decision reached, she made an appointment for her first gynecological examination. After her appointment, she reported the following conversation.

Semantha told the doctor that she had decided on the diaphragm, and he told her that he discourages girls from using them. He described the diaphragm as not as effective as the pill and told her that girls today find it old fashioned. She was not convinced and said that she was afraid of the pill, having heard so many stories about its negative side effects. The doctor claimed that the media has given the pill a bad press and proceeded to persuade her. He said that the majority of users find the pill a very satisfactory method of contraception and suffer no side effects. Semantha was still not convinced. She told the doctor that she didn't feel she needed such a constant method of birth control. He responded by telling her it is better to be safe at all times. She capitulated and left the clinic with a three month supply of low estrogen birth control pills.

Semantha's experience is one example of the numerous tales we have heard and interactions we have observed. Our research suggests that persuasion is more the rule than the exception in the delivery of health care. For doctors, persuasion is often seen as part of the job they have to do. It is their responsibility to insure medical care that is in the patient's best interest. Since patients live in the same social world and frequently share a reciprocal view of the appropriate roles for doctors and patients, it is not too surprising that patients often concur.

This is the functional relationship described by Parsons (1951) as benefitting both doctor and patient. The reciprocal benefit of the doctor-patient relationship has been challenged, however, by patients as well as by those studying the delivery of health care (Waitzken and Waterman, 1974; Freidson, 1970). More specifically, those in the women's health movement have argued that doctors' use of persuasion, while friendly, may not be in women's best interests.

The Context of Persuasion

The moral, political and economic context for the prescription of contraception can be best understood when placed against the background history of the development of the medical profession. The growth of a predominantly male medical profession during the 19th century was closely tied to a redefinition of women's reproductive needs (Barker-Benfield, 1976; Gordon, 1976). Prior to the 19th century, reproduction was seen as a natural process. Women midwives attended and supported but rarely intervened in the birth process. The regular doctors of that time were urban based members of the upper classes who were competing for legitimacy and financial resources. To gain income and status, physicians redefined themselves as male midwives, promulgated a view of female midwives as dirty and ignorant, of birth as dangerous and in need of medical intervention and management, and of women as sickly, irrational individuals always at the mercy of their reproductive organs and in need of medical ministrations (Wertz and Wertz, 1981; Ehrenreich and English, 1978; Gordon, 1976; Barker-Benfield, 1976). As Conrad and Kern (1981) point out, this view of women served a dual function--it made women incapable of providing medical care or getting a medical education while at the same time converting them into an ideal population of patients.

The consolidations of a predominantly male medical profession was more the result of power and privilege than of the development of medical expertise (see Conrad and Kern, 1981, for a more complete discussion of this point).[1] The professional monopoly of regular doctors was enriched by its ties to the monies of the newly formed foundations (e.g., Carnegie) as well as to state and government, ties cemented in class and gender interest (Ehrenreich and English, 1978; Stevens, 1971). These ties when combined with an erroneous and demeaning conception of women and a mood of social reform shaped the medical profession. As Friedson (1970) suggests, one of the organizing features of the profession of medicine is its autonomy. Autonomy combines with a professional monopoly and state support to give physicians top position in the medical hierarchy. Physicians have state supported control over every aspect of their training and practice. They monitor the education, licensure and conduct of their fellow practitioners. By so doing they have nearly total control in determining health care practices and policies. The consumer often has little voice. In more recent years the power of the AMA has been replaced by what Ehrenreich and Ehrenreich (1970) call the "medical industrial complex"--the tremendously profitable corporations that produce drugs and medical supplies, the hospitals, insurance and nursing home industries as well as the medical profession.

This health care system is oriented toward technological cure for acute disease. The medical model is organized to treat dysfunctional body parts. Women seeking reproductive control do not fit easily into that model. Contraception is a preventive measure, not an acute or chronic disease. Once in the medical system, a biomedical framework is laid on. Women are encouraged to manage a situation that is psychosocial and biological in nature within a technological model. This technical fix for a social problem engenders a conflict, which has the potential to have an enormous impact on women's lives, for contraception use can be closely tied to women's sexuality, and family relationship, as well as other moral, political, and economic issues (Todd, 1982; Luker, 1975).

Those who are reaping the benefits from the system as it is currently organized are hesitant to see it change. Their vested interests and financial resources support powerful legislative lobbies which have been successful in resisting and limiting change while maintaining the status quo--a health care system largely under the control of a predominantly male American Medical Association and medical corporate establishment. The male medical profession continues to function as an agent of social control using definitions of health and illness (Freidson, 1970), prescriptions for drugs and contraception (Todd, 1983; Prather and Fidell, 1975) and recommendations for reproductive surgery (Fisher, 1982; Morgan, 1978) to promote and maintain the "proper" roles for women. This control is not the brute force of the police enforced with guns and jail, but rather the much more subtle control of knowledge and skill, supported by institutional authority and used to persuade (Fisher, 1983). Since this control is exercised in the name of alleviating hurt and promoting health it is all the more difficult to perceive. While there have been some changes, women are still underrepresented in the medical profession, overrepresented as medical consumers and dominated by predominantly male physicians (Fisher, 1983; Todd, 1983; Scully, 1980; Ehrenreich and English, 1978; Ruzek, 1978; Corea, 1977; Scully and Bart, 1973).

The organization of the health care system is reflected in medical interactions which are social and, borrowing a phrase (Henley, 1977; Waitzkin and Stoeckle, 1976), micropolitical. They reflect and sustain larger cultural, structural and institutional factors and, in turn, are shaped by them. While medical decisions are interactional accomplishments, the interactants--medical practitioners and patients-- are not equal partners in the decision-making process. Doctors have medical knowledge and technical skill which patients lack. By virtue of their authority they have the ability to act as gatekeepers controlling patients' access to and understanding of contraceptive information.

In this paper we examine doctor-patient communication during the medical interactions through which decisions about contraception are reached and discuss how these interactions are characterized by a style we call friendly persuasion. We analyze how this style is social and micropolitical--how it is accomplished through communication during face-to-face interaction and how the authority of the doctor's role and gender stereotyping combine, contributing to the decision to prescribe birth control pills even when they may not be in patients' best interests. Since it is our purpose to display the intricacies of how contraceptive decisions are accomplished, we use a case study method analyzing three cases in depth.[2] Based on our research, women persuaded to use birth control pills fall into three categories: new users, continuing users claiming side effects described in the medical literature as "nuisance" problems, and continuing users with medical problems acknowledged as potential contraindications for continued use.[3] We chose an illustrative case from each of the categories in which persuasion was likely to occur.

The Research Context

The data for this paper were gathered in five settings in two disparate geographical regions across a combined period of six years. Our observations and data gathering techniques were grounded in the commitment to systematically study a language event, in this case medical interviews. In addition, our research had a similar focus. We were both interested in women's health care. While there is much written about the politics of health care for women (see, for example, Scully, 1980; Ehrenreich and English, 1979; Ruzek, 1978; Corea, 1977; Dreifus, 1977), the actual discourse which expresses and maintains the doctor's authority has received much less attention (see Fisher, 1982, 1983; Todd, 1982; West, 1982; Silverman, 1981; Strong, 1979).

Doctor-patient discourse was recorded on audio and video tapes and transcribed for later analysis. We analyzed eighty-four transcripts of medical interviews, blending taped discourse with more impressionistic ethnographic data. It seems reasonable that neither practitioners nor patients say aloud all that contributes to the medical interview process. For example, patients rarely say aloud that they feel unheard, manipulated, and dissatisfied with the medical care they have received. Similary, neither private physicians, staff doctors, nor residents say aloud that patients look like poor women or talk like uneducated women. They do not say that the way patients talk, act, or dress leads them to believe that patients are not responsible, influencing treatment recommendations. Practitioners do not usually say aloud to a patient that she is not smart enough to use a diaphragm. Yet while not said aloud, our observations and interviews with doctors and patients suggest that these factors, and a host of similar ones, contribute to the diagnostic-treatment process.

One of the main benefits of ethnographic research is derived from the time spent in the field. While we were sociologists in medical settings to gather data, we neither began to gather data immediately nor occupied all of our time taping. We spent time talking informally with various staff members asking questions about values, attitudes and practices. We spent time watching interactions and overhearing conversations, as well as consultations. We spent time participating in the functioning of a clinic and a residency training program. This time provided a sense of the social world and made us privy to the beliefs and practices of the participants. But perhaps most importantly it provided a richer background from which to interpret the data.[4]

We observed highly trained specialists--a physician in the private practice of obstetrics and gynecology, staff physicians and residents in the Department of Reproductive Medicine and the specialty of gynecologic oncology (cancer of the reproductive system), and residents in a model family practice clinic. Residents were observed in teaching hospitals where they were under the supervision of attending staff physicians, and in a community health clinic, where they were hired by the hour from nearby hospitals to staff the women's clinic. The medical providers were gynecologists, oncologists (cancer specialists), and family practice providers who were prescribing birth control. They told their patients and reported to us that they considered the birth control pill the most efficient method of contraception available. Their opinions are consistent with general prescription patterns in the U.S. The birth control pill is the major interventionary form of contraception prescribed in the U.S. today.

In our data regardless of the setting, who the practitioners were, what they were doing, or how they were paid the diagnostic-treatment process was characterized by friendly persuasion. We have identified three interrelated persuasive patterns that cut across our data and are exemplified in the cases to be presented. These patterns include: 1) the selective use of science, 2) the selective presentation of information, and 3) the selective use of authority. They are the interactional mechanisms which function to produce decisions about birth control.

1. Scientific information provides medical practitioners with a double edged sword. On the one hand, it supports the institutional authority of medical providers and legitimizes their presentation of contraceptive information. On the other hand, scientific findings can be ignored to make a case for one method over another. Scientific information is used selectively in another way as well. When used in the

service of the doctor,it reinforces authority. When used in the service of the patient, it is overwhelmingly dismissed as a media scare tactic.

2. In the cases to be discussed, the selective presentation of information takes several forms: a systematic downplaying of the negative side effects of the pill, deleting contraceptive options from some discussions while coloring the presentation of contraceptive options in other discussions.

3. The selective use of authority is harder to see. Patients rely on medical practitioners as authorities and medical providers act like authorities. Since none of the patients came to the clinic certain that they wanted a prescription for the birth control pill, the reliance on and use of authority functions to persuade.

It becomes apparent in the analysis which follows how these strategies interweave across the flow of the medical event producing contraceptive decisions and placing patients in a double bind. While medical literature documents many potential health hazard with both the pill and the IUD, doctors in our data systematically pushed for the pill and against the IUD, while ignoring or downplaying all other contraceptive methods. If doctors give information using their directive power to persuade or withhold vital information, the consequences for patients are often similar. Patients are systematically denied the information they need to participate actively in the contraceptive decision, yet this decision-making has the potential to affect their lives. This process can be seen in the first case.

The New User

Sarah is a rather plain looking, quiet spoken, shy Anglo woman dressed in a conservative, middle class style. She is 23, unmarried and has only recently become sexually active. While her stated reason for coming to the family practice clinic is for a Pap smear and a pelvic examination (her first), it quickly becomes apparent that her motivation for coming to the clinic includes a prescription for birth control. During the opening phase of the medical interview the patient brings up the topic of birth control and toward the end of the medical history phase she returns to it.

Patient: Would you be able to prescribe an oral contracep-

tive for me, since you don't know my family history?
Doctor: Well, I was going to talk to you about that. See, you want a birth control pill for birth control?
Patient: Uh huh.
Doctor: Alright, well we ought to talk a little bit about all the different types of birth control and I could tell you about some of the side effects and what are the good effects. First of all, do you want children?
Patient: Yes.

The doctor begins with a discussion of the birth control pill.

Doctor: Ok, well, let's go through them all. There is birth control pills which is a little bit over 99% effective. Which is pretty good odds. If you take them right and don't miss your pills you are going to be in pretty good shape. Uhm, and of course, everybody uses birth control pills. But as you know, anybody that reads the paper knows, that there are some side effects from them. The short term side effects, the biggest one that everybody worries about is the likelihood of blood clots. It's very uncommon, I haven't myself seen one. I haven't had a patient to have it but, of course, everybody knows somebody who's had a patient who's had a blood clot while they were on it and it usually forms in the legs and the reason it's bad is 'cause sometimes it can get into your lungs, cause that kind of problem we see in girls that smoke.
Patient: Uh uh (shakes head no).
After establishing that the patient does not smoke and is not overweight, the resident continues by discussing the side effects of the pill.

Doctor: ...The short term studies look pretty good but// [5]
Patient://What are the short term studies? How long does it run? 5 years?
Doctor: 5 or 10 year studies. You know, uh, the, I think the cancer that everybody worries is the endometrial cancer. Not necessarily cervical cancer, it doesn't appear to be related. Now if you told me your mama had cancer of the womb and my aunt had breast cancer, and my grandmother died of female cancer, then maybe we should talk a little bit more. But that sounds like cancer runs in the family. It doesn't sound like uh, you have any, you know, predisposing uh

factors with cancer, so you know I think we can feel safe on birth control pills. So they're, they're 99% effective and all side effects short term, but there are a lot of little nuisance problems, some ladies have that we can blame on birth control pills. Some ladies seems to have headaches, uh, that never had headaches before. Uh, but I'm talking about this as what has been recorded and this is not you, not just going on birth control pills and gets headaches.// (Patient://uh huh.) Uh, that's happened that some ladies get skin rashes. Uh, some ladies complain that they feel different on these, you're in a worse mood. Uh, I guess that's probably the three biggest complaints that there are.
Patient: Are those short term, are you just suggesting to me what they are?
Doctor: Yeah, usually if you just ride it out in that short term, that means that some ladies get . . . short term headaches... headaches are so common and so many people have them, it is hard to say whether or not birth control pills uh, cause, I mean, if you never had a headache and two weeks after you started taking the pill, you get a horrible headache, we got some (headaches) that the birth control pills start and I think if you uh, hang in there a little bit they will go away, and sometimes we can just adjust the medication in the pills, try a new one and it doesn't cause them. And we can do the same thing with the other little problems ladies get// (Patient://Um hum.) and I think every complaint that has ever come up has been blamed, at one time or another on the birth control pills, so we just hang in there, but most ladies that I prescribe birth control pills for, they, they take them and they go away and they never have problems//(Patient://Um hum.) One thing I will tell you is really not a long term problem, it's sometimes a short term problem. When you decide, I want a child, I think it's good to get off of them six months before you wanna start trying because there's such a thing called post-pill ammenorhea. Which means after you quit the pill there will be several months interval in some ladies where they don't have a period.

At this point the doctor goes into quite a lengthy explanation about how birth controll pills work and what happens physiologically when the patient goes off of them.

He then moves on to the next type of birth control, the IUD (intrauterine device:)

Doctor: The other type of birth control is the IUD. Now what that is is a little coil that we put inside of the uterus and...uh, we're not sure exactly how they work... but they are pretty effective, about 99% effective. Now, but, I don't recommend them for anybody that's never had a baby. Their side effect is that they occasionally cause a pelvic infection which can get into your tubes and cause scarring and infertility. So I never recommend it for someone who definitely wants children, too much risk, and I won't use it. Some doctors may use it, but I don't not on// (Patient://when) not on you, someone who wants babies. Now if you had three children and don't want two more, I think it is pretty well worth the risk.

The doctor moves on to a discussion of barrier methods of birth control (the diaphragm and condom).

Doctor: OK, now you are down the diaphragms. Diaphragms are reported to be anywhere from 85% to 95% effective and what it is, it's a rubber shield that you put over your cervix. You slip it in before intercourse. It's kinda like a guy wearing a condom. Here what you're doing is blocking the pathway of the sperm way to the cervix. You're keeping it on the outside and keeping the egg and the womb on the inside and also you punt a little jelly on it that's fairly effective. When somebody is intelligent and that would take time in putting it in. A lot of people won't take the time to put it in, so if it's not in, it's in the drawer next to the bed, it doesn't work, so that's a reasonable form of birth control. Now the birth control pill is safer uhm, and of course you've got condoms, which are very effective as long as they are intact. They are effective, there's no way, uh, just according to you feelings are toward them// (**Patient:** //Uh hum.) If it's, intercourse, is just as pleasurable for you and your mate well there's no reason not to use it. It's safe as long as you're sure there's not a hole in it.// (**Patient:**// Uh hum.)

And finally he discusses over the counter birth control remedies.

Doctor: OK, and then there's foams and jellies and uh they are anywhere from 70 to 85 percent maybe. I don't think they are as high as 85 and there are a lot of failure rate on foams and jellies. So I don't recommend them to anybody // (**Patient:**// Uh hum.) I mean if you're playing with fire, you might get pregnant before long, but eventually I think it will catch up with you. Uh, o.k., so that's it.

Patient: OK, let me ask you this, it's kinda a personal question, if your wife had to use a form of birth control what would you give her? What would you recommend?

Doctor: Well my wife, we uh, have used birth control pills in the past, but she doesn't use them now. We have a child, and we want some more. We use a diaphragm. It has been very effective for us// (**Patient:**// Um hum.) and its no side effects, and if she got pregnant accidentally it wouldn't be any great problem, because we want some more children// (**Patient:** //Um hum.) but then I have one couple uh, whose wife has caesarians and the physician feels that there's no way that she should have another child... and she had used a diaphragm for 30 years and she is still fertile... and I feel safe using that. You know I never had a lady get pregnant on the diaphragm, course I don't have a 1000 patients with a diaphragm// (**Patient:**// Um hum.) but as far as I know no one's come back pregnant// (**Patient:**// Um hum.) But you know, for a short period, I don't have see anything wrong with the birth control pills. I don't like them but I don't hate them. Uh, its a hard decision to make. You know that there are a lot of birth control methods around, but they all have their drawbacks. There's not a perfect birth control yet. Well when you decide not to have any more children you are, yours could have your tubes cut, either a vasectomy or have a tubal ligation for you// (**Patient:**/ / Um hum.) that's nice//(**Patient:**//Would take care of it.) it sure does, but you're really gonna have to be the one to make your decision on that// (**Patient:** Um hum.) You plan to get married soon, or...[6]

Patient: Uh huh// (**Doctor:**// OK) it wouldn't be until I get out of school which should be next summer.

Doctor: Well, what would be perfectly acceptable for me, if I was in your shoes, is to be on the birth control pill until next summer for sure, and, uh, that time see how you did on them and if you don't like them you know you can always switch over to a diaphragm or he can switch over to a condom.

Sarah wants information about birth control. Early in the medical interview she brings up the topic and while the resident is taking her medical history, she returns to it. In response to her questions the resident provides quite a detailed description of the available contraceptive methods. Since she exhibits none of the medically excepted cautions for avoiding the birth control pill, there is no family history of cancer, she does not smoke, and she is not obese, she leaves with a prescription for oral contraception (the Pill).

Sarah's interest in contraception coupled with her desire to avoid an unwanted pregnancy is evident in the transcript. Thus, at first glance, the decision reached had qualities of an interactional accomplishment jointly produced by doctor and patient. But while Sarah, and patients in general, do have some input into the decision-making process, it is the doctor who has the authority to persuade. We have included large segments of this transcript to display the persuasive way language is used to influence the patient to choose this method of contraception, persuasive strategies which we have observed frequently in our research. Information is presented selectively. The IUD is efficient but risky, infection and infertility are possible outcomes. A diaphragm is all right if you are intelligent and it is inserted properly, the condom is ok if it is intact, and foams and jellies are not recommended. The doctor explains that foams and jellies are not as safe (in preventing pregnancy) as the birth control pill.

Scientific information is used selectively. Despite several noted risks the birth control pill is advised. When the birth control pill is pushed, the more negative aspects of its use are systematically downplayed. Blood clots and endometrial and breast cancer are all called "short term side effects" and their dangers are qualified. Blood clots are declared uncommon. And, while the evidence is not in yet, endometrial cancer and breast cancer are said not to appear to be related to pill use.[7]

The selective use of authority, while running through the transcripts, becomes more evident as the resident qualifies the major contraindications for taking the birth control pill, and dismisses the minor ones as "nuisance problems." These problems include headaches, mood changes and skin rashes. He tells the patient that if these nuisances appear, all she has to do is "hang in there a little bit, they will go away." He further implies that women often blame problems on the birth control pill when other sources are the culprit. However, studies have shown that these "nuisance problems" can be serious contraindications for taking the pill (see Seaman and Seaman, 1977). Further, when patients come back to doctors with problems they associate with the pill, medical providers can blame the patients, not the pill, for the problems.

Toward the end of the presentation of information about birth control methods, Sarah asks for a recommendation. It is here that the selective use of authority is clearest. She asks: "...if your wife had to use a form of birth control what would you give her?" In response, the resident recommends birth control pills and grounds that recommendation in the patient's status as an unmarried woman who cannot risk pregnancy. This recommendation provides an example of how the doctor, while providing information, also expresses more subtle assumptions about women, family arrangements, childbearing, and birth control.

The Continued User: Nuisance Problems

In the second case, as in the first, the doctor's presentation of information about birth control methods moves the patient toward birth control pills. However, this patient is somewhat different than the last. She is not a first time user of contraception coming to the doctor to learn about the available methods. Rather she has taken birth control pills for five consecutive years, has vague complaints but no strong medically accepted indications for discontinuing them and has come to the clinic to investigate alternative contraceptive methods.

A gynecological resident hired by a community clinic is talking with the patient, Donna, in the examining room. She is a low-income, 22 years old, Anglo woman who is plainly dressed in a skirt and blouse. She has never married, never been pregnant and has given no information in this interview as to how she envisions her future reproductive life. While her birth control pill history has been uneventful, she presently feels a growing dissatisfaction with this method. Recently she has been vaguely uncomfortable. She has occasional headaches and feels "bloated" much of the time. Her concern is that oral contraceptives can have a cumulattive effect on the body. She thinks a break from this method would be advisable and is potentially interested in the intrauterine device (IUD) but knows little about it. In her first question to the doctor she asks:

Patient: What about IUD? I'm really interested in um changing...
Doctor: I, I have a very negative opinion of the IUD, particularly for young women who haven't had their family yet, because if//
Patient://Um, they give it to girls who have abortions and miscarriages. Why, why is that?
Doctor: I think that's because it's, the, the women don't feel that they could take the pill, and it's some, it's some form of birth control, at least. For women who just can't remember to take the pill or won't, that need protection, then the IUD is some you know, is second best. But you're really taking a big chance of infection. We're seeing at least I'd say five in a hundred IUDs that we put in are coming back with some, some sort of infection, often not serious, but it can be very serious. It can mean hospitalization and antibiotics into your veins, and some of them even have their organs operated on or removed because they get so infected, it can even result in death, then, you know, so it's, again, a remote possibility the same as blood clots are with birth control pills, although it's not as remote as that. It happens, it really, you know, much more frequently. Uhm, I think the scariest thing, even if, you know, you don't get an overwhelming infection, with the IUD is that we don't know what we, what your future fertility would be like. The IUD works by causing a little infection inside your uterus and it can climb up inside the tubes and it may destroy the normal structure of the tubes enough so that the egg, which is very small, and the tube, which is also very small, don't fit, and they can get hung up. There's a // (**Patient:** // I see.) higher incidence of ectopic pregnancy, tubal pregnancies, when the egg stops in the tube and then tries to grow into a baby there, with women who've had IUDs. So I, I really think, unless you're really adamant and you, you're willing to take all those chances. I really wouldn't tend, wouldn't recommend it.// (**Patient:**// Oh, I see.) So it sounds like maybe the pill really is the right thing.
Patient: (laugh) Okay, that answer...
Doctor: Do, do your legs swell, is that part of your

problem or do you just feel kinda bloated?
Patient: My, I don't know, my stomach just feels really, like it's out here, you know, very//
Doctor: //uh hum. Sometimes things get blamed on the pills that aren't always the pills' fault so, like// (**Patient:** //What?) women who say they gained weight because they're taking the pills when ordinarily they're expecting to gain weight, so maybe they eat a little bit more, and, uh, then they gain weight, and say, look at the pill made me gain weight.
Patient: But it makes me hungry. When I'm not on the pill, I don't feel hungry.
Doctor: I've never heard that one before (laughs).

Donna, like Sarah, wants information about contraceptive options. Her question about the IUD triggers a response from the doctor which stresses a concern for her reproductive capacity while also reflecting how interactional mechanisms function to persuade. First, scientific information is used selectively. While the resident expresses concern about the IUD, there does not seem to be an equal concern about the birth control pill or the physical complaints the patient associates with taking them. Then information is presented selectively. After discussing the problems associated with the IUD the pill is recommended with no discussion of the diapraghm, condom, foam or jelly, all methods which are available in the clinic. Finally the selective use of authority is evidenced as the doctor's presentation makes it seem that Donna has two contraceptive choices, the IUD or the pill. Whatever the doctor's motives (he may in fact believe that it is in the patient's interest to continue using the birth control pill) he has used the authority of his role to persuade. He provides scientific information selectively by explaining that infections, hospitalization, surgery, and death are all possible effects of the IUD. While blood clots are presented as a remote problem with the pill, they are not dealt with in the same depth as were the side effects of the IUD. Further, the resident declares that while infection and death from the IUD are serious, the "scariest" outcome is infertility. By stressing infertility as the most serious possibility, the doctor[8] uses the authority of his role to reinforce a traditional assumption: young women center their life priorities around motherhood. By omitting detailed discussion of contraceptive options, by excusing the pill and blaming the patient, the case for the pill is made. The patient leaves with another prescription for birth control pills and a conviction that the problems she is experiencing with hunger and bloating are hers. If she could only diet more effectively, her problems would be relieved.[9]

The Continued User: More Major Problems

In the third case, as in the first two, the doctor does not take an active role against the pill. This patient is different than the last two. She is neither a first time user seeking contraceptive information nor does she have vague "nuisance problems" which she associates with birth control use. Rather, she is representative of the category of patients who have medically acknowledged risk factors which raise serious questions for remaining on the pill.

The patient, Amy, is a young, unmarried, sexually active VISTA worker. She is a gregarious Anglo woman dressed in jeans and an embroidered Mexican shirt. Her stated reason for coming to the model family practice clinic is because she needs a prescription for birth control pills. However, throughout the medical interview she expresses her ambivalence about being on the pill, her knowledge of the scientific information about their side effects, and her concern over what she sees as potential contraindications for continuing to use them. In response to the doctor's opening question, the patient states her reason for coming to the clinic and voices her ambivalence about the birth control pill.

Doctor: Nice to meet you. What are you doing here?
Patient: I'd like maybe to get a prescription for the pill. I'm on it now and I'm just about at the end of the month and ah I'm not sure I want to continue taking it but I do want a prescription for it.
Doctor: Ok, what alternatives do you have in mind if you don't continue taking the pill?
Patient: I don't know yet, that's why I'm probably going to take it.
Doctor: Do you think that//
Patient://But I want to get a prescription, but I'm not sure if I want to keep taking it or not. I don't like taking 'em you know.

Doctor: Have you any problems with it before?
Patient: No, I haven't had any problems.

While the patient claims not to have had any problems on the birth control pill, she discloses a concern-- a possible contraindication for continuing on the pill.

Doctor: Well, are you having any other problems or things we need to direct our attention to today?
Patient: OK, there is another thing that has been weird. I don't know what's causing it. I've been getting these cramps in my legs. Once in a blue moon I'll get 'em, just out of the clear blue sky, and I always thought that on the pill there's a sort of relation, you need to know about that and smoking too, you know. But I was on the pill, I've only been on the pill for about five months.
Doctor: Never before that?
Patient: Yeah, I was off it. I was on it, I was off the pill for over two years.
Doctor: When did you start taking the pill?
Patient: I don't remember the year. I was on the pill for two years or so, I went off it a little more than two years and I just started again. Now I am usually in perfect and never feel a cramp in my body whatsoever, but I was about four weeks ago, or something like that I was in Nashville, and I got the strangest, it won't go away, it was all the way up along in here in my leg and it lasted all day, hurt like anything. It wouldn't do like this. It felt really tight. I didn't know if it was my circulation or my muscle and then last week the same thing happened on this leg. But it wasn't near so bad. It didn't last as long and like I worry so I don't like, but that's all there was just that weird cramping sensation in my leg.
Doctor: I worry too, ah cramps, muscle cramps are a reason or a caution like in birth control pills. Uhm, it's, ah, one thing that makes doctors think that maybe it shouldn't be taking birth control pills.
Patient: Um hum, well that's why I'm here, to check into that.
Doctor: And the fact that you smoke and take birth control pills increases your risk of cardiovascular disease// (Patient: //Um hum, I know that.) about ten times and you're skirting several risk factors. There you really have a backing on that. You're young and have a lot of reserve and

all that sort of stuff. The longer you take oral contraception the more chance// (**Patient:**//uh hum) of some of the side effects and that happen to you ah, if there is a reasonable alternative to birth control pills for you, I would urge you to give it serious consideration.

Patient: I do really get bad cramps (menstrual) when I don't take the pill.

Doctor: When you don't take the pill?

Patient: When I don't take the pill. When I am on the pill everything is under control. No cramps whatsoever, a very light flow. It's nice and comfortable. When I'm off the pills it's like unusual cycles// (Doctor:// um hum) terrible cramps (menstrual).

Doctor: Which string of pills are you taking now?

Patient: Norlestrin or something, they call them.

Doctor: Norlestrin, right.

Patient: Is that mild?

Doctor: Uh hum.

Patient: That's what they told me.

Doctor: So you haven't had any problems you can relate to the pill?

Patient: They do, when I was off for two years I never had one cramp in my legs, you know or whatever, cause (unintelligible) I'm really, you see, I know facts about some of the pills that's why I kind of ask for this mild one and they said

Doctor: What facts about the pill were you...

Patient: Just the facts that you read on that I know there could be a chance of a problem, you know, side effects with them// (**Doctor:**//yes) I don't care to get a blood clot or you know// (**Doctor:**//yes) stuff like that, but then again I don't want a baby. But there's other birth control methods, I'm sure. But like I was saying, I get very sick when I am on my period and ah my cycle is always irregular, you know so I//

Doctor://You kind of have to weigh the benefits of bad things about it and come to a decision about whether the good outweighs the bad// (**Patient:**//I know.) Uh, your risk factors are **annual**. The longer you take the pill, the more you start, and if you have leg cramps it's kinda worse.

Patient: Well like with that leg cramp, I know that's not the part for I went through. Now as soon as it went away, nothing ever happened to my leg, and it scared me, you know and I said well, I want to stay on the pill, but if I get a lot of cramps, I mean that's I don't think I will.

As the medical history continues, the patient disclosed a history of hypertension in her family. In fact her mother has high blood pressure, another possible contraindication for staying on birth control pills. At the close of the medical history portion of the examination the doctor asks:

Doctor: Can you think of anything else that I haven't asked you?
Patient: Trying to think, just cramps at the bottom of my legs that is a concern of mine.
Doctor I think we all occasionally have leg cramps// (**Patient:** //um hum) occasionally is not anything to worry about if it gets to be a pattern then we start to worry.
Patient: Then I'll have to stop taking the pill like I said I probably would sometimes, but...
Doctor: I would be thinking about stopping birth control pills or stopping smoking within the next couple of periods, give a little, OK?
Patient: uh huh.
Doctor: That's, that's, I'm beating my wife in the head trying to get her to stop one or the other.
Patient: She doing both of them too?
Doctor: Yeah.
Patient: I noticed that with two it's really bad. One is bad enough, you know. I know that.
Doctor: Both of them are atrocious, really increase your risk of having problems.

At this point the doctor gets a nurse and the physical examination is performed.

While this medical interview sounds different on the surface, the results are much the same. Amy, like Donna, comes to the clinic concerned about continuing to use the birth control pill. Unlike Donna her complaints are not vague, "nuisance problems" which can be easily dismissed by the medical provider. She has at least three medically accepted risk factors, risk factors that at least signal caution for her remaining on oral contraception. She smokes, has a family history of hypertension, and recently has experienced leg cramps which may indicate cardiovascular problems. Doctor and patient acknowledge these to be serious problems with grave potential consequences, yet, when all is said and done, the patient leaves on the birth control pill.

Why, then, does the patient remain on birth control pills and how is her continued use of them an interactional accomplishment? The transcript gives us several clues. First, Amy tells the doctor more than once that when she is not on birth control pills her periods are irregular and she has severe menstrual cramps. Second, Amy indicates at various intervals that she has come to the doctor for advice, perhaps even for direction. When telling the doctor about the leg cramps and about smoking she says, "You need to know." When the doctor tells her that muscle cramps are a reason to be worried and that such symptoms make doctors think about taking patients off the birth control pills, Amy responds, "that's why I'm here, to check into that." Yet, by the end of the interview, the resident selectively uses his authority to suggest that she stop smoking or stop taking the pill within the next couple of periods. He selectively presents scientific information by telling her, "...we all occasionally have leg cramps", and even more subtly, by acknowledging that his own wife is a smoker and a birth control pill user. By so doing he encourages the patient to stay on the birth control pill. More obviously, the doctor selectively presents information. He does not give Amy the facts she needs to reach an informed decision. He does not discuss with her the seriousness of continued use of the birth control pill nor does he give her information about other forms of contraception. He uses the authority of his role to withhold information in another way as well. He does not share his medical knowledge about ways to manage menstrual distress other than the birth control pill.[10] While there is no completely satisfactory contraceptive on the market, the patient does have choices beyond the birth control pill or getting pregnant.

Friendly Persuasion

Each of the patients came to these doctors concerned about contraception and each left with a prescription of birth control pills. While all three patients were young, unmarried Anglo women, their experience with the birth control pill and their lives were quite different. Sarah was sexually inexperienced and inquiring about contraception for a relationship that she portrayed as premarital. Neither Donna nor Amy presented themselves with the same innocence and neither of them were first time users of birth control. Both Donna and Amy reported the pill for five years, complained of headaches, bloating, and weight gain. All these are vague but well documented side effects of the pill. Amy, used the pill for two years, rested for two years, and then returned to it, but complained of leg cramps. During the medical interview she disclosed that she also smoked and had a family history of high blood pressure. (Recent medical research has disclosed a long suspected linkage between oral contraception and cardiovascular problems[11].)

In each case doctors used the authority of their role to selectively present information about the available contraceptive methods and influence the patient's decision. While Sarah was given the most thorough review of contraceptive options, the presentation was colored by the doctor's preference. Information was used selectively to make it quite clear that at this time the doctor preferred the birth control pill for her. The presentation of options to Donna was more limited. She was given information on the IUD and the birth control pill; however, the information on the IUD was presented so negatively that the birth control pill seemed to be the only reasonable choice. With Amy, the lack of choice was even clearer. Although both resident and patient expressed concern about the continued use of birth control pills, no alternative methods of contraception were discussed.

These cases display three women with differing contraceptive problems receiving health care in very different medical settings. Whether the practitioners were private practice physicians or residents, in the practice of Ob/Gyn or Family Medicine, earning a fee-for-service or on salary, in our data scientific information was presented selectively to favor the birth control pill. While this occured in each case discussed, it is more conspicuous with Sarah (the first case). In discussing birth control options, the resident first stressed the effectiveness of the pill and claimed that the data from the studies about the side effects of the pill were either inconclusive or not in yet. He then established that if patients try hard enough they can get used to the side effects of the pill. In so doing he displayed his attitude, and we suggest a widely shared medical assumption about pill users and the pill. This belief system provides the grounds to treat patients' complaints about the pill as neurotic, to dismiss the side effects of the pill as nuisance problems, and to keep prescribing oral contraceptives.

In the second and third cases scientific information was ignored or downplayed to make the case for the pill. Donna's complaints were dismissed, and she was accused of erroneously blaming the pill for her problems. If she was gaining weight, it was because she was eating more. She only thought she was hungrier while taking birth control pills. The presentation of scientific information about contraception displayed a blame-the-victim-attitude which shifted the fault away from the birth control pill and toward the patient. It also dismissed as unimportant, problems that affect the quality of women's lives. In the third case, even when Amy presented "bonafide" risk factors, they were subtly downplayed, and by the end of the medical interview birth control pills were again prescribed.

Discussion about contraception was couched in terms of safety and efficacy. Again scientific information was presented selectively. Birth control pills and the IUD were presented as 99% effective (a fact that many would disagree with, see Seaman and Seaman, 1977). While the IUD was dismissed because it can cause infections and infertility, the problems associated with the birth control pill were deemphasized even though death has been a documented consequence of its use.[12] With birth control pills the only problem that was treated seriously was described as "short term infertility."

Again the selective use of information is clearest with Sarah. The discussion about contraception began with the question, "First of all do you want children?" Why was a question about children first? Why not ask how much interest do you have in protecting yourself from possible iatrogenically produced illness? This seems to us to be the more critical question. Yet neither of us has ever heard it asked.

Barrier methods of contraception were only discussed with Sarah. When information was presented about them neither their efficacy nor their safety was stressed. When the doctor discussed the diaphragm he focused on the commitment, intelligence, and marital status of the user. The implication was that most women were neither intelligent nor committed enough to use the diaphragm effectively. With the condom, pleasure with intercourse and intactness of condom were stressed. The messages sent were subtle and potentially frightening for the patient. She had clearly stated that she wanted a safe method of birth control. If the diaphragm was presented as less safe, it was unlikely that she would risk its use. And given the assumption in this society that intercourse with a condom is akin to taking a shower with a raincoat, she was equally unlikely to risk her partner's pleasure or her reproductive security by using them.[13]

The selective use of authority in our data is evident over and over again. When prescribing the birth control pill we have each frequently heard doctors explain that even the more dangerous methods of birth control are safer than an unwanted pregnancy. In our opinion this is like comparing apples and oranges. How can the known risks of pregnancy be compared with the as yet unknown risks of the birth control pill? The pill was relatively untested before it went on the market and what testing was done was either directly or indirectly under the control of the pharmaceutical industry. Such a persuasive strategy assumes that there are only two choices for women, the pill or pregnancy and that all the risks are known for both.[14]

The selective use of authority is evident in another way as well. These cases highlight traditional understandings of women's roles by reflecting the twin medical concern: to perserve the reproductive capacity of these women while protecting them from unwanted pregnancy. Traditional understandings lead to the assumption that it is a higher priority to protect women who are single from pregnancy than it is to protect their married counterparts. This assumption is displayed in the resident's statement that his wife could use a diaphragm because she was married, but Sarah would be safer with the birth control pill. Someday she will want to marry and reproduce. It is also discernable in the bias against the IUD. This bias was evident in all these cases, but was perhaps clearest in the presentation of information to Donna. She was told that the IUD was an inappropriate method, "particulary for young women who haven't had their families yet." While the doctor explained that death was a possible outcome of the IUD, the "scariest thing, even if, you know, you don't get an overwhelming infection..." is the possibility of infertility. This was all explained to a young, single woman who had not even mentioned her reproductive plans.

Conclusion

It is medically well accepted today that no organ system of a woman's body is unaffected by the birth control pill (Seaman and Seaman, 1977). The risks associated with the pill take ten to twenty years to mature and are too varied to enumerate here. Yet despite this information, doctors continue to prescribe them. Several factors make this possible. First, the practice of medicine is very time consuming, and most doctors do not spend a lot of time keeping up with the latest developments in their fields. More specifically, they receive most of their information about drugs such as birth control pills from drug salespeople and medical journals. The pharmaceutical industry has reaped tremendous profits from the birth control pill. They have a history which demonstrates a greater commitment to profit than to humanitarian concerns like patient safety. They are, therefore, biased teachers. This same bias is evident in medical journals. Most journals are dependent on advertising dollars. The pharmaceutical industry is a heavy advertiser. Editorials and articles as well as advertisements reflect the journal's dependence on the pharmaceutical industry's continued good will.

Historically the American Medical Association and the American College of Obstetrics and Gynecology have been hesitant to explain the side effects and risks of the pill to pill users. It has been argued that to do so would confuse and alarm many women patients, and to have others do so would interfere with the doctor-patient relationship. These are male dominated, sexist assumptions based on a view of women as emotionally unstable and unable to understand complex explanations. While to a large extent the medical profession lost this battle in Senate hearings and information about the risks and side effects of the pill are included in each packet of birth control pills, doctors still have the upper hand. As we saw in the data, patients look to doctors as the final arbitrators of contraceptive information, and the ways in which the information is presented function to persuade. Feminists argue that to the degree that discrimination toward women is pervasive in our society, it is also deeply embedded in the field of medicine (Scully, 1980; Ruzek, 1978; Ehrenreich and English, 1978). These cultural and institutional values toward women and reproduction, patriarchal values and attitudes, play an important role in the medical treatment of women.

The persuasive communication patterns medical providers use in precribing birth control are social as well as micro-political phenomena. They are social in that they are produced and constrained in a social context and accomplished by the activities of the participants. They are micropolitical in that they reflect and help to sustain the status quo. The social and political factors woven into the fabric of society and mirrored in the shape of the health care delivery system are embedded in the practitioner-patient communication through which medical decision-making is accomplished.

In the prescription of birth control, the selective use of scientific information legitimizes the dominance of the medical profession. Medicine is a technological approach which addresses itself to physiological or biological aspects of health and illness. Medical practitioners are separated from the social or contextural lives of patients (Todd, 1982). We did not hear medical practitioners ask women what different forms of contraception meant to their lives. We rather observed medical providers prescribing birth control pills abstracted from the social lives of their patients but embedded in their traditional assumptions about women. The technology of reproductive control developed, promoted, and found profitable by the drug companies creates a demand for its use and leads to the prescription patterns and the persuasion strategies we have discussed. Medical providers using the institutional authority of their role provide information in ways that function to persuade and the birth control pill becomes an institutionalized, self-serving, standard medical procedure. While the persuasion may be friendly, it denies patients the information they need to be active participants in their own health care and in so doing, especially in the area of contraception, cannot be in their best interest.

NOTES

[1] The neophyte medical profession would have been hard pressed to demonstrate its skill. Medical knowledge and technique at the time was limited and often dangerous. While today the medical profession is heralded with having improved the health of the population and especially with controlling infectious disease, others (see Dubos, 1959)

argue that these improvements preceded medical advances and were the result of social reforms = e.g., better sanitation and nutrition as well as a rising standard of living. Nevertheless such discoveries as small pox and polio vaccines do give modern medicine a basis for asserting its skills, skills that 19th century doctors did not have.

[2]We neither provide nor seek statistical relevance in this paper. We present and analyze discourse between medical practitioners and patients. It is our contention that the kind of data, analyses and findings in this paper contribute toward a preliminary examination of connections between macro systems and micro communication (see also Knorr-Centina and Cicourel, 1981, for a more complete discussion of this point).

[3]Logically, there is a fourth category: continuing users showing no adverse side effects. While it is obvious that such patients exist, their medical interactions were not the topic under discussion in this paper. Such interactions were not characterized by a continued discussion of birth control methods. A choice had been made at an earlier time and if it involved persuasion, we were not in the examining room to observe it.

[4]While our interpretation is perhaps only one of the many that are possible, it is nevertheless grounded in a way that others cannot be. It is grounded in our experience in the settings under study, backed by audio and video tapes available for study. Corsaro (1982) does an excellent job of reviewing the pros and cons of AV recording, stressing the need for additional ethnographic data to provide a broad enough picture for sociological inquiry.

[5]Double slash marks (//) are used to indicate simultaneous speech overlaps or interruptions.

[6]A series of dots (...) are used to indicate that the speakers voice is trailing off, providing juncture into which the next speaker may insert an utterance.

[7]If the doctor had favored the IUD, we believe we would have observed reverse persuasion concerning the pill and the IUD. Our point here is that doctors selectively use scientific

information to persuade.

[8]We have data on both doctors and residents interacting with patients. To minimize confusion in this section we use the term "resident" and "doctor" interchangeable.

[9]There is an interesting continuum between this case and the last. When discussing the side effects associated with the pill, contraindications are dismissed as "nuisance problems . . ." In so doing the doctors displayed their attitudes about pill users and the pill.

[10]There are a range of nutrition remedies such as vitamin B_6 and calcium as well as the more medically accepted aspirin-like drugs which, if taken correctly, have been found to inhibit the prostaglandins which are responsible for some types of menstrual cramps (see Seaman and Seaman, 1977). Further, there is current debate in medicine about using the birth control pill to manage menstrual disorders. It is felt that while there may be short term improvement there is long term damage.

[11]Sloan, et.al., (1981) have found in their hospital based, case-control study, that long-term use of oral contraceptive increases the possibility of myocardial infarction even after discontinuation of the pill.

[12]It is not our intention to imply that birth control pills are never an appropriate prescription. Nor is it our intention to suggest that any of the providers were "poor" medical practitioners consciously providing "bad" medical care. Rather our goal is to use these cases to illuminate how persuasive techniques are used during medical interviews to accomplish contraceptive decision-making as well as to illuminate the moral, economic and political context in which decisions take place. The data discussed in this paper raises two questions. First, how doctors and patients communicate to reach common decisions about contraceptive methods, and second, why, despite considerable evidence to the contrary, birth control pills continue to be the most widely prescribed method of birth control.

[13]In Japan, condoms are the leading birth control method. They are sold in an array of colors and textures and

presented as safe as well as sexually stimulating.

[14]There is also an important difference here in the gathering of statistics for pregnancy-related and birth control pill-related problems. When complications arise with pregnancy, the relationship between the two are generally clearly recognizable and recorded into the statistical records. The relationship between the birth control pill and potential complications, however, are much harder to identify. Blood clots, strokes, cardiovascular problems are often recorded as just that, a stroke, rather than a birth control pill-related complication. Further, drug companies are often involved in the compiling of statistics around drug complications and their interests are in low problem rates. This difference in record keeping distorts the data, making such comparisons all the more meaningless.

Paper prepared for the 1983 American Sociological Association Meetings, Detroit, Michigan

We would like to thank William Corsaro, Donna Eder, Hugh Mehan, and Samuel Wallace for their helpful comments on this paper.

3

A quatitative pragmatic analysis of discourse

Some theoretical and practical implications

T. van der Geest

"From a scientific point of view therapy cannot be more valid than is indicated by its system of ideas. It is irrelevant in this respect that therapy is now and then successful, as it is clear that also before Galileï stones fell down to earth" (Kropf, 1976).

This quotation from the German therapy-researcher (Kropf) may serve as the motif for the talk I would like to present here. In this talk I will try to answer two related questions:
1) whether or not linguistics is able to justify or indeed, if necessary, to correct any system of ideas; and if this happens to be the case 2)what this finding may imply for the role of linguistics in society. For the answers to these questions I shall make use of some investigations in the domain of doctor-patient and of therapist-client conversation, in which I was involved.

A first study I want to deal with here in order to get a clearer picture of the problems involved in the questions as formulated above, concerns therapeutic communication in a client-centered non-directive therapy. In this project we were confronted with the superficially surprising fact that on the one hand therapeutic experts - both therapists and researchers - who had to pass broad judgement on the quality of a client-centered therapy, were very positive with respect to the discourse procedures used in this special therapy, although on the other both the therapist and the client indicated that the results of the therapy were rather disappointing. After a confrontation with this apparent contradiction, the therapists (i.e. both the actual therapist and the researchers) were not able to explain this contradiction in the research data but persisted in their opinions and judgements.

By carrying out a linguistic analysis on randomly chosen parts of the whole therapy we found some remarkable differences between this special therapy and some other more successful client-centered therapies. One of the more important differences to which I will restrict myself here concerned the combinations of kinds of verb and person of the subject. It appeared that both the therapists and the client in the non-successful therapy used far more state and process verbs especially in the combination with a third person subject than the participants in a more successful therapy did. Furthermore, the client in our special case used far fewer action verbs with a first-person subject and the therapist in this case far fewer action verbs with a second-person subject. Finally, it appeared that these differences between the non-successful therapy and the other ones increased markedly from start to finish of the therapeutic intervention.

According to experts the reported differences could not be considered to be theoretically disadvantageous for the therapy that interests us here. On the contrary, they told us, both therapist and client demonstrated a great degree of symmetry by their use of verb and subject type, which is of special importance in a client-centered non-directive therapy (see also Lennard & Bernstein, 1960; and Jaffe, 1964 for empirical evidence). In other words, according to experts the reported differences between the successful and non-successful therapies could not be used to solve the contradiction, as the conversation was within the system of ideas of client-centered therapy.

On examination of the texts of the problematic therapy we found that the client is of the opinion that all kinds of negative facts and events have happened to him in his personal history and that these were caused by other people or by fate; he was having problems at home, at work, with colleagues, with friends and relatives.

Furthermore, he spoke about himself in strongly negative terms and about others in rather positive terms. In the psychological literature this personality-type is described within the theory of "Locus of control" (Lefcourt, 1976). Within this theory it is assumed that people can be subdivided into two groups, viz. people with internal and people with external control. By internal control is meant that a person thinks and acts from the standpoint that his life is essentially determined by this own decisions and actions. In external control the opposite is the case. It will be clear that the client in our therapy belongs to the last group of people with external control.

As a layman in matters of psychotherapy one could be of the opinion that the client's problems that caused him to look for therapeutic help are occasioned by too negative a self-image to be characterized by external control. The client's conversational contributions, at least, seem to confirm this opinion.

As a therapist, one may tell him this with a view to finding a strategy with the client as to how to develop a way out of this problem. This is not the practice in client-centered therapy. It seems that client-centered non-directive therapists are not allowed to take the initiative. They apparently have to play a dependent role, do not direct their clients and have only to react to problems that are introduced by the clients. Although a number of modifications of client-centered therapy have been proposed during the past twenty years (see amongst others, Van Kessel, 1976), to cope with such problems as outlined above client-centered therapeutics is still generally practised so that initiatives of the therapist are avoided in the conversational process. What we see here is that ideology, i.e. the system of ideas, dominates over reality. There is another point that deserves our special attention here, viz. the result of theanalysis in which it appeared that initial differences became stronger at the end of the therapy. In other words, the client's contents in the conversation at the end are rather more determined by external control. It is therefore not only the case that therapy did not solve the problem, did not cause a change in mind in the desired direction but it also appeared that the therapeutic process strengthened the client's false opinions; a process reinforced by the therapist's congruent understanding of the client's problem and by making his opinions in his conversational reactions. We must conclude therefore, that the conversational conduct in non-directive therapy does not always contribute to the solution of the client's problem but that this solution is indeed influenced negatively by the conversational conduct. To put it provocatively: in some cases it is not so much understanding as help that is asked for.

Although a case study as reported here in a nutshell cannot have the status of conclusive evidence, it nevertheless illustrates how linguistic analysis may contribute to the determination of how a system of ideas functions in everyday practice. Suppose we find that in a number of cases everyday practice corresponds with the system of ideas; we would then be able to determine on the basis of knowledge about therapy success or failure of these cases whether this system is correct or has to be changed in one or more respects. Linguistics and pragmatic analysis will have a central position in such a research program, given the following conditions: Firstly a linguistic and pragmatic analysis should be able to determine whether or not the therapeutic system of ideas is translated correctly into daily practice. Secondly, linguistic and pragmatic analysis must be able to detect which conversational features are related to or interact with therapy success. Thirdly, if both conditions are fulfilled, it can be decided whether or not both the scientific system of ideas and daily practice have to be changed and in what respect.

1. Behaviour therapy

I shall now report some research findings as to conversation analysis in institutional contexts, of which more empirical evidence has become available. It will be clear that I shall try to demonstrate that if linguistic analysis is not merely interested in deepening our linguistic knowledge of conversation, but on the contrary is also willing to apply available linguistic knowledge to matters of social relevance, linguistics can be of great help to ensure better functioning of the institutions under investigations. The three points mentioned above regarding diagnosis, evaluation, and development will be of central interest to the discussion.

If we direct our attention to behaviour therapy it should be recognized at once that it is extremely difficult to cope with, as its system of ideas is less clear with respect to the conversational conduct. Therefore, we do not have, from the onset, a clear picture of how to determine whether or not the system of ideas is translated correctly into everyday practice. In psychotherapy there is a debate going on between intervention techniques, in which the conversation itself is a substantial and most essential part of the therapy on the one hand, and therapies in which other techniques are available and of central interest, in which communication is not the central issue, on the other. Psychoanalysis and client-centered therapy belong to the former group and behaviour therapy to the latter. It is therefore not surprising that in the former group of therapy-forms conversational theory, training and practice is (and has to be) much more sophisticated than in behaviour therapy. One of the topics in the debate concerns the claim of non-directive therapy of being more humane than behaviour therapy is.

This assumption is supported by the acceptance of non-directness, congruency and symmetry as the starting-points of the system of ideas and the central claims for conversational conduct. As behaviour therapy is directive and possible authoritarian in the sense that the therapist takes the initiative with respect to treatment procedures and techniques to be used.

With qualifications such as 'more or less humane' the discussion does not take place so much on a scientific level but rather on an ideological one and depends on what kind of assumptions concerning human beings and society one has in mind. The question that should interest us here is: what kind of treatment is more apt to solve which kinds of psychological problems. Ideological starting-points that probably influence therapeutic practice and therefore its effects are relevant to our research program as independent variables. In order to get a clearer picture on how such independent variables may influence therapeutic practice it seems to be relevant to mention that client-centered therapy defines human relations on a one-dimensional continuum, a continuum that is also utilized in modern sociological research on power and solidarity (see also Van der Geest, 1985a). At one end of the continuum authority, competence and power is placed, at the other end we find warmth and solidarity. Now it is claimed in client-centered therapy that therapists should function in the solidarity part of the continuum, which leads to non-directness, symmetry and congruence. If we accept this view of client-centered therapy, it cannot be maintained, however, that behaviour therapy, although clearly directive, operates on the opposite side of the continuum, as therapeutic warmth and solidarity with the client will also be claimed here. Apparently we need a less primitive model to describe human relations in this sort of conversations. It is not unrealistic to define human relations - as is done traditionally in socio-psychological research - on a two-dimensional scale, in which one continuum gives indications from 'emotionally distant' to 'emotionally warm' and the other dimension informs us about authority/competence and the like. Brown & Levinson (1978) came to be the same two-dimensional model for sociolinguistic research on independent grounds, so that now also linguistic research can be done with respect to these different dimensions. We may conclude, that as to behaviour therapy it is impossible to deduce mandatory communicative styles that can be used as independent variables beforehand. Instead the correct research question should be: are there any differences in communicative styles in behaviour therapy that can be related to therapeutic success or failure.

Although one might get the impression that Behaviour Therapy has a rather primitive status as to mandatory communication styles, this should not lead us to the conclusion that communication is a neglected area in theory and research. At least during the past twenty years the claims with respect to conversational conduct have changed markedly. This, however, seldom led to changes in therapeutic procedures and in therapist-training, and to empirical verification in daily practice, at least not for all I know. Initially it was simply assumed that communication style is to be considered a therapy-external variable, as it does not participate in therapeutic processes as represented in the different therapeutic techniques. In the early seventies we find all kinds of suggestions to consider it one of the initial tasks to teach the client the language of behaviour therapy as an important condition for therapy success. In later studies (e.g. Morris & Suckerman, 1974 a and b) it appeared that emotional warmth affected therapy success positively. These studies, together with the reproaches by client-centered therapists, as dealt with earlier, led indirectly to a change of insight as to the influence of communication style on therapy processes and success. A number of publications in the late seventies (Fiedler, 1976; Halder, 1977; Lutz, 1978) depart from the assumption that many aspects of conversational style should be taken over from the style that is practised in client-centered non-directive therapy. This latter point will have my special interest, as will be clear from what precedes. For it seems rather strange to me that behaviour therapy with fairly directive techniques and procedures should make use of instrinsically non-directive conversational procedures. The techniques call for asymmetry, the conversational style departs essentially from a symmetrical standpoint.

In order to get a clear picture of this problem, conversational data of eight behaviour therapies (using Jaconson's relaxation technique and systematic desensitization for clients suffering from severe non-social phobias) were investigated. Mind that the techniques are already programmed in the research design, which amongst other things implies that treatment is decided upon without discussing it with potential clients. Clients can refuse to cooperate or accept his treatment. From these data we selected from each therapy eight fifteen-minute samples in which the conversation was directed most of the time to the life and problems of the client. A large number of linguistic, pragmatic and conversational variables were taken into account in the analysis of the data. Considerations of space make it impossible to discuss these variables into detail. Those who are interested in such matters, may be referred to the discussion in Van der Geest & Fehlenberg (1982) and the literature mentioned there. I shall restrict myself here to summing up the most important groups of variables of the present investigation: a large number of different speech-act types; directness vs. indirectness from which conclusions can be drawn as to politeness, warmth and authority; aspects of propositional and attitudinal content, e.g. type of verb and subject, modal verbs, positive or negative feelings; explicitness and redundancy of content; concrete vs. abstract; conversational conduct more or less of the type discussed in Schwitalla (1979) van Van der Geest (1978); and finally thematic responsiveness according to Lennard & Bernstein (1960). All these aspects were analyzed as to the questions 1) what kinds of speech styles have been used by the different speakers, and 2) with what kinds of speech styles the different participants of the therapies are addressed. Finally a questionnaire was developed to be filled out by both therapists and clients after each session to estimate the interpersonal relationship with regard to the two-dimensional scale discussed earlier on, with a subdivision into eight different mental aspects. The participants have not only been subdivided with respect to therapist and client, or success as against failure, but also with respect to a combination of both. Subjects are furthermore subdivided with respect to sex and education of the clients. The therapy dyads, finally, were subdivided into same sex dyads (M/F) and different sex dyads, and into male or female therapist with female or male client respectively. What concerns us most of all is the opposition succesful versus non-succesful. The following results have a crucial bearing on our study:

1. Succesful therapists used more directives than non successful therapists. Successful clients were more often addressed with directives than non-successful clients were.
2. The directives that were used in successful dyads by the therapist are more often indirect, conventional or unconventional in the sense of Brown & Levinson (1978). This indirect use of language was apparently possible as these therapists did not lack authority, so that a wish uttered by them may function as a distinct imperative. This was in sharp contrast with the non-successful therapies in which the less frequently occurring directives were most often bald on record.
3. Successful therapists stuck more closely to facts, actions, to reinforcement by positive evaluation, and to exploitation of the positive feelings of clients.
4. Emotional warmth strategies are more often used in successful therapies.
5. In successful therapies fewer discussions took place with respect to therapy planning, procedures and matters of diagnosis. It seems reasonable to admit that such discussions are signals of non-acceptance by the client of the authority of the therapist.
6. In successful therapies clients and therapists demon strated clear differences in terms of conversational roles to be played. These differences appeared amongst others things from differences with respect to speech act types, from themes to be introduced (e.g. client's life and past by the client and therapy matters by the therapists), from the contents of the utterance (e.g. past events against future action), and from the conversational conduct.
7. In successful therapies so-called responsiveness decreases from the first to the last session. This means that participants slowly but surely react less frequently to the central theme of the preceding utterance of the other participant in the dyad.
8. The decrease of responsiveness is almost exclusively caused by the successful therapist.
9. Whereas successful therapists show low, successful clients demonstrate high responsiveness. This result can be seen as another indication for asymmetry in successful ther-

therapies. The therapist and client role are typically complementary.
10. If we abstract from different roles and from beginning and end of therapy as dealt with in the two previous points, successful therapies show far less responsiveness. Points 8, 9 and 10 demonstrate that there are great differences between behavior therapy and psychotherapies such as client-centered therapy. As can be deduced from e.g. Jaffe (1964) and Lennard & Bernstein (1960), psychotherapy in general, but psycho-analysis and client-centered therapy inparticular, show a growing similarity of therapist and client roles with respect to contents, interpersonal relations and responsiveness.
11. Length of turns taken by therapist and client were less comparable in successful dyads.
12. Interpersonal relationships, as determined by means of the above mentioned questionnaire to be filled out after each session by both therapist and client, appear to be significantly higher for both types of participants in the successful ones. If we keep in mind that both authority- and warmth-questions had to be filled out, it is remarkable from the view of client-centered therapy that, even if there was much more authority and asymmetry in the successful therapies, these conversations were considered to be relationally much better.

There are some additional findings to be mentioned here that on the one hand appear to be of particular interest to therapeutic practice but from which some additional evidence for the two-dimension discussion can be deduced on the other:
1. Same sex dyads appear to be more successful than different sex dyads. Since in our society conversation is generally of a more confidential nature at least in so far as personal psychological problems are concerned if the other participant is of the same sex, and since authority also appears to be less questionable in such dyads, this result was to be expected from the start.
2. In different sex dyads male therapists appear to be more successful than female therapists.
3. The third result is implied by the former one, viz. female clients seem to be more successful than male clients in different sex dyads. These latter two findings reflect society rather nicely. Especially male clients did not

accept female authority, as can easily be demonstrated by the conversational data.

4. A final interesting result is that less-educated clients tend to be more successful in therapy than higher-educated clients. This is in contrast with the generally held belief in psychotherapy that the yarvis type - i.e. young, attractive, intelligent etc. type - should be more successful. Our results may support the assumption that authority or at least the acceptance of therapist-authority is a necessary precondition for therapy success. A medical student, for example, did not accept the techniques as proposed by a discipline which, according to him, was lower qualified than medical science, as appeared from the conversational data.

From the results of our analysis on a linguistic, pragmatic and interactive level it may be deduced, that the conversation in the successful dyads must be qualified as two-dimensional in the sense that the interpersonal relation in the investigated successful behaviour therapies were emotionally warm and authoritarian in an indirective way. Therapists and clients played different parts which were complementary/asymmetrical; and these differences became progressively more explicit. The results of the data confirmed these conclusions. The non-successful therapies on the other hand were more or less one-dimensional in the sense of the concepts used in client-centered non-directive therapy, viz. that the relation between therapist and client was warm but somewhat conflicting and lacking in therapist authority.

Furthermore, in the latter therapies assimilation of roles took place during the intervention period, which is also in agreement with conversation-based humane therapies.

We should be careful not to overestimate the value of these results, as the findings are restricted to just the analysis of eight therapies in which only one kind of psychological problem is dealt with, viz. non-social phobia.

As far as the number of therapies is concerned, it should be mentioned that the linguistic analysis of conversation in which the explanation of underlying processes is emphasized and not so much the measurement of all kinds of linguistic and communicative capacities, is a rather time-consuming business. In such a research program one has to maneuver between the Scylla of superficiality in linguistic terms on the one hand and the Charybdis of a slender basis of data on the other. In our case we decided on eight therapies, as Lennard and Bernstein (1960) did, in which a number of interesting independent variables, such as sex, could be varied. The argumentation with respect to the results and their implications for the institution under investigation cannot in such cases be merely based on statistical principles, but should seek its power of conviction in a chain of empirical data that is in accordance with the results of the present investigation. In our case, it may be stated that the one vs. two-dimensional approach in institutional conversation is not only found in behaviour therapy but also in the illustrative case of non-directive and client-centered therapy as dealt with at the very beginning of this paper and also in the analysis of classroom conversation (Van der Geest, 1985b). In the latter case it appeared that the teacher's authority combined with a congenial climate in the classroom led to better pupil achievement with respect to some central aspects of the curriculum. Communication theory - based on Roger's ideas as it evolved during the last 20 years - developed symmetry-claims with respect to all these institutions and their conversation. Our analysis of all these types of discourse demonstrated clearly that if conversation is just a precondition for doing things and reaching aims at other levels, like solving phobia-problems, achieving better mathematics results or even teaching language skills and training them, a conversational concept in which the two dimensions as dealt with above are integrated turns out to be more successful.

If we now return to the three starting-points as mentioned earlier in this paper, the following conclusions should be drawn:

1. The analysis demonstrates clearly that two different systems of ideas were correctly translated into daily practice (consciously or unconsciously), viz. the more traditional two-dimensional system and the new-fashion one-dimensional system that has been taken over from client-centered therapy.

2. The analysis is apparently able to detect the conversational features that correlate with success and failure in therapy.

3. On the basis of the former two points it may be concluded, that the system of ideas in which therapeutic techniques concur with conversational principles from client-centered therapy, as has been recommended by recent

literature, must be rejected. From these three points it may be deduced that linguistic and pragmatic analysis of conversation may be of great relevance to problems of public life.

2. Doctor patient communication

A problem not dealt with so far in this paper, concerns the phenomenon of adaption. By adaption is meant that speech is not only determined by speech characteristics of the speakers, but also by the person spoken to. One of the findings from our research on behaviour therapy, that I did not mention, was that the therapists adapted their speech as to the sex of the clients. This could be investigated easily, as each therapist in the investigation had both a male and female client. This was, furthermore, of special interest as female clients appeared to be the more successful ones. With these results in mind, we investigated doctor-patient communication. Intuitively, it is generally held that the influence of conversation on therapy success can be more easily investigated than its influence in the convalescence of the patients. There is, however, a striking correspondence between behaviour-therapy and medical communication. For in both cases, the quality of conversation is just a precondition for the proper therapeutic treatment. In this sense the therapeutic techniques and advices correspond with medication in doctor-patient cooperation. If this assumption is correct, it means that therapeutic communication should establish an interpersonal basis of trusting each other, on which a fruitful cooperation in terms of compliance by patient or client could become possible. For both types of therapy, finally, it is uncertain whether the prescribed therapeutic techniques or medications are effective.

Formulated in this way, it may be hypothesized that two-dimensional communication, especially with female patients is most fruitful for treatment. To investigate this problem, we had 32 conversations at our disposal from eight patients during warding rounds (the data were taken from the Ulm-project on doctor-patient interaction). Of the patients 5 are male and 3 female. Four patients were terminally ill (2 male and 2 female). The linguistic variables of this investigation consisted of a representative selection of the variables used in the former investigation. The following adaptations by the physician to the sex of the patient were found:

1. **Duration of the visits:** significantly longer visits for female patients.
2. **Number of contributions:** the number of doctor contributions depends on the diagnosis of the male patients. He speaks a lot if the patient is terminally ill and less if not. For female patients this is not the case.
3. **Speech acts:** the physician is more informative and less directive and puts questions to female patients.
4. **Conventional indirectness:** the physician is less direct to male patients, as was evident from the analysis of modal verbs.
5. **Involvement:** the physician is much more involved in the conversation with female patients, as appeared from the analysis of the grammatical subject.
6. **Action perspective:** the physician is much more preoccupied with action in the case of the female patient, as appears from the analysis of the combination of grammatical subject with verb type.
7. **Time perspective:** conversation with female patients is much more concerned with the here and now, with male patients, however, with the past as appears from the analysis of grammatical tense.
8. **Quality of information:** the larger number of informatives to female patients consists of a larger number of contributions that can or should be interpreted as unconventionally indirect directives, suggestions and indications of medical action, as may also be evident from the previous points.

In brief, it may be concluded that interaction with female patients can be described as more concrete, more to the point, and from the standpoint of medical care as more relevant.

Another point that deserves our special attention in terms of interaction, concerns the question of what are the sources in conversation for the adaptation by the physicians? I am dealing here with adaptation both to the sex of the patients and to the diagnosis. I have dealt with this question in more detail in two different studies (Van der Geest, 1982; 1985a), so that I can restrict myself to the most interesting results here.

The first source (see Van der Geest, 1982) concerns the physician's possible prejudice as to male and female patients. Such a prejudice has been found more than once testpsychologically. In these investigations therapists and (or) physicians were asked to make attributions with regard to male or female and in a later investigation with respect to health. The results show that attributions with respect to women correlate significantly and positively with lack of health as male and health attributions do. In our analysis we found the same kind of behaviour on the part of therapists and doctors. Restricting us here to the latter category: we found correlations for duration of visit, number of contributions, unconventional indirectness, and speech-act types.

A second source for adaptation was the institutional setting. The ward round also appears to be used by the physician to inform the patient on planned physical examinations and treatment procedures. As the degree of examination and treatment possibilities is also determined by diagnosis, prognosis and the attitude of the patients towards medical care, the different adaptation to the different types of patients is also determined by the institution.

A third source to be mentioned here concerns the role of diagnosis. This type of adaptation is most apparent in cases in which diagnosis and the patients' initiatives contrast with each other. This is, incidentally, most often the case with female patients. In such cases diagnosis determines the physicians' contributions more than the initiatives of the patients do. Action verbs and future tense are more often used by doctors in their conversation with non-terminally ill patients than could be expected from the patients' contributions. The situation is more depressing in the case of dyads with terminally-ill patients. Their questions are responded to with questions rather than with answers. Their rather frequent use of action verbs with second-person pronouns as grammatical subjects is responded to with frequent use of process verbs with third person subject, instead of action verbs with a first-person subject: Doctor, do - you..... etc. is responded to with utterances that things are changing. The patients' future perspective is adjusted to the present tense, etc. It is noteworthy in these cases that especially female patients make an opposite contribution to the physicians' turns. This leads directly to the last source of adaptation to be discussed here. The most essential source of speech adaptation by the doctor is the conversational activity of his partner in the dyad. It appears that many variables that pointed to adaptation by the physician as to the patients' sex can be explained from the differences in contribution between male and female patients. The female patient is converationally active (e.g. puts many more questions), which has its consequences for the duration of the visit and the number of informatives by the doctor. She is less conventionally indirect, uses more first and second person pronouns in grammatical-subject position, in combination with more action- and process-verbs and with more present tenses. This means that her contributions in the dyad deal with actions in the here and now, even more than is the case for the doctor contributions. In comparison with male patients female ones are more initiating, more concrete, and more directed towards action. Both the doctor's conversational style and that of the therapists on the one hand and that of the female patient and client on the other are quite similar. In spite of all kinds of similarities between doctor- and patient contributions, there is a clear asymmetry present in each dyad-type as can easily be demonstrated from the data (see also Van der Geest, 1982 en 1985a). Essentially this asymmetry corresponds with the one found in our investigation on behaviour therapy.

In this case too, I have to admit that the actual data base is too small in order to generalize the results. On a different level, however, we have additional evidence for the fruitfulness of the two-dimensional conversation model. In the female dyads there is asymmetry of the fruitful sort, but this asymmetry is also warm in the sense that the directives are most of the time unconventionally indirect: viz. a lot of suggestions, hypotheses on possible actions etc., and emphasis on concrete medical action. In this sense it may be expected that more effective medical communication takes place in the female-patient dyad than in the male-patient dyad. It may therefore be hypothesized that in an additional investigation dealing with the relation between compliance and conversational style, a cooperative warm but authoritarian conversational style, as could be demonstrated especially in the female dyads, will appear to be more successful in terms of compliance.

We should, however, be careful in not overestimating the contribution of conversation to medical and therapeutic success. In our experiment in behaviour-therapy the intervening variable 'therapeutic techniques' was controlled. Differences in the professional capacities of the therapists could therefore be excluded in the analysis. Such capacities, however, are more essential for success. Conversation is but a very interesting condition for success of treatment. The same goes for the kind of diagnosis and prognosis as to the patient's or client's situation. A third point is more relevant to our discussion here and concerns the quality of the information exchange that is hardly dealt with in this paper. The problem of investigating the quality of the information flow is that linguistics cannot make strong claims in this direction, as the medical/therapeutic relevance of information is also at stake here. This expertise largely belongs to the medical discipline. In most cases linguistics can only conjecture about such matters. In our investigation of behaviour-therapies we could control this factor by using a professional diagnostic scheme (Schulte's diagnostic scheme) and by a professional guidance and control of the application of this scheme.

3. Some final remarks

In sum, if we accept the conversational adequacy of the two-dimensional models for conversation in the institutions referred to we should not close our eyes to the restrictive power of these models as to medical expertise, diagnosis of the patient's physical conditions, and the medical relevance of the information flow.

To clarify my standpoint I shall now deal with some topics in the literature.

Fisher (1982) and Todd (1982) have very clearly demonstrated that the authority of physicians with respect to female patients may lead to false or at least less optimal medical treatment in a large number of cases. Unfortunately for our purpose they carried out their research within the power-solidarity paradigm, and therefore, we are uncertain whether only too big an authority or indeed a lack of interpersonal emotional warmth may have caused the false decisions by the physicians observed. In their data, I could find a number of clues that are indicative of the latter cause. In my opinion misconceived views of authority combined with the neglect of socially relevant information about the patient, or indeed not asking such information of the patient can only be explained by a lack of interest in the conversational partner. Interviews and other indirect evidence seem to indicate that patients are aware of this.

Recent sociolinguistic publications seem to stress the relevance of the power-solidarity paradigm. As for the studies of Todd and Fisher I will try to demonstrate that a two-dimensional model gives a clearer picture of what is going on during the conversation, so that a more valid interpretation and evaluation can be made. The following passage from Conte (1981) is illustrative: a mother tells that her two-year-old daughter Veronica does not eat. Veronica's weight is, however, not incongruent with her development. After the interview it has become clear that the child eats enough and that the real problem for the mother is that she does not eat Mexican food at night, made by herself. That this is so may be due to the fact that the child ate enough American food, cooked for her during the day by a baby-sitter. But the mother fears that she will not eat Mexican food when back in Mexico. The doctor gives as his opinion that the child will eat when they are back home. Apparently the mother accepts this medical standpoint. Not so, however, the researcher, who is of the opinion that the doctor does not take this problem seriously, and should have gone into this problem. There are two possible interpretations here. The first is that the medical authority judges this problem as medically irrelevant and therefore does not care about the mother's psychological problem. In that case we have to do with an emotionally cold authority. This is not in agreement with his description given in the paper. A second interpretation starts with a combination of medical authority and a strategy or advice not to care about things that might happen in the future. Such a strategy may be fruitful in dyads in which a trustful, cooperative and warm atmosphere exists. From the data we may conclude that this is actually the case here. Why did the investigator stress that the doctor had to go into the problem? This may be explained by the widespread conviction in modern one-dimensional communication theory, that every contribution of participants has to be taken seriously in order to arrive at symmetrical, non-authoritarian (Rogers) or **Herrschaftfreie Kommunikation** (Habermas). It is stressed in the literature that this has to be the case especially in therapeutic, medical, classroom and family communication. Although I can agree with such an opinion, at least in principle, I would like to warn against too strict an application of this claim. From cognitive learning (e.g. Meichenbaum, 1976 or Bandura, 1976) it may be deduced that the way participants react to a person's opinions may influence these opinions. By taken cognitive and mental problems (including non-realistic, hypothetical and phantasmic mental ideas) seriously, therapists and doctors may reinforce such problems. The consequence may be, that, if a client was uncertain about the reality of his thoughts before the conversation, afterwards he becomes more certain about the reality of them on false grounds, e.g. because the doctor went into them. At this point I ask myself if therapists are not often trying to cure problems they caused by reinforcing the client's opinion about which they were - at least initially - uncertain. The problem as outlined above, fits into a larger asymmetry problem of institutional conversation. Participants do not only have knowledge (e.g. medical against complaint knowledge) but also different viewpoints as to shared knowledge: a complaint like cold extremities is experienced in a painful way by the patient; for the doctor, however, it is on the face of it only a symptom of a deeper problem, viz. diabetes. This problem comes to the surface in an investigation of White & Robillard (1982). A first and most important contribution of a female patient deals with "still cold hands and feet". The doctor does not go into that problem but concentrates on checking urine, pill-taking and the patient's physical condition. The conversation ends as follows:

Dr. Any other trouble since last time I saw you; any problems you want to ask about?
P. Mmh no I don't fill. I mean I cold, that's all.
Dr. So, feelin pretty good other than that?
P. Yah.
Dr. Okay. (follows physical examination.)

Also after this last reminder, the doctor does not go into the actual problem of the patient. Although the medical task may make reordering of the complaint information necessary, I think that the doctor's avoidance of the "cold-hands" topic that is so essential for the patient, cannot be explained from asymmetry but rather from a lack of interest in the patient, as might also be deduced from the many interruptions and topic changes by the doctor. From my own data (Ulm project) it also appeared, that doctors do not always immediately respond to the patient's complaints. They apparently reorder conversation and conduct according to certain medical routines. In contrast with the former illustration, however, there was always a retarded reaction during which they went into the complaint mentioned earlier on. Only in a few instances did I find that the doctor indicated that the information was relevant to him immediatly after the topic had been introduced by the patient and that he would come back to it later. Such a type of conversational behaviour is necessary in order to arrive at mutual understanding in institutional contexts.

A last point I would like to go into in this paper concerns asymmetry in the sense that both participants have different tasks: the patient has to be cooperative in the description of his problem and complaints, the doctor on the other hand has to diagnose, to inform the patient as far as relevant to the therapy, to prescribe correctly and to conduct the process of medication. The next example is taken from Lacoste (1981):

Dr. How long have you had this pain in your stomach?
P. I've never had pain in my stomach, I have a pain in my spleen.
Dr. Listen, the spleen you are not supposed to know where that is, you had a pain in your stomach.
P. I have a pain there.
Dr. That's in the stomach.
P. If you say so.

The medical problem whether the stomach or the spleen hurts is irrelevant here. It is interesting, however, that a conflict arises as to the doctor's competence. It is clear that in the sociolinguistic literature the doctor's contributions will be criticized. It is remarkable that the conflict is introduced by the patient, who denies the medical diagnosis by the doctor. The protocol is uncertain as to whether her utterance was pronounced in a surprising fashion, or as a simple rebuttal. The doctor's reaction is not friendly and makes the impression of being authoritarian, which means that the patient was not surprised but that she did not accept the medical diagnosis. The subsequent utterances of the patient also make clear that she still is not convinced of the diagnosis. The problem here is not so much that the doctor was not correct in his contributions, even though he sounded rather unpleasant, but the patient was not. On the other hand, the doctor could easily have prevented this clash to occur. He really has to prevent it, viz. by informing the patient he brings it into the conversation as something given. A conversational style by doctors in which it is taken into account that patients are lacking in terms of information, requires both a conversational conduct in which the necessary information can be given in the right place of the conversation and for insight into the patient's situation during the conversation. The first task requires authority, the second empathy and emotional warmth. But it may be feared that medical treatment is seriously impaired from the onset here.

A last example concerns the way a patient experiences a specific complaint, and how the doctor reacts to it. In this volume this problem will be discussed in more detail by Bax. I took the following illustrations from the data appearing at the beginning of the interview after an invitation by the doctor to tell him what the complaints were.

P. I had a dreadful headache.
Dr. You had a headache?
P. I have had a small cold for more than a week, nothing serious but.....
Dr. A cold. Fever?

It is interesting to see that physicians tend to leave out of the contents of the patients' complaints the subjective degree of the symptoms. Although more interpretations are possible, I think that it is correct to state that the way in which patients are alive to their complaints, at least at the beginning, is irrelevant to the physician in order to plan his examining activities. As such the objectification by the doctor is correct, but it depends on how the patient reacts to it whether it has consequences for the interpersonal relationship. If, for example, a patient reacts with "Yes, doctor, indeed an awful headache" it seems appropriate to show more empathy. What I am actually trying to say with these examples is that an objective and medical approach as illustrated here should not be condemned beforehand.It has to be related to the question as to how such an attitude is experienced by the participants. What is demanded of authorities in institutional settings is that they have an open eye for the conversational needs of their participants in the interaction with him.

participants in the interaction with him.

4. Conclusions

In this paper I have outlined a research program which from a linguistic point of view is not at first sight so much interested in deepening theoretical insight into conversation but rather in the application of theoretical linguistic knowledge to socially relevant problems. This standpoint does not, however, necessarily imply that the results of the investigation are of no interest to linguistics itself. Theoretical knowledge is empirically tested and verified and new kinds of hypotheses can be developed within this field. The main interest of the research program is, as mentioned above, concerned with the contribution of linguistics to other scientific disciplines and to institutional settings, in this case doctor-patient and therapeutic communication. Departing from the question whether or not linguistics is able to justify or correct some or other system of ideas, client-centered therapy, behaviour therapy, and doctor-patient communication have been investigated. It was found amongst other things that client-centered therapy may fail to succeed in some cases by shortcomings inherent in its system of ideas.

As to behaviour therapy it was found amongst other things that a communication theory taken over from client-centered therapy is not appropriate in terms of therapy success.

As to linguistic conversational theory it was found that two models with respect to conversational style and conversational conduct can be distinguished in institutional contexts, namely a one and a two-dimensional model. Linguistics should go deeper into this problem by determining the exact differences between them. In doctor-patient communication it was not only found that the conversation was basically two-dimensional, but also that all kinds of adaptation and its sources with respect to sex and diagnosis of the patients occur. The adaptations were similar to the ones found in behaviour-therapy.

Findings such as these mentioned above may - if generalizable - lead to changes in the scientific systems of ideas concerning psychotherapy and doctor-patient communication and to changes in communication theory. Such changes may then lead to changes in daily institutional practice. Not only this indirect way via systems of ideas, can linguistics influence daily practice in society. Above I already mentioned some rather general results of the program. There are, however, other results that may be translated more easily into advices for daily practice, e.g. as to pairing off therapists and clients and as conversational conduct in institutional settings.

Summing up a research program in linguistics as described in this paper may be of help both of the further development of linguistics, and to that of other disciplines and indirectly to a society that today is a more communicative one than it appeared to be in earlier decades and centuries.

COMMENTS ON TON VAN DER GEEST

J.H.M. Ettema

As a psychologist I would like to express my admiration for the contribution of the research conducted by Dr. Van der Geest to the practical field of psychotherapy and to the understanding of the main dimensions of human communication. The linguistic approach is of great help in reviewing or adjusting our crude ideas about psychotherapy. Very often the field lacks an explicit theory of the relation between language, communication and the impact on, or from, psychopathology. In recent years, the counselling approach in particular has had considerable influence on the very broad field of medical care such as in general practice, medical education, community psychology and social work. Under the influence of a general-purpose definition of the counselling approach, the question "Which treatment for which individual?" at times seems to have been answered in advance. For this reason a two-dimensional model of human communication may help to differentiate between proper therapeutic goals and simple goodwill taken for therapeutic competence.

In the case of behaviour therapy, linguistic analysis cannot only help assess the relevant conditions for successful therapy, but, as behaviour therapy is growing more complex with the cognitive approach, it can clarify the operation of the concepts involved as well.

Psychology has tried to emancipate from philosophy and has consequently eliminated concepts which were derived from introspection. A behaviouristic approach was advocated to ensure a "realistic" assessment without ontological presuppositions of the process under study. However, a conceptualization of relevant behaviour presupposes the interpretation of social or psychological reality, which is grounded in, and supported by, descriptions of situations, feelings, attitudes, cognitions, symptoms or complaints, and so on. Every assessment of psychologically relevant behaviour contains a theory which always implies a certain concept or model of language. In this way the system of ideas in psychology or psychotherapy conceals a system of descriptions and reports, or rather, a system of discourse.

Apparently, the problem which arises concerns the relationship between and delineation on the one hand and translinguistic social or psychological reality on the other. Hence, it is important to know whether at present the two-dimensional model is the result of a merely naive empirical observation or, conversely whether it is the product of a more fundamental theory of human interaction as Brown and Levinson (1978) have pointed out. In addressing this issue I would like to formulate some remarks and pose two questions which are induced by Van der Geest's paper.

Briefly, these questions are:

Firstly, what is the nature of the relation between the "therapeutic interaction" and the proper therapeutic techniques and goals? Is the explanation of conversational behaviour by the two-dimensional model to be considered the exploration of the non-technical part of the aiding-relationship? In other words, does this approach exclusively affect the therapeutic climate and not the therapeutic intervention itself?

Secondly, and related to the first question, what is the status of the two-dimensional model as a theory of the structure of human communication in relation to the (psychological) problem communicated about?

In a first apporach of the problem outlined by Dr. Van der Geest an analysis is made of a so-called client-centered non-directive therapy. It is suggested that, according to the judgement of experts, symmetry is the only criterion at hand. In this way, an antithesis can be constructed between the (obviously wrong) ideas (or ideology) and the "real" linguistic observation. The system of ideas offered by Rogerian therapy is rather loosely formulated. Nevertheless, it is not possible to neglect the Rogerian theory, even though the experts fail to comprehend it!

A central task of the Rogerian psychotherapist is to understand and empathize with the unique and experiential world of the client. An earlier stage of the Rogerian theory did in fact prescribe a purely non-directive approach. Acceptance of the client, establishment of a non-judgemental climate, permissiveness and clarification of the client's world were the main goals and techniques.

In a second stage, however, Rogers centered on redirecting the feelings of the client, resolving incongruities between ideal self and real self, etc.. This second approach is called client-centered.

Later on, Rogers moved increasingly to an approach of personal involvement. For instance, he emphasized present-tense experience. What I would like to state is that empathy (in relation to symmetry) is not to be considered as a simple mirroring of the content of the client's verbalizations. After a stage of encouragement, paraphrasing and so on, it is essentially an interpretation and reflection of feelings. In short, it supposes the activity of the psychotherapist. The therapist calls the client's attentions to an as yet unclear, partly cognitive and situational complex which is concretely felt by the client. So, "healthy" or experiential speech places the locus of experience on the "self".

This can be made plain in a linguistic approach. As an example, to the question: "How would you feel if you were caught telling a lie to your wife?" one may answer:

a) "I'd feel terrible, bad and guilty" or

b) "You'd feel bad, terrible and guilty" or even more generally

c) "It would feel bad".

As Alban and Groman (1976) indicated: In the first example the subject answers in the first person singular. The subject of speech indicates that he recognised the possibility of being in such a situation and also acknowledges personal responsibility. The locus of responsibility is the "self", (i.e., "I").

The linguistic analysis given by Dr. Van der Geest, is rather an example in the negative of therapeutic understanding. The client under study did not talk about negative facts and events which had happened to him at one time or another. Actually, during the therapy, he did not present himself as acting (and as a responsible) subject.

In other words, not only the content of his speech (the world referred to, the story) was externally controlled (according to Lefcourt, 1976) but the actual presentation, (i.e. the discourse itself) as well. So, I cannot see why this reasoning should discourage translating the ideas of the Rogerian client-centered approach into the linguistic results as reported in the paper of Dr. Van der Geest. In addition, I'm not sure whether therapists are following such sketchy systems of ideas. On the other hand, I have to admit that Rogerian theory is not always very suitable for the explanation of the therapeutic process. However, although the relation between ideas and therapeutic understanding, explanation and practice may be very loose, it is difficult to understand why this system of ideas should actually prescribe dependency and merely understanding. Moreover, in psychotherapy, in which the conversation itself is the essential part of therapy (the proper talking cure), the problem is how to conceptualize the "authority-function", which evidently plays an important role. Psychoanalysis might say that the client-centered approach lacks a view on transference, i.e. the recognition of one's own position in the actual identification with the position of the other.

In conclusion, I think that the widespread vulgarization and the obscure implications in using the adjective "human" in theoretical discourse are in the main causative of conceptual difficulties of Rogerian theory and interpretation. In addition, the idea that this style of counselling is good for all purposes may lead to the above-mentioned problems. Nevertheless, the ideational systems of the verbal therapies can be investigated as well.

In contrast to these talking therapies, behaviour therapy does not incorporate a proper communication-theory. Following De Voge and Beck (1978) in their review of the literature on the therapeutic relationship in behaviour therapy, friendly submission should make the ideal client for therapy. However they add that these patients, from a theoretical perspective (from psychopathology), should be most able to assume nonaversively a compliant role with a dominant other. The often suggested warm, empathetic and guiding style of behaviour therapists has an inherent difficulty. It might very well be limited to those clients who present themselves initially as friendly and submissive (for instance phobics). A question is, whether various types of individuals, preferring otherwise to engage in particular tactics, can actually be manoeuvred into a friendly submissive position vis-a-vis the therapists. In other words, the elaboration of the two-dimensional paradigm asks to take into account the type of problem or psychopathology that is treated in therapy.

This leads me to a last remark about the connection between the therapeutic relationship and the proper therapeutic technique. In the paper of Dr. Van der Geest it is suggested that the therapeutic technique can be distinguished from the style of communication. This idea is reinforced when Dr. Van der Geest says that we should not "close our eyes to the restrictive power of these models as to medical expertise, diagnosis of the patient's physical condition, and the medical relevance of the information flow". One can easily get the impression that in the therapist-client relation a rather strong distinction is made. As Goffman (1961) puts it, a technical part (the giving and getting of the relevant medical or psychological repair or construction information) on the one hand and a contractual and sociable part on the other. Does this approach conceive the conversation essentially as only instrumental for the proper (technical) aim of the professional contact?

In psychotherapy it is assumed that there exists an adequate conceptualization of the technical part. However, this is not necessarily so! For instance, systematic desensitization has first been considered as a technique based on biological, neurophysiological foundations. After the profound critique of Breger and McGaugh (1969), the learning theory basis of this behavioural technique has been seriously questioned, and a cognitive explanation was given, in which the influence of the belief of the patient was accentuated. This turned out to be more adequate! However, this belief is rather a result of communication.

Complementary, my second question shortly deals with the two-dimensional paradigm.

In their study on "Politeness Phenomena" Brown and Levinson (1978) mention the relationship of their basic interaction structure with the Lévi-Strauss "kinship atom". Like Radcliff-Brown, Lévi-Strauss assumes that the kinship system is governed by two antithetical systems of attitudes. In one case the maternal uncle represent family authority. In the other there exists warmth and familiarity in the relation between the nephew and the maternal uncle.

In a lecture at an interdisciplinary seminar, organized by Lévi-Strauss, the French psychoanalyst A. Green (1977) constructed a very interesting connection between the kinship system of Lévi-Strauss and the attitudinal movements inside the Oedipal structure as outlined in psychoanalysis. As is assumed in psychoanalytic theory, it is precisely the identity of the subject that is at stake. The subject that marks out separation between itself and its own surroundings in order to find a place for itself; the subject that on the one hand relates to the other which is an imaginary reflection of its own desire, on the other hand to the other which is totally different. Would it not then be possible to relate the two-dimensional model in a more dynamic manner to the different positions that are articulated in psychotherapy?

Contrary to a perspective in which the guiding, authoritarian dimension is identified in advance with a technical institutional pole, authority and asymetry may turn out to be a more dynamic dimension of conversation therapy.

4

Feeling for feelings

Expressive information and its role in doctor-patient communication

M.M.H. Bax

I aver that my favourite doctor is Dr. Watson; but I hasten to add that my preference for this MD is based on his human qualities in general rather than on his achievements as a general practitioner. As to this professional functioning, we receive little information from the many chronicled recollections of his adventurous life in the company of Sherlock Holmes. But the few examples we do have can be reduced to a common denominator: in the alleged stories, it sometimes happens that a new client, while relating what has befallen him or her, is overcome by emotion and has a fainting spell. At such moments the physician in Dr. Watson - who is nearly always present at these narrations - is awakened unfailingly, he hurries with brandy to the patient's side for the sufferer's lips - in order "to bring back the colour to the cheeks".

The point of bringing this typical behaviour of Watson's to your attention is that it is in stark contrast to what Sherlock Holmes does; it is, paradoxically, the performance of the latter, especially the way he participates as a conversational partner, that is most informative of the way doctors talk to patients. As a rule, Holmes's achievements as a detective draw, at least in part, upon the outcome of a conversation with his client that in many respects resembles the anamnesis stage in the medical interview.

In short, what happens, during the Baker Street interviews, is that the client presents his case, telling Sherlock Holmes all he thinks that is relevant, while the detective sometimes asks questions or only encourages the client to go on (by typical phrases like "Please proceed" or "Pray continue your most interesting narrative").

It is characteristic of these interviews that Holmes is rather passive in his rôle of conversational partner, but most active in his rôle of listener: while listening to the client's narrative, he is busy constructing an interpretative framework. The client provides any fact that may possibly have a bearing on the case (a murder, a theft, an abduction); against the background of rigorous laws of deduction[1], Sherlock Holmes is constantly evaluating elements of the client's flow of information, deciding whether or not the information is useful or the facts relevant. Thus he sets up a hypothesis as to what has 'really' happened. In the process of this verbal interaction, the hypothesis begins to function as a kind of filter: as a 'model' of what has happened, as a frame of interpretation, it sorts out what is relevant and what is not. All the information that the client supplies which is irrelevant from the perspective of Holmes's theory, is given no further attention, but is assembled in a 'waste-paper-basket'-like category, from which only Watson can profit to enliven the descriptions in his casebook.

This digression enables me to develop somewhat further my suggestion that the conversational practices of Sherlock Holmes resemble those of doctors during the anamnesis routine. It is, notably, the notion of 'filter of interpretation' that allows for the assessment of the point of convergence.

At the risk of overgeneralization, it seems common feature of doctor-patient communication that during the anamnesis or the explorative stage the medical model functions as a filter with regard to the flow of information that the patient offers. Just as with the detective's approach, a doctor (D) evaluates what a patient (P) asserts from the perspective of medical theory, thus selecting bits of information that can contribute to a correct or plausible diagnosis (cf. fragment 1).

(1) D: what can I do for you?
P: well I come for my stomach because it's getting worse and worse.
D: yes. how's that?
P: when I get up in the morning then I feel so sick that I just have to sit down for half an hour, uh, to get better and I just don't know anymore where it is. whether it's my stomach or my belly.
D: what do you mean by 'feeling sick'. of course it sounds a bit vague doesn't it feeling squeamish?
P: yes not really squeamish. that I would have to vomit. it's just cramps.

D: cramps. in the belly right?
P: stomach belly. it's everywhere. sometimes in my back.
D: yes?
P: and uh if I press my stomach then it really hurts.
D: yeah well then shall I have a look? (...)[2]

"What a doctor is looking for", Haberland and Mey recently noted (1981, 106-107), "is symptoms, so that he or she may be able to classify, and treat, the illness as best as possible, according to the training received in medical school and to the tradition of the profession". They complete their picture of what I have just called the medical model by stating that "in this, the doctor bases himself or herself on previous experiences gained in treating cases of the particular disease, as well as on other doctors' research and experiences as reflected in the literature".

This picture of D sifting out information that has a diagnostic value according to the medical model, may well seem an exaggerated version of what really happens. One may be inclined to believe that the alleged reductionist approach of D is rather the make-up of critical outsiders (e.g. linguists like Haberland and Mey) than well-established fact of doctor-patient communication today. It might be argued that medical reduction applies to the practices of bygone days, but - just as the methods of Sherlock Holmes are not illustrative of modern police work - it certainly cannot be a characteristic of conversations in the medical context, since nowadays full attention is given, in the curricula of medical schools, to the training of the communication skills of medical students. It may therefore surprise the reader that in a recently published textbook, entitled **Medicine as a Human Experience**, the editors, the medical educationists Reiser and Rosen, think it is still worthwhile to stress the importance of communication 'in simple English', as they call it, not in the "usually dispassionate language of medical science. In four years", they say (somewhat inaptly from a linguistic point of view), "medical students learn more than 10,000 new words but often do not learn how to talk to patients, or how to listen. They 'do' things to patients, such as tests, or 'get' things, such as blood or a history, without considering what the patient does or gives, or how to let the patient in on the process".[3] This characterization also applies to the Dutch situation, cf. Geldrop (1978); Gevers, Kapsenberg, and Straatman (1980); van Aalderen and Hollenbeek Brouwer (1982).

To put it strongly, something is still wrong with D-P communication, notwithstanding the fact that since the 1960s the importance of effective communication is acknowledged among medical professionals and that interview courses are now required aspects of the education of doctors.

The question then is: what factors are responsible for the fact that, in spite of the positive attitude that most doctors have as regards the communicational aspects of their profession, D-P communication is still largely unsatisfactory, or that, to use Haberland and Mey's phrase, "doctor-patient relations are, almost per definition, potentially strained" (1981, 105).

At this point, I would propose to avoid trendy criticism (pertaining to the unwillingness of D to really listen to patients, to his or her exercising power for power's sake in a situation that ought to be free of dominance, to his 'white coat magic', and the like); from my contacts with doctors and from my reading of medical textbooks dealing with D-P interaction, I gather that among practitioners there is a sufficient awareness of the importance of 'language' as one tool that doctors must use in the process of healing.

So I would prefer instead a closer look at the conversational genre under discussion, and try to ascertain what may be problematic properties of this communication, see what textbooks have to say about those aspects and, subsequently, present an evaluation of these from a linguist's point of view. Finally, I would try to offer some insights that may be profitable for those who engage in these interactions on a professional basis, i.e. doctors.

As a first step in analyzing D-P communication, generally an endeavour subsumed by what is called, in the medical literature at least, micro-sociology, I must point out that since the development (in the 1960s) of the sociology of medicine as a scientific discipline (Foets and Peeters 1982, 55), due emphasis has been laid on the fact that D-P relations are social relations (Henderson, Freidson), thus making possible a more precise characterization of the communicative context and of the differences in rôle behaviour of D and P (Armstrong 1981, 94). Several theories have been proposed as to these social rôles and the type of relation between them. We need not go deeply into these theories in order to conclude that there are considerable discrepancies in the expectations of both D and P about the interaction and, consequently, about their approach and their actual behaviour. As Persoon notes, "It is a characteristic of P that he is highly dependent on a situation in which he feels threatened and uncertain, but which he is strongly emotionally involved in" (1978, 230).[4]

Merton and Barber (1963), both sociologists, refer to 'the character of crisis' that defines D-P relations; according to Freidson (1962), D-P interaction connotes the fundamental concepts of life and death, hence its fear-ladenness.

What I find remarkable in the descriptions of the P-rôle, is the emphasis on the emotional aspect; this preoccupation of P constrasts strikingly with a certain rôle-feature of D: it is repeatedly explained that the prominent D-attitude must be one of 'detached concern' (Fox 1959). According to Persoon (1978, 231), doctors are taught to be aware of the fact that they cannot possibly solve all of P's problems, that it is undesirable that they become emotionally involved with P or his problems, and that is impropable that they can take away all of P's fears and worries, is stress or despair. As he concludes, "this attitude guarantees (..) an adequate discharge of the medical profession, yet it allows (..) for shortcomings and deficiencies in the interaction between individual patients and their doctor" (1978, 231). Reiser and Rosen (1984), though insisting that they in no way want to play down the importance of medical skill and scientific training go so far as to state that showing compassion is a lost skill in the medical context. It is their conviction that the modern professional attitude of detachment - which, they believe, is developed during medical education - has brought about the situation in which present-days doctors have to face 'a hostile and distrustful public'.

Even though this may be too severe a judgement, it is certainly true that D and P operate from different structures of expectation. While P favours or expects complete interest and full understanding of D, D is preoccupied with the medical, technical, and instrumental aspects of the case; these differences, however, have little to do with personal characteristics of P and, especially, D, since they are, as Persoon observes, a concomitant of the nature of the D-P relation itself. As he adds, "My investigations showed that there is a considerable discrepancy between the normative expectations and the actual behaviour of D; that is to say, that patients are noticeably more demanding with respect to the quality of the communication than doctors are" (1978, 234; he also mentions social stratification as a factor in the prediction of satisfaction, but this must be left aside here, cf. Persoon 1975). Since several researchers agree as to the reality of the different frames of expectation, opposing for instance 'professional referral systems' and 'lay referral systems' (cf. Touw-Otten and Verbeek-Heida 1978, 243), it may be supposed that, at least in part, the problems of D-P communication can be stated in terms of a divergence of attitudes as a structual property of that communication, or, if you will, as a generic feature of this form of talk.

Attitudinal divergence leads, among other things, to a situation of potential conflict; although manifest conflict is reported to be exceptional (since 'social withdrawal' is not feasible, as the medical system in the Netherlands does not allow for 'shopping around', one possible outcome of such a situation is the 'psychological withdrawal' of P, which manifests itself in non-compliant behaviour (Persoon 1978, 232)). So, the consequences of the problematic status of D-P communication are far more serious than mere dissatisfactions on the part of P: if it is indeed true that communication failures enforce non-compliance, D-P interaction contains elements that are nothing less than counterproductive.

The analysis of D-P communication so far is of a rather global character, certainly from the perspective of the linguist. Some important problems of D-P communication can be acknowledged and partly classified on the basis of global analysis of the macro-sociological sort, yet not, I believe, fully understood. Such problems call for a far more detailed analyses of actual verbal interactions between doctors and patients. It must be conceded, however, that it is possible and worthwhile to make use of macro-sociological analysis, since they allow for the ascertaining of the relevant issues or for the determination of aspects that deserve a further linguistic analysis.

Insum, D and P are in agreement as to the general outcome of their interaction (e.g. a prescription, advice, a medical treatment); but they have different opinions about the procedure that leads to that outcome, and especially about how the other participant is going to behave, or should behave. D-P interaction draws upon conflicting cognitive 'realities', and it is predictable that this will manifest itself in the actual verbal behaviour of both participants. There must be deficiencies, so to speak, in the coordination of the language that is used and the speech actions that are performed; linguists should be able, on the grounds of a more or less exhaustive analysis of the verbal interaction, to state precisely what goes 'wrong', where and how in D-P communication, and how individual samples of verbal interaction between individual doctors and individual patients reflect a more general and 'impersonal' structural problem.

As for the latter category, the discussed differences in approach that hamper D-P communication suggest that it is worthwhile to focus on one aspect of the multi-layered phenomenon, namely P's expression of emotions and D's dealing with this information.

As noted earlier, P is emotionally involved with the interaction: he is ill, he has some problems with his health, and it is only natural - at least for a normal person, if we may use that term here - that he worries about his disease, ailment or disorder. One major task of P, when consulting D in order to be medically attended to, is to present his case, to make his problem known. This is realized by the act of complaining: P offers D insight in the nature of his case by giving him all kinds of information, by presenting him with all the details that are relevant according to the lay referral system that P necessarily uses. As explained, D filters this stream of information in that he evaluates the information that P gives from the perspective of the medical model or the professional system. What P feels in physical terms is all-important; what P feels in emotional terms is far less indicative of the kind or type of illness that he is suffering from. D's approach may seem appropriate from the medical viewpoint: on the basis of information about where the pain is, what kind of pain it is, when it comes and goes, how long P has been suffering from this particular pain, etcetera, D can set up one or several hypotheses leading to a physical examination. But D's viewpoint is not necessarily congenial to that of P: for P his disease is not a 'thing' that he possesses - or that possesses him -, his disease modifies his existence, and it may even threaten it (or P may believe so). P experiences his disease, he lives with it, feels it, thinks and speculates about it - it is, for a longer or shorter period, a most important aspect of his daily life. His disease

becomes, not surprisingly, an 'object' that is liable to the formation of attitudes of the evaluative sort, which are likely to be experienced as emotions, and which, also, lead to a variety of concomitant actions and activities (including non-activity).
Thus P's complaint becomes integrated in his personal history; therefore, when it comes to presenting his case, P is disposed to include, perhaps in great detail, aspects of his personal experience with 'living the illness'. And moreover, since these experiences and emotions eventually relate, consciously or not, to the conditions of his very being, P may be expected to highly value an expert's opinion, also with respect to these aspects. Or, to put it less dramatically, when P describes his case, also highlighting a lot of attitudes and emotions, it may be assumed that he wishes to be 'ratified, understood, approved of', to use some of the qualifications that Brown and Levinson utilize to characterize the notion of 'positive face' (cf. 1978, 67).

It now seems that this expressive information is not always adequately responded to in D-P communication, as fragment (2) will show. And, in fact, I suggest that the way this D reacts to this P's evaluative utterances is more or less prototypical.

(2) (P has informed D that he often suffers from feeling puffed, especially after eating sauerkraut; one method, he has found out, to feel relieved is to drink a glass of mineral water containing carbonic acid).

P1: ...and then uh once in a while I drink a glass and then I can belch
D1: that can also help of course. yes.
P2: yeah that's relieving.
D2: yes.
P3: for it's such a lousy pain.
D3: hmm.
P4: though I am used to it because I've always suffered from rheumatism.
D4: yes.
P5: so I am used to it.
D5: yes.
P6: but then again I absolutely cannot remain laying down in my bed.
D6: no.

It will be observed, that P explicitly complains about the seriousness of the pain (that he feels before belching) (P3); furthermore, he corroborates this emotive statement by thematising that - as regards the suffering from pain - he is competent to judge (P4); this corroboration is repeated in P5; in P6 he describes the seriousness of his pain by referring to the fact that he cannot stay in his bed and has to undertake some activity to ease the pain. Although P is emotional enough, D's minimal responses do not constitute the hearty proofs of compassionateness that P supposedly favours. That, at least, is how I see it; of course, I am aware of the fact that this type of D-behaviour is consistent with the questionable doctrines of Rogerian therapy. As suggested, D's behaviour is in no way exceptional;[5] neither does this sample of verbal interaction illustrate a unique phenomenon, nor am I the first to draw attention to the non-committal nature of such responses as D gives (cf. Berenst et al. 1985, forthcoming; see also Van der Geest's contribution elsewhere in this volume). In short, the observation is trivial. Yet this trivial observation deserves further consideration, since it violates what one might expect on the basis of our reading of the more recent normative literature pertaining to D-P relations. As mentioned, studies in the sociology of medicine, which are descriptive in nature, stress that structural characteristics of D-P interaction further or beget conflict. Different frames of expectation cause friction, and, as I have argued, some friction (or a special type of friction) can be the result of divergent opinions about the rôle and status of expressive information.

Textbooks that are normative in nature, however, and that primarily prescribe how doctors should behave and which contain suggestions and advices as to how to perform this desired behaviour, are pertinent about the importance of expressive information offered by P and about the relevance of an adequate response by D to such a display of emotions.

Usually, these texts distinguish (and stress the importance of distinguishing) various stages or 'rounds' in the interaction; they single out the anamnesis or the 'explorative stage' as the locus of emotional information (cf. Gevers et al.1980, 102ff; Van Aalderen and Hollenbeek Brouwer 1982, 5ff).

Van Aalderen and Hollenbeek Brouwer argue against medical reductionism and advocate a position that utilizes an

'integrational model' of illness, giving due weight, in addition to somatic, to psycho-social and societal components of a case (o.c., pp. 67-68). The way in which P experiences his complaint, and his emotional involvement, can be particularly revealing of the non-somatic aspects that influence the clinical picture. Therefore, the anamnesis or the 'intake' (as they also call it) should be thus conducted that it grants P ample space to express his opinions, worries, emotions, and the like (o.c., p. 70).
A similar position is defended by Gevers et al. (1980, 103ff). As they assert "at this (explorative) stage, it is important that the doctor not solely pays attention to the 'content' of patient's complaint, but also to the way the problem is stated: it is especially the manner of presenting the problem that informs him about the patient's feeling and attitudes pertaining to his complaint, or to his expectations and aims" (o.c, p. 104).

This philosophy of medicine contrasts sharply with the practices that I have just been describing.

Several considerations may serve to explain (or to explain away) this lack of balance between theory and practice.

One extra-linguistic factor - one that may well explain, though only in part, D's restraint with respect to P's emotionality - is that it can be assumed that D is overly preoccupied with a tangible outcome of the interaction: what he wants (and has learned to want), above all other things, is to cure; what he believes is all important is to achieve something practical, to bring about something concrete (such as a recipe, a good advice, a medication). As to P's emotions, there is little he can 'do', except for sympathizing (and for hoping that medical treatment will take care of the emotions as well). Obviously, D tends to ignore the importance of showing sympathy and understanding, cf. fragments (3) and (4).

(3) (P complains about his swollen feet)
P: ...but I've had it for yea:rs for I've worked till uhm january 16. january 30 I became 65 and I had some
D: hmm.
P: days off. so I've worked till I became 65, yeah, I've been working for 35 years
D: and that's really finished now I see.
P: always hard labour that's why my muscles. that of course they uh and from my neck. it comes from my neck.

D: yes hmm.

P: I was treated for that and uh this spot here was treated with a sunlamp and uh my ankles they treated

D: hmm, hmm.

P: them too but well they told me/ I had to come to doctor V. then and he told me uh I had to learn to live with it.

D: hmm, hmm.

P: well so that's what I tried to do for the last 10 years or so.

D: hmm. hey tell me how does it feel that you quit working?

(4) (P consults D with respect to his suffering from erysipelas; D describes the use of a shampoo, but P doesn't seem satisfied)

D: ...and then twice a day you use the shampoo and you do some massage with your fingertips and then you'll be rid of it soon.

P: well yes uh uhm that's uh. last time you talked about shampoos that uh/ there is so many people that try to get rid of it. they use this shampoo and that shampoo, so uh

D: hmm hmm, well then you should certainly try this one it is rather/ there are indeed shampoos against it. but I think that first you should uh. I know of some pretty good results of this hair lotion (name) so I mean

P: it simply is a problem, what is it, well one had this recipe and the other that lotion. All those people messing around with uh with them shampoos

D: but well that is

P: and then again something else and they never find it (= a proper treatment), good heavens no. but there are many problems like that.

D: that uh. it's a commercial product you know but that is uh there is a lot of uh

P: yeah like going to the drug store and asking 'do you have anything against dandruff?' then they will

D: what did you say your number was by the way

P: uh 346.

It has also been proposed - and that is another factor - that because interview courses during which medical students train their communicative skills, are usually taught by psychologists and other non-physicians, many students are apt to conclude that it has little to do with 'real medicine' (Reiser and Rosen 1984).

As to the latter object (interview courses), I think it is important to note another defect, one that is far more serious (and has more to do with linguistics). When one evaluates the assumptions and theories that form the basis of the instructions, the advice, the considerations, and the practical trainings and excercises that are offered in the context of such courses, one must conclude that, by and large, these instructions can but be vague if not inept. It is my contention, then, that the nature of the object of training, verbal interaction, is not fully understood or is underestimated. Human verbal behaviour is richer and far more complex than that it allows for the simple and global directions we find in the deontic textbooks. "(..) D makes use (..) of the skills that belong to the 'open listening model' (..). He listens to what P says, to how he says it, and expresses, at a well-chosen moment and if necessary, his own feelings and desires" (Van Aalderen and Hollenbeek Brouwer 1982, 26). And a similar citation from another book: "By his approach, D must give P every opportunity to state the real reason of his consultation, either by letting him talk spontaneously or - if the conversation falters - by stimulating him by means of asking (open) questions. (..). So D must be non-directive, put aside his own (medical) frame of reference, go into what P says, for instance by requesting clarifications, by summarizing, or by giving (emotional) reflections" (Gevers et al. 1980, 104).

All this is easier said than done; vacuous deliberations of this kind only roughly relate to communication in actu, and I fail to see how anyone armed with these truims can improve the quality and the functionality of the interactions in which he participates. The effects of this type of prescriptions, if any, draw heavily, if not exclusively, upon the student's communicative competence as developed during primary socialization; the alleged prescriptions can only reinforce D's judgements about communication and language use. If indeed verbal skills can be developed in training programmes, it is only a deeper knowledge about how people communicate, together with an adequate integration of this knowledge into the context of the training programme (a task of educationists rather than linguists), that can help to bring about the intended improvements.

anything practical was one of the lame consequences of being a linguist (if I may thus playfully allude to the title of a well-known article of Labov's). Today linguistics, not solely focusing on the language system but also paying full attention on the systematicity of language use, can possibly contribute to effect improvements in verbal communication processes. A sweeping statement indeed, and one that saddles me with the burden of proof. For briefness' sake, I cannot go deeply into the particulars of the linguist's contribution. Let me point out, first in general, what I would propose with respect to the problem of D-P communication that I have circumscribed, i.e. the rôle - or rather the fate - of expressive information. I believe that much can be gained by an accurate description, based on linguistic analysis, of the various ways in which people, including patients, do in fact express their attitudes and emotions. This, together with a display of the options that are feasible and occur in the communicative community to verbally respond to evaluations in a cooperative and coordinated manner, should constitute in part the subject-matter of an interview course. If teachers in verbal training programmes would be able, on the grounds of more detailed insights, to create in their (medical) students at least a greater sensibility of, and more affinity with, the different and sometimes subtle strategies that speakers use to express their evaluative judgements and their emotional states, including the devices that serve to obtain a positive reaction to this expressive information, this could result in a situation in which due respect is shown to P as a 'competent member' or, if you will, as a human being.

At the risk of your suspecting me of mere verbosity, I must now confine myself to an outline of the research-topic under discussion, i.e. expressive information.

Until recently, the expressive function of language has not been treated in great detail by linguists. Searle, in his classification of the five basic functions of language, i.e. the five categories of illocutionary acts (1976), deals but briefly with 'expressives', and his characterization of this type of speech action is largely incorrect. One thing to be noted is that under the category of expressives rather different types of language behaviour are subsumed. Whereas it is possible for a person to be expressive of a mood or a psychological state, a desire or a sentiment, I would now single out the subcategory of evaluations as the expressive single out the subcategory of evaluations as the expressive speech actions that are indeed relevant to the communication problem under discussion. Evaluations are best characterized (and distinguished from other types of expressive language) by proclaiming that they attribute a value to an object that does not coincide with the speaker, at least not in his rôle of evaluator (if the reader appreciates this analytical difference). By means of an evaluative utterance, the speaker predicates of an evaluatum that, as far as he is concerned, has a certain value. Evaluation is synonymous with value judgment, to put it apodictically.

When it comes to analysing utterances, and, subsequently, discourse that to a lesser or greater extent contains utterances that ascribe values to things, states, events or persons (including the speaker), such as narratives or the anamnetic stage in D-P communication, a first and fundamental step is to distinguish between entities that are entailed by, or co-occurrent with, evaluation processes, since these entities are reflected when value judgments are expressed verbally. Therefore, a conceptual analysis of the evaluation process may serve as a categorization device with respect to evaluative language. Without even summarizing the arguments in favour of it (cf. Bax 1985) I maintain that the concept of evaluation is best characterized by this prototypical scheme:

(5) The Concept of Evaluation

categorization device for the semantic analysis of evaluative utterances

```
E : X Xs  Y Z A
    1
    R
```

Whenever a value judgment is formed - regardless of the various ways in which psychologically speaking a subject may in fact arrive at such a conclusion - the evaluator relates the evaluatum (E) to an evaluation standard (X); applying a set of rules, he ranks or grades the evaluatum, thus arriving at a value judgment (Xs) (Cf. Taylor 1975, 9ff). It is important to realise that Xs is in principle object-oriented (and only secondarily subject-oriented): when a value judgment is uttered, it counts as the speaker's of value, regardless of the evaluator's saying so or not (cf. Ross 1968).

Yet this does not affect the plausibility of the fact that the evaluator, having arrived at a value judgment, is liable to assume an attitude (Y) towards the evaluatum. As Taylor suggests, such an attitude is entailed by the (logically preceding) value judgment. Skipping the reasons now for this being indeed the case, I further aver that an attitude may manifest itself as an emotion in the subject (Z), although not by definition. Lyons has convincingly shown that emotions are characterized by both cognitive (i.e. attitudes) and physical aspects (bodily feelings such as those caused by physiological changes associated with adrenaline flow, blood circulation, respiration, muscular tension, temperature, or secretion; cf. 1980, 60). It is a matter for conjecture how mind and body interact in this respect, how cognitive attitudes of the evaluative sort can cause the bodily changes that define a particular emotional state, but this is something that has to be left aside (cf. Popper and Eccles 1977).

In conclusion I can only say that both attitudes and emotions may connote an appetitive aspect that is responsible for overt actions of the subject (including speech actions) or for the planning of such actions (A).

Leaving much unsaid, I suggest that evaluative utterances, expressing the speaker's judgment of a state of affairs, are based on this conceptual structure, and can be described and classified in terms of that model. I have found that there are three basic modes of encoding expressive information; the notions of attitudinal mode, emotional mode, and actional mode refer to the nature of the propositional content of an evaluative utterance. More often than not, this propositional content is amplified and modified; that is, the evaluative proposition is uttered together with a lot of 'other information'. Without going into details, I may say that this additional information results from the speaker practising certain linguistic devices that serve to indicate his personal involvement with his evaluative standpoint. To give an indication, besides stating what he thinks of something, the speaker may realize an elliptic formulation, use exclamations or prosodic modifications, repetitions, particles, illogical demonstratives, marked lexical and stylistical choices, etcetera, in order to allow for his evaluation to have a definite personal touch. Furthermore, the tical choices, etcetera, in order to allow for his evaluation to have a definite personal touch. Furthermore, the conceptual model can be used to analyse devices that are rhetorical in character; that is, to describe phenomena of language use that are predominantly hearer-oriented (in that they serve to achieve the dimension of 'projected agreement', cf. McLaughlin et al. 1983; see also Bax 1981).

These remarks must suffice to illustrate our point that the expression of attitudes and emotions constitutes a multi-faceted phenomenon of language use. But in order to fully understand and appreciate the ways in which people express themselves expressively, linguists must (as I believe they can) account for the details of evaluative language. Figure (6) summarizes the options speakers have in order to be 'expressive'. (see page 117)

Within the scope of this article, which may be criticized for its lack of substance as regards the linguistic aspect, I find it impossible both to discuss the expressive function of language with a sufficient amount of detail, and to make out a case for the importance of the rôle of expressives in D-P communication.

Having performed the latter task, I must confine myself to merely indicating the different kinds of expressive signals, although much more could be said about expressive information in D-P communication (as the above display implies). Fragment (7) shows several of the alleged options: (see page 118)

(6) Display of Options to express Evaluations

A) From a semantic viewpoint:

- explicit
  - direct —— attitudinal mode
    - object-oriented - value judgment (Xs)
    - subject-oriented - appraisals, appreciations (Y)
  - indirect
    - emotional mode (Z)
      - emotion labels
      - descr. of emotional symptoms
    - actional mode (A) —— (concomitant)
      - actions, speech actions
      - action plans
- implicit (utterances in which the expressive function is merged with other functions; implicit evaluation formally marked by strategies as subsumed under B; besides, there are textual strategies like climax or contrast)

B) From a pragmatic viewpoint:

- explicit evaluations
  - apodictic
    - propositions according to Y, Z or A mode
    - (ditto +) personal involvement stressed*
  - justified
    - argumentative strategies**
    - interactional strategies***

* e.g. realised by:
- performatives
- prosodic modification
- adverbs, adjectives (measurement)
- superlatives, comparators
- ellipsis, exclamatives
- demonstratives
- lexical, stylistic choice
- particles stressing S's certainty
- repeats

** realised by
- verification
- validation
- vindication

*** e.g. realised by
- thematizing S's sincerity
- thematizing S's competence to judge
- pronominal shift, time shift
- tags, particles projecting agreement

Within the scope of this article, which may be criticized for its lack of substance as regards the linguistic aspect, I find it impossible both to discuss the expressive function of language with a sufficient amount of detail, <u>and</u> make out a case for the importance of the rôle of expressives in D-P communication.

Having performed the latter task, I must confine myself to merely indicating the different kinds of expressive signals, although much more could be said about expressive information in D-P communication (as the above display implies). Fragment (7) shows several of the alleged options:

```
[D: how are you doing?
[P:                 Well not too well. since last sunday I do have this terrible pain in my muscles you know
[D:                           fine. we'll do something about it
[P: I get completely chagrined                               Yes? at night I just cannot stay in bed because of
[D:          and in the daytime?
[P: the pain                  as long as I am busy and moving about it's more or less okay. but as soon as I sit
[D:                                         did you catch a cold lately?
[P: down or lay down then it's terribly bad                                well doctor honestly I've had it for years
[D:                                    that didn't help,                                 I see. some people have it
[P: I did get that massage at Dr. X's                   no. the muscles are so very tight.
[D: every winter   but never in summer tight?
[P:              yes                      in the summertime I have it less I have to admit that. and now this.
[D:                                                   okay.  I'll give you some pills. three times a day
[P:Week again. I can still/ my breasts hurt all over
```

In this paper, I have focused on extra-linguistic features of D-P communication in order to stake out with sufficient rigour one particular problem area. I admit that linguistic research, if it is to be applicable, cannot be conducted without a thorough survey of the problem areas involved. The next step, of course, would be to carefully analyse, on the basis of a linguistic theory of evaluations, samples of spoken interaction in the medical context, and to consider where and how the problems become manifest which are favoured by the superimposed structure of the context. The next step (though I am not sure whether this would be one for a linguist to take), would be to translate the findings of the research into a form that is manageable in an interview course. Exploring emotions, however, is no easy thing, neither for doctors nor for linguists. But both may profit from doctor-linguist communication.

NOTES:

[1]What Holmes terms 'the science of deduction' (cf. for instance Chapter I of The Sign of the Four) is actually the reasoning process that is usually referred to as 'induction'. The semiologist Eco, however, claims that what Holmes practises is 'abduction' in the sense of Ch.S. Peirce (cf. U. Eco, 'Lecture de Sherlock Holmes: l'abduction dans les sciences naturelles et dans les sciences humaines", lecture (Groningen, May 24, 1984)).

[2]This fragment (and the other ones too) stem from an extensive collection of transscripts of D-P interactions made by HIVU (Huisartsen Instituut Vrije Universiteit) in Amsterdam. Part of this collection has been placed in the hands of an interdisciplinary research group of Groningen University (i.e. WG Taalgebruik in de Medische Context).

[3]When the present article was written, this textbook was not yet obtainable in the Netherlands. I took my insights in the book from an extensive review (by F.M. Hechinger) in the New York Times of August 7, 1984. The quotations are from this review article. It is, in my opinion, particularly revealing of the doubtful reputation of D-P communication that (a study of) this subject is given full attention on the education page of a leading daily.

[4]For the benefit of the reader, I have translated, as literally as I could, all quotations of Dutch text fragments, including the transcripts of consultations (cited below).

[5]As background reading for the present article, I studied about fifty transcripts in the corpus mentioned in note 2.

COMMENTS ON M.M.H. BAX

M.Fahrenfort

I quite agree with Bax that "much can be gained by an accurate description, based on a linguistic analysis of the various ways in which people, including patients, do in fact express their attitudes and emotions". It could even be true that a training programme in doctor-patient communication could benefit by such an undertaking, although to me as a trainer in communication skills, this is not nearly as sure as Bax makes it out to be.

As his paper deals primarily with non-linguistic aspects of the matter in question, I will address myself to these also, limiting myself to a few remarks that can be made on his analysis of doctor-patient communication.

Bax tries to show that notwithstanding training programmes, doctor-patient communication is still unsatisfactory, largely because doctors do not pay the right kind of attention to emotional aspects of the patient. His "typical" example does not, however, convince me as being typical in this respect for several reasons. Firstly, it may well be that non-linguistic elements (i.e. bodily posture, tone of voice) are much more important in this respect than the utterances themselves.

It has been shown in psychological literature that precisely these elements account for the relational, emotive aspect, whereas the linguistic content of the communication plays a relatively minor rôle. Secondly, to be sure of this example as a "typical" one in relation to Bax's argument, we need to know whether the doctor involved really thinks communicative skills are important for doctors. Training programmes have been slow to start and only marginally important in the education of new physicians, and many of them still do not have any training in this respect. To be convincing, his example would have to be typical of the behaviour of a well-trained, well-informed doctor like the ones he cites from the literature.

Moreover, Bax's argument on the causes of the defects in doctor-patient communication is sadly lacking in sophistication for the following reasons:

He does not draw distinctions between the personal characteristics of the participants (e.g. doctor's lack of communitative skills), characteristics of the situation (e.g. medical necessities, time-constraints), sociological characteristics (e.g. differences in position of the participants). Some of these, notably in the first category, could be modified by adequate training, many others, however, not at all.

- Showing compassion is not the same as being emotionally involved: on the contrary, to be efficient in compassion a certain detachment (i.e. non-identification), is necessary. It would not do at all for the doctor to shake with the patient's fear and pain while dressing a wound, but the psychological complexities involved here are far beyond linguistics.
- To make his point on the deficiency of communication training, Bax cites Haberland and Mey on doctor-patient relations as being almost by definition potentially strained. "Almost by definition" in this respect means, however, that the strain is a structural property of the different positions involved, and in this way independent of the personal skills of the participants, and not amenable to training.

There is more, but I believe the foregoing is sufficient to show that when linguists try to follow in the footsteps of trainers in communication skills, they are at least as likely to fall into the trap of "vacuous deliberations" that constitutes Bax's reproof to trainers. Straying into a field that is not one's own, involves running the risk of inaccuracy and overgeneralization.

I really think linguists and behavioural scientists have much to learn from mutual contact, the linguists providing linguistic expertise, the others their own (not always vacuous) deliberations.

Maybe this could lead to better training programmes, though thus far I doubt it, on account of the complexities involved. It could certainly lead to fruitful reciprocal fertilization of research, leading to more comprehensive and sophisticated analyis by mutual contributions from different disciplines to the same research subject.

5

Conversational control in doctor patient interaction

J. Berenst

There seem to be quite a lot of problems in the interaction of doctors and patients, if the amount of interest it attracts from sociologists, psychologists and linguists means anything. But if the attention paid by physicians is anything to go by, there seems to be hardly any problem. In the literature on the subject, I have often come across complaints about the lack of interest in interactional aspects shown by medical workers (nurses and psychiatrists excepted). Is there any explanation for it, apart from other priorities they set themselves? I think we can find one if we study their conversations with patients: physicians hardly ever come up against any interactional problem because of their dominant position in the conversation, save perhaps the language use in the answers of some patients which is not very clear. Even if patients feel unhappy about the treatment by their doctor, they often do not tell the doctor, this being caused by a discongruency of what happened. (Cf. Cicourel 1982). In the following fragment (1) we see a patient reporting to his family doctor the former's dissatisfaction with his previous doctor's behaviour. The stretch of conversation[1] is preceded by the advice of the doctor to see a urologist for a prostate operation.

(1) D1: normally speaking it has no consequences. none at all you know. none at all. You don't need to worry about either sexual or urinary uh in respect of the passing of urine not any consequences.

P1: I don't think of worries I'm thinking more of the/ so uh well yes that's the interaction with doctor X. at that time I have already. so I have at that time already brought that complaint to his attention and fairly early too but it was not given any attention all the time in that sense, he did listen, certainly, but it was not examined. and so as a patient you don't know when you have to put it forward.

D2: yes. yes I think it's very wise that you put it forward and I think it's very worth while just to ask the urologist what he thinks about it, you know.

The patient is resentful of his former doctor because he did not pay enough attention to his complaints. The doctor listened to the complaints but did not investigate them. The patient had expected a serious medical examination, when he presented his complaints for the first time. So if the doctor does not come up to this expectation, it makes him uncertain about the adequacy of his complaints. Although there is no recording available of the conversation with the previous doctor, I would not be surprised if there should not have been the slightest indication of disharmony. Patients and doctors may hold different views about the implications of complaining in a medical setting, the conversational outcome of this activity is nearly always that the doctor becomes the master of the game.

In this paper I will try to make clear that doctors and patients do not exert equal control of the conversation and that this situation is mostly brought about by patients, but can be reinforced by certain conversational strategies on the part of doctors. Firstly, however, I would like to make some statements about doctor-patient communication as a special kind of discourse.

1. To be clear from the outset, I do not think that there is much reason to consider D-P conversations as a very special type of discourse. There are many task-oriented conversations between an expert and a layman who seeks help, which are to a very large extent similar, and possibly have the same communication problems. This position does not mean, however, that I want to deny the uniqueness of D-P conversations seen in the light of the topics and the goals of the discourse. Nor will I deny that there are sometimes utterances and sequences which can only be interpreted with references to the 'higher predicates' (Cicourel 1980) of the 'activity type' (Levinson 1979). But I think we are engaged in a great many activity types every day, which call attention to their proper goals, and mostly we succeed in coming through, unless the situation is unclear or we are not familiar with the activity. Consulting room conversations

with a general practitioner are neither uncommon nor unclear. That is why I said they do not constitute a very special type of discourse.

However, not everyone seems to agree with me on this point. Shirley B. Heath (1979) views D-P communication as a kind of discourse where Gricean conversational maxims are exchanged for another set of maxims, which are conflicting with the cooperative principle and are therefore only valid for one of the participants. She suggests that doctors and patients have different sets of rules, while they are each thinking that only one set is operative. Others (Conte 1980, Cicourel 1982) suggest that the essential problem in D-P communication is the fact that doctors and patients possess different cognitive schemes for the achievement of the interactional goal. The arguments which are adduced in support of this position may be found in educational advice handbooks for medical practitioners (Heath), in the confusion which sometimes seems to exist about the relevance of new contributions to the conversation (Cicourel), and in the often signalled conflict about the information given by the doctor concerning the Quality- and the Quantity-maxim: what is the truth the doctor has to tell and how much information is adequate (Heath 1979, Conte 1981, Bliesener & Siegrist 1981, Fisher 1984a).

These observations however, do not tell us anything which is unique for doctor-patient communication. Aside from completely ritualised interaction, conversations are not predictable in detail, not even in institutional settings. The implicit agreement about conversational goals can be more or less rough, as the congruency in cognitive schemes which specify the sequence of activities in view of the achievement of the ends.

In consulting room conversations all participants know that one of the very likely 'reasons for call' of the patient is a physical or mental discomfort on the patient's part; and everyone expects that the doctor will try to account for the complaints and then give some advice as to how to handle them. I do not think their aims are different in this respect, and so there is no reason why they should not be oriented towards the cooperative principle. But it does not mean that both participants externalize their behaviour in the same way; the interpretation of what is relevant, or how much information is sufficient or clear and unambiguous, or even what is true, to a certain extent depends on how they are positioned in the situation. A great many clarification sequences (initiated by the doctor) signal the discongruency in assessment by doctors and patients of what exactly is a relevant and adequate response. But that is quite different from intentionally abolishing the cooperation, as may happen in an interrogation (Hoffmann 1980) or in a quarrel (Apeltauer 1978). Such an abolition may give rise both to questioning strategies that do not provide any opportunity for escaping the recognised relevance points (e.g. in a court trial) and to conversations where people only trust logical and conventional implications, but no conversational implicatures. As far I have seen there are not many D-P conversations which must be interpreted from this non-cooperative point of view.[2] This means that misinterpretation in the way of satisfying the conversational maxims is sometimes due to the unequal distribution of knowledge, especially concerning the medical aspects of the complaint, which can be characterised as medical frame knowledge.

When there are problems concerning the goals of the interaction, these are mostly related to the social-emotional aims and need of the patients. These aims are not strictly bound to the activity type but vary among patients. Some require the doctor to declare them ill, others are afraid that they may hear that it is something serious: a few only wish to be alleviated of the pain, others only need reassurance, etc. These goals are difficult to recognize in the conversation because of the indirect or even hidden ways in which they are brought forward. So if doctors do not react (or react in the wrong way) to the concern of the patient, or to his shame, or to his sorrow etc. it may be the result of the ambiguous way in which those aspects are conveyed. I will give one example of this functional ambiguity, in fragment (2); the first turn is realised by a patient who is preparing for a physical examination:

(2) P1: I come here quite often.
D1: I beg your pardon?
P2: I come here quite often.
D2: O, that's nice. so we see a good deal of each other, don't we?

The doctor reacts to P2 with a move which can be characterised as a minimization (Goffman 1971), an acceptance of an apology; so the doctor presupposes that the patient has started a remedial interchange with an **account** by stating his intruding behaviour, which often includes an apology (cf. Owen 1983). This interpretation by the doctor is in accordance with other interactional behaviour of patients which is found frequently: accounts, apologies or justifications when doctors do not find anything serious, and complaint descriptions with strengthening hedges, which can be (and are) interpreted as account strategies (cf. Berenst et al to appear). P1 and P2 could however also be interpreted as an expressive act of concern by the patient about his physical functioning, and in this way as a **request for** account by the doctor. This interpretation rests on the assumption that it is not a good thing to see the doctor too often. It is most likely that the patient refers to this assumption, becaause of his frequent consultations with the doctor concerning several complaints which cannot all be explained - and he is only twenty-one years old! In that case the reaction of D2 is inadequate.

We will dwell on this example for a moment with another point in the relationship between doctors and patients: Why does not the patient clarify his intentions? It can be argued that he is asked for a clarification in D1, considering the possible double-duty function of this type of subsequence (cf. Springorum 1982). But the patient chooses just to repeat his former utterance. There are many reasons why someone prefers indirect or even hinted communication, but it nearly always concerns the possibility of being able to deny the interpretation by the communication partner. Clarification excludes this possibility, so it may mean that one has to choose not to convey the act if there was no intended uptake by the hearer (cf. Brown & Levinson 1978). An often defended contention (e.g. Streeck 1980) that the meaning or function of an utterance depends on the sequential negotiation in the conversation, consequently presupposes an 'Herrschaftsfreie Diskussion' (Habermas 1971) between participants who are completely open to each other and are not aware of any taboos or impositions. The utterance P2 is taken as an account/apology as appears from D2, and the patient does not disagree. But does he agree? Students of discourse analysis may say "we can't answer that question", but if they should have anything to say to professional conversationalists - in this case to doctors - they should point out the possible misinterpretations of the utterances of their patients, resulting from the perceived unequality on the part of the patients. This unequality is closely tied up with the professional differences, but may be extended to status aspects of their relationship (Hauser 1981), which causes style differences between the participants in the interaction.

So the point is that doctor-patient communication in the consulting room of a general practitioner is an activity type which has much in common with other institutional (and even informal) activity types in considering problems of adequacy and interpretation: It presupposes the cooperation of both doctor and patient, an agreement on the ultimate goals of the interaction and the components of the activity type. There may be confusions about 1) the manners of adhering to the conversational maxims because of the differences in framing the complaint, 2) the social and emotional goals of the patient and their importance, 3) the interpretation of the interpersonal aspects because of differences in the perception of their relationship.

But what are the constraints on the contributions in the conversation which define doctor-patient communication in this setting, as an activity type? I will point out three speech activities of the interaction[3], which may be described by performative verbs, but which are seldom realized in only one utterance:

1. Presenting the physical or psychological problem
2. Diagnosing the problem
3. Advising on the treatment of the problem.

The first is the task of the patient, but the other two are activities which are included in the doctors rôle. I do not see any other constraint on this activity type, but these three activities can explain much of the language usage in doctor-patient conversations. The explanatory power of these three essential functions especially pertains to the distribution of initiatives during the conversation. After a ritual opening, which may include greetings but consists essentially of a Summons-Answer sequence, where the doctor indicates in the Answer that the channel is free for the initiative of the patient, the patient Presents his problem to the doctor. At this time the doctor contributes by hearer-signals and/or contingent questions which do not affect the right of the patient to continue his description of the complaint. The next stage, which consists of the Diagnosis by the doctor, may be realized by a single act; but usually there is a special kind of pre-sequence which can be very elaborate. It contains many topics which are not mentioned by the patient and are presented now as questions by the doctor. These questions not only check whether some precondition obtains for the Diagnosis to be made (as Levinson (1983) characterizes the function of pre-sequences), but also calls for extra information which may be helpful for the doctor to establish a more exact diagnosis of the kind of disease. I prefer to call these question-answer pairs (with the possible inclusion of the physical examination) a pre-sequence because of its contiguity to the main act Diagnose. Moreover, this analysis makes clear why the doctor has to take control of the conversation after the Presentation of the complaint: it is his responsibility to make an adequate diagnosis. In addition to this - it explains the usual absence of questions[4] from the patient during the investigation by the doctor, apart from questions indicating that the former utterance was not understood: his contribution to the Diagnosis is to deliver the information needed to create or check possible hypotheses.

After the Diagnosis has been made it is again the doctor to lead the conversation because he has to formulate Advice for the patient concerning the treatment of the problem. Sometimes this Advice is preceded by a pre-sequence too, concerning specific conditions which must be fulfilled if the Advice is to be suitable for the patient. Obviously it is again the doctor who initiates such a pre-sequence. After the Advice of the doctor has been given, there can be a subsequential discussion on the implications of the advice, initiated by the patient who is asking for explanations. Questions at this stage of the conversation can, however, easily be interpreted as challenges to the professional competence of the doctor, and therefore they often contain hesitations, false starts (cf. West 1983) and hedging formulae like 'perhaps' and 'I don't know, but...', indicating the scruple and uncertainty of the patient who is trying to provide a challenging interpretation.

Finally, it is nearly always the doctor who initiates the closing section of the conversation, using a routine like 'If it doesn't clear up in a few days, I'll see you again', or a minimal response utterance with rising intonation, following a minimal response by the patient. The explanation for this can be found in the structure of the Advice-stage: the patient is the respondent to the Advice and so he is not in the position to introduce the closing section. He can only create an adequate transitional point by not starting or not continuing a subsequential discussion.

This crude analysis of the structure of doctor-patient conversations may have made it clear that the control of the conversation is usually completely exerted by the doctor. But it is important to understand that this control is implied by strategies which are functionally adapted to the three main functions of the activity type. In the next section we will discuss some conversational phenomena which may be analysed as strategies to increase the existing control differences between doctors and patients.

2. Firstly, there is variation in the relationship between the Presentation and the Diagnosis stage: the Presentation can be very short and immediately followed by pre-sequential Diagnosis questions, it may also last much longer and even make those questions redundant. It depends on the manner of Presentation and on the reaction from the doctor how long the initiative of the patient will last. Let us first look at the patient: he may conclude his complaint description after a few utterances with a statement indicating that he will abandon the floor, leaving it to the doctor, as we see in P2 in fragment (3):

(3) P1: and so as a matter of fact I spent friday through sunday in bed and on the couch

D1: Yes

P2: But now and eh:: yes, I want to do something about it.

D2: Yes. it is still the same?

A minimal response and a short pause in D2 did not encourage the patient to continue his complaint, so the doctor starts asking questions. In other conversations patients present their helplessness in just mentioning the area of the trouble, which forces the doctor to ask for explanations. This failure of initiative is striking because of the preceding move of the doctor, the availability formulation, which in general presupposes conscious patients, who are able to determine their own lives; for example:

(4) D: what can I do for you?
P: Well, I'm coming for my stomach. it's becoming very peculiar.

But even when a patient does react to the literal content of the available declaration by the doctor, he may immediately turn over the initiative:

(5) D: What can I do for you?
P: Well, perhaps just examine me. because I don't feel so good.

As said before, the availability formulations of the doctors are quite routinized: Just tell me, just tell me what's the matter with you, just tell me what I can do for you, why did you come here? What can I do for you? Although there is a style difference between those formulae, they are handled by the patient all in the same way. Unless the motive of the visit is periodical control of blood pressure, or anticonception pill use, most patients do not seem inclined to state their expectations of the doctor. They present their trouble, mostly even without any suggestion as to the diagnosis. So it sometimes seems that patients react to the availability of the doctor just as they would have done if it was the initiative move of a question-answer sequence; this means, they seem to observe the chain maxim (as Churchill (1978) has refined Sacks's chaining rule): When you are asked a question, respond with a direct answer, and then give the turn back to the questioner. And it is not amazing to find Fisher (1984b) remarking that the asymmetry of the doctor-patient relation is already reflected in the "doctor's opening questions", among other things, because it enables the doctor to control the floor. I would like to say, however, that patients often choose immediately to establish an inversion of the original conversatonal roles, bringing themselves in the respondent-rôle by interpreting an available expression as the first pair part of a question-answer sequence. When a patient does not wait for an available expression in the form of a request for information, it is more than likely that he will present intentions or a suggestion for the diagnosis. In a corpus of 46 D-P conversations[5] (not including control visits), I discovered 9 conversations without a request for information in the opening; in 44% of these conversations the patient formulated in his Presentation a request or a suggestion about the diagnosis, while this was observed only in 16% of the conversations where the doctor made a request for information in the opening stages. An example of this alternative opening is found in :

(6) D: Mrs. I
P: Hello doctor. yes I feel so miserable and I think I might have a bit of flue, I think.

This example shows that such an alternative opening still does not guarantee a long lasting initiative of the patient. He creates a turn transition point, by using among other things, a tag (in Dutch a tag particle) and becomes dependent on the next move of the doctor regarding his continuance possibilities. Let us now look at the strategies which may be used by the doctor to increase his control of the conversation. To begin with he can stop the patient's presentation by asking non-contingent questions, which have an initiative character, thereby introducing new topics which could be relevant for the diagnosis. For example:

(7) P1: I have here, well yes, a lump. It is becoming a little larger and it also bothers me.
D1: Yes.
P2: It does, uh/ it is painful.
D2: Yes.
P3: This week I thought everything turned over or something like that I felt and towards the shoulder and
D3: =yes. how long has it already been troubling you?

After two minimal responses from the doctor, which did not affect the initiative rights of the patient but encouraged him to continue, the doctor interrupted, responding to the preceding move, but immediately continued with a question.[6] So he exchanged the conversational roles, thus starting a pre-sequence for the diagnosis.

An other example of exchanging the roles is found in (8):

(8)P1: I'm here because of my cold. this evening I had a performance which I had to cancel because I tried to sing this morning at nine and when I sang a note it was stopped half-way due to the phlegm.

D2: Yes. yes.
P2: Do you have something which clears up phlegm quickly?
D2: Don't you cough or isn't it that too bad?
P3: Yes awful.
D3: Shall we listen then?
P4: Yes okay.

The critical moment was P2-D2: The patient concluded the complaint description with a request, maintaining the initiative position. But the doctor started his diagnosis questions, without even answering the patient, just as in the other conversations where the patient gave up his initiative. Mishler (1975) called this mode of connecting questions, arching, and stated that it is a strategy for a respondent "attempting to gain control over the conversation", and mainly used by participants who have authority.

These two cases might be clear, the difference between contingent questions, which do not follow the Chain Maxim, and initiative questions which do, is, however, not very exact. Particularly requests for explanation which are not realised by a minimal response with a fall-rise intonation, or by the repetition of a previous utterance, seem to have the same consequences as initiative questions, and create a role shift in the conversation.For example:

(9)P1: Well, I've been having a lot of trouble with my back lately.
D1: Trouble with your back, what exactly?
P2: Well, down here you see.
D2: Yes, in the lumbar region or higher up in your back? Trouble with my back, when? In the morning, in the evening, all day?
P3: All the time.

So when the doctor starts asking questions it seems probable that he will continue to do so, partly because the patient forces him into that position.[7]

What are other strategies of doctors to consolidate their control of the interaction? I will briefly mention three of them:
1. The down grading of previous utterances of patients in repetitive or paraphrase responses or interactive moves[8], cf. D1 in (9), and the following examples:

(10) P: (   ) and I have to pass water so terribly often.
D: Often pass water.

(11) P: (   ) I have awful stabbing pains in my chest and sometimes it gets very severe. now at this moment=
D: = stabbing pains in your chest.

(12) P: Well then I have a very strong feeling that my ankle gives way under me.
D: Then you're a little unsteady on your legs, it twist a little as it were.

The doctors are not only ignoring the emotional elements in their recapture of the contribution by the patient, but in this way they are also pointing out to patients their obligation to justify their visit to the doctor: The doctor avoids the intensity components in the descriptions of the patients which could be interpreted as account strategies. (Cf. Berenst et al. to appear).
2. The avoidance of verbalizing the Diagnosis. We see an example of this in conversation (13). The doctor requested some information, and the patient delivered the information to contribute to the Diagnosis; but at the very moment the patient is treated like a child who was considered not interested in conclusions concerning his own health, nor in the ultimate result of the activity he was to be involved in:

(13) P1 : Good morning.
D1 : Good morning. come and sit down. how are you?
P2 : It's all right, but now I have come yet.
D2 : What can I do for you?
P3 : Well it's so. last week I am troubled very much by dizziness all week long=
D12: When are you so dizzy, is it as if the whole world is spinning round as if you are sitting in a round about or is it something else?
P13: No, it's nothing like that. and uh::I feel pressure on my eyes.
D13: Yes.
D14:and then it gets a uh, my vision gets a little blurred
D14:   yes   yes
P15: Yes, uh and then I don't take much notice of it

then I just go on with my work. but yes uh not really in the way I'm used to, you
D15: not like it should. be right. and it has been like that for one week now.
P16: That's since last week. I have had it since last week I haven't been friday I haven't been to work since friday.
D16: No?
P17: But well yesterday. I had a lot of trouble with it.
D17: Just let me see your health insurance certificate.
P18: Yes.
D18: Uh ( ) number ( ) isn't it?
((D. writes prescription))
D19: With this note you just have go to the laboratory. we just prick some blood. we just look what's the matter with you now.
P19: Yes.
D20: You just have to go to the pharmacy with this prescription. you'll get some tablets to make you feel a little bit better.
P20: Okay.
D21: But uh, it would be best if you go along to the laboratory this morning
P21: Yes?
D22: for uh:: then I will have the results back on wednesday morning in any case. it's of course convenient that we will settle it, as soon as possible.
P22: Okay.
D23: Yes?
P23: May I come back for the results on thursday then?
D24: O yes, you can.
P24: Well, I'll do that then.
D25: Okay.
P25: Thank you doctor.
D26: Good luck.
P26: Yes.
D27: Bye.

3. The Advising without information. In many studies on doctor-patient communication it is noticed that doctors often fail to inform their patients adequately. (Cf. Hauser 1981). Advice presupposes a positive effect of the suggested

activity on the existing situation. If patients are neither informed about the effect nor about the motivation for the advice as related to their situation, it all depends on the authority of the doctor. In (13) no reference is made to the previous conversation in the advice, and only a very general reference is made to the consequences (D19, D20). The patient seems to accept this demonstration of domination; only in P21 he does try, in a very careful way, to get some explanation, which is given in the next turn, but not very substantially.

3. Finally, what is the function of this analysis of speech activities and sequencing phenomena for practice in the consulting room? It is my contention that doctors can learn from it that they do not need to be blamed for their control of the conversation, because of the constraints which are created by the goals of this activity type, and because of the way in which patients generally realise their right of initiative.

In this context I am inclined to query the adequacy of the way in which some doctors try to be more 'patient centred' in their conversations, uttering only minimal responses or requests for confirmation after the opening ritual, for a long time. This listening position of the doctor, which can create a long Presentation stage, is only justified, however, if the framing of the complaint by the patient is congruent with the relevant points for the doctor. If that is not the case, the doctor still has to put his questions forward, because it is he who has to make a diagnosis. The advantage of not controlling the conversation (by not requesting) could be -as is often said- that the patient supplies more information about the social and psychological circumstances surrounding the complaint. However, this does not appear to be the case, according to an evaluative Dutch study of the effects of 'listening training' for doctors: no relation between the amount of listening or questioning behaviour (of D) and the amount of psychological or social information (of P) could be established (Bensing & Sluijs 1984). But even if that effect would be established, it does not guarantee that the doctor wants to or can use this information in his diagnosis. The control by the doctor comes through the selection of information, and this selection process is demonstrated ultimately in the diagnosis and the resulting advice. Creating room for patients' 'complaining stories' can for this reason merely be a disguise for what is really going on (see fragment (1)).

This scepticism does not mean, however, that I would like to defend authoritarian behaviour of doctors. I just hope to have made clear that conversational behaviour of doctors which increases their control and domination has to be viewed in connection with the structure of the activity type and the encouraging behaviour of many patients.

NOTES

1. Legend for the transcriptions of the conversational fragments:

´	: simultaneous speech overlaps
/	: abrupt termination of the intonation contour
::	: prolongation of the prior syllable
=	: no interval between the first speaker finishing and the next starting
,	: continuing intonation with a short pause
?	: rising intonation
( )	: part of text skipped

2. Bliesener & Siegrist (1981) have shown that sometimes non-cooperation is used as a reproach or protest strategy by patients in hospital who feel neglected by the doctor.

3. I will consider only the prototype of conversations with a family doctor. Consultations to check the effects of a treatment will be omitted as a secondary matter.

4. Cf. West (1984) and Fisher (1984b).

5. This corpus is used by an interdisciplinary workinggroup on 'language use in medical contexts' at the University of Groningen.

6. Todd (1984) reports having found these two elements in one turn of the doctor very often, following the response move of the patient.

7. Cf. Mishler (1975) who argues that the probability of extended chaining sequences is dependent on the perceived status differences between the conversation partners.

8. **Reactive moves** are considered to be the third part of a sequence which acknowledges or evaluates the previous response.

Appendix : Dutch originals of the quoted fragments of conversation

(1)

D: dat heeft normaal gesproken geen konsekwenties nee. nergens voor hè. helemaal/ u hoeft zich daar geen zorgen over te maken noch sexueel noch wat de urine eh de urinelozing betreft konsekwenties.

P : ik denk ook niet aan zorgen ik denk meer aan dat/ dus eh nou ja dat is die wisselwerking met dokter X, ik heb destijds dus al die klacht naar voren gebracht en ook vrij vroeg maar er is dus steeds geen aandacht aan besteed in die zin heeft hij dus wel geluisterd maar 't is niet onderzocht. en je weet dus als patient niet wanneer moet je hier komen.

(2)

P1 : ik ben wel veel hier

D1 : wat zeg je?

P2 : ik ben wel veel hier

D2 : o dat is gezellig, dan zien we mekaar nog eens hè

(3)

P1 : en ik heb dus vrijdag tot en met een eh zondag dus in bed en op de bank doorgebracht

D1 : ja

P2 : maar nou en eh:: ja ik wil er wat tegen doen.

D2 : ja. is het nog steeds hetzelfde?

(4)

D : wat kan ik voor u doen?

P : nou ik kom voor m'n maag. dat wordt steeds gekker

(5)

D : wat kan ik voor u doen?

P : nou me misschien even onderzoeken. want ik voel me niet bijster goed.

(6)

D : mevrouw I.

P : dag dokter. ja ik voel me zo belabberd en ik denk dat ik een beetje griep heb hoor

(7)

P1 : ik heb hier zo ja een knobbel hier. is wat dikker en ik heb er ook last van

D1 : ja

P2 : het doet eh/ het is pijnlijk.

D2 : ja

P3 : van de week dacht ik dat alles m'n omkeerde of iets dergelijks voelde ik en het zo naar de schouder toe en=

D3 : =ja. hoelang heeft u daar al last van

(8)

P1 : ik kom voor m'n verkoudheid. vanavond heb ik een voorstelling die heb ik af moeten zeggen want ik heb vanmorgen om negen uur geprobeerd om te zingen en als ik een noot maak dan wordt die halverwege afgebroken door het slijm.

D1 : ja ja

P2 : hebt u iets wat snel slijm oplost?

D2 : hoest u niet of valt dat wel mee

P3 : ja verschrikkelijk

D3 : zullen we eventjes luisteren?

P4 : ja okee

(9)

P1 : nou ik heb de laatste tijd erg veel last van m'n rug

D1 : last van je rug. wat precies?

P2 : nou onderin hè

D2 : ja. bij je lenden of hoog in je rug? last van m'n rug. wanneer? 's ochtens 's avonds? de hele dag?

P3 : altijd

(10)

P : ( ) en ik moet zo ontzettend vaak plassen

D : vaak plassen

(11)

P : ( ) en ik heb ontzettende steken in mijn borst en soms wordt het heel hard. nu op dit moment

D : steken in je borst

(12)

P : nou dan heb ik heel erg het gevoel dat ik door m'n enkel ga

D : dan ben je wat onzeker op de benen. het zwikt als het ware een beetje

(13)

P1 : goedemorgen
D1 : goedemorgen. kom zitten. hoe is het met u?
P2 : 't gaat goed maar nou ben ik toch gekomen
D2 : wat kan ik voor u doen?
P3 : nou 't is zo. vorige week had ik heel de week had ik erge last van duizeligheid
:
:
D12: als u nou zo duizelig bent hè is het dan alsof de hele wereld draait alsof je in een draaimolen gezeten hebt of of is het iets anders
P13: nee dat niet. en eh:: ik krijg een druk op mijn ogen
D13: ja
P14: en dan wordt het een eh/ het zien dat wordt dan een beetje wazig
D14: ja ja
P15: ja eh en dan let ik er niet op dan eh: werk ik gewoon door. maar ja : toch niet zo als hoe ik gewend ben hè
D15: niet zoals het hoort. goed. en het is nu sinds een week eigenlijk
P16: dat is sinds 't vorige week/ ik heb het sinds vorige week maar ik ben dus vrijdag ben ik dus toen niet meer gaan werken
D16: nee
P17: nou maar gister had ik er veel last van
D17: ik wil nog even uw ziekenfondskaartje erbij
P18: ja
D18: hh( ) nummer ( ) hè
((D schrijft recept)) (22)
D19: met dit briefje moet u even naar het laboratorium. prikken we even wat bloed. kijken we even wat er nou aan de hand is
P19: ja
D20: met dit recept moet u even naar de apotheek. krijgt u wat tabletten waardoor u zich wat lekkerder voelt
P20: okee
D21: maar eh 't fijnste zou zijn als het vanmorgen nog lukt om even langs het laboratorium te gaan
P21: ja?
D22: want eh: dan heb ik in elk geval woensdagochtend de

uitslagen. dat is natuurlijk plezierig dat we het dan zo snel mogelijk even afwerken
P22: okee
D23: ja?
P23: kan ik dan donderdag terugkomen voor de uitslag?
D24: ja hoor dat kan
P24: nou. dat doe ik dan maar
D25: okee
P25: bedankt dokter
D26: sukses
P26: ja
D27: daag

COMMENTS ON BERENST

Dick Springorum

There are a lot of interesting points in the presentation and interpretation of doctor-patient interaction, given by Berenst. In general they really refine the approach to interactional problems, and I agree on most of them, especially with the way Berenst approached the symmetry-asymmetry 'problem' in doctor-patient interaction, recognizing that asymmetry in itself is not a rejectable form of interaction. I would like to follow his line, and if possible, to go just one step further.

Let me start in the presentation of the well-known sequential ordering in doctor-patient interaction:

D opening
P presentation of complaints
D diagnosis
D advice / treatment
(closing)

On this point Berenst seems to follow the common interpretation that it is the doctor who opens the process of interaction, and who gives the floor to the patient in and by this process of interaction. Then the patient may use his conversational or interactional position for presenting his complaints. Berenst calls this position an initiative position; elsewhere he wonders why patients in a rather systematic way do not use, or seem to refuse to use their conversational rights: in his sample he has found a great many small turns, as if patients were eager to hand back the floor to the doctor as soon as possible, contributing also to the picture of inequality or asymmetry. Then the question arises: why are patients so timid in exercising their full rights, or their full initiatives?

In my opinion speaking of patient-initiatives in presenting complaints is in general rather confusing and seems to be a misuse of the term 'initiative'. I would like to present a slightly modified act sequence, one that takes into account the answer-like behaviour of the patient in presenting his complaints that Berenst has pointed at, as well as the full act of diagnosis on the doctor's part.

1. Entering the consultation room is, that is counts as a request for help. In entering the room the patient hands the initiative to the doctor, thus making himself available for all kinds of investigations on the part of the doctor, verbal as well as non-verbal.

2. Diagnosis is not an act or an activity that follows the verbal presentation of complaints; from the very moment P enters the doctor's room, the doctor is diagnosing: by observing the patient, by looking into his papers, by reconstructing previous complaints, by consulting his amount of medical knowledge, by making inferences, and often, though not always, by asking questions, and by asking the 'open' question: "Well, tell me what the problem is".

3. In presenting his complaints, the patient is answering this question, in a more or less detailed way, according to his diseases, his knowledge of the medical frame, and the knowledge of his own body; and not seldom as a layman impeded by feelings of uncertainty about the seriousness of his complaints. So for many patients it is the doctor's job to construct the disease by verbal and/or non-verbal investigations.

To speak of 'initiative', or 'initiative position' when the patient is invited to tell something about his disease, is, in my opinion, to speak of a pseudo-initiative. Why blame the patient for not demonstrating initiatives in conversational positions in which he prefers to give short answers?

In relation to this point I should like to stress another one: the phenomenon of the 'hidden complaints'.

I fully recognize the possibility that in the course of the consultation the patient is or becomes more or less uncertain about the adequacy of his own presentation, or of the interpretation or investigation or advice of the doctor. In such a case he has to break in on the ongoing action sequence, or on the doctor's action plan. I should think that a favourite strategy to break in without giving the impression that one is breaking in, is 'dropping' comments in appropriate positions, e.g. sequence 2 in Berenst's paper. He has pointed to the doctor's move in D2 in which the doctor gives a so-called 'superficial' interpretation of the preceding move; or, in his terms, a 'misinterpretation'. My point is: does his sample contain any sequence in which the doctor in such a position reacts in the 'right' way? And has he found any evidence in the ongoing sequence or elsewhere that such an interpretation was indeed a 'right' one, or 'the right' one. And in what way could the rightness of such an interpretation or continuation be tested?

6

Notes on 'privacy' in conversations with schizophrenic patients

D.M. van Bijsterveld

1. Preliminaries

1.1. Several types of studies on language and schizophrenia

There has been a long tradition of interest in language and schizophrenia, mainly because a disruption or a disturbance of speech was considered indicative of a disorder of thought.

The tradition of research starts more or less with the assumption that the 'language disorder' might provide information about the disorder in thought: research in this area has focused on the syntactic and semantic structures of sentences of schizophrenic speakers. The data were collected through experiments, like Chapman's (1964 and 1976) multiple-choice tests on the meaning of ambiguous sentences. Tests of the understanding of proverbs were carried out as well as experiments on the sensitivity to syntactic sentence structure (Carpenter 1976, Gerver 1967). In all these studies a certain degree of difference between schizophrenic groups and non-patient groups was found in their carrying out of the tasks set, but not significant enough to warrant the conclusion that there was a definite case of language disturbance which is part of the condition of schizophrenia.

In 1970 Salzinger formulated his so called 'immediacy hypothesis', according to which schizophrenic speakers are able to connect only immediately adjoining sentences coherently, which leads to their incoherence in any longer stretch of text. Since then researchers have also been concentrating on monologues. These monologues were judged on their coherence, sometimes indirectly via the 'Cloze Procedure', where each n-th word was systematically left out and had to be reconstructed, in some experiments by non-patients, in others by schizophrenics (Salzinger 1970, 1973, Portnoy 1973; for a criticism of the method see: Maher

1982). Another method was to disconnect all the sentences of a monologue and then have it reconstructed, as was done by Rutter (1979).

They mostly found that it was more difficult to reconstruct monologues of schizophrenic people than of non-patient or other control groups, but there were contradictory findings as well.

The results of the various types of research might well be due to the fact that 'language' -and consequently language disturbance- is considered an isolated phenomenon and not an interactional activity. Very few investigators have paid attention to the discourse problems which may arise in conversations with schizophrenic people. I shall discuss some aspects of this type of research below.

1.2. Towards an interactional approach of the language use of schizophrenic people

The discussion of Chaika (1974) and Fromkin (1975) also concentrates on the discourse problems of the schizophrenic speaker. Chaika mentions for instance 'idiosyncratic' utterances as typical of schizophrenia, while Fromkin argues that precisely such utterances are merely 'slips of the tongue', because they are not uncommon even amongst people "working at the White House".

Both Chaika and Fromkin seem to overlook the fact that there is always the possibility of asking for clarification of an 'idiosyncracy' or of anything else that the addressee did not understand. Whether a participant in a conversation actually chooses to do so depends of course on his opinion concerning the relevance at that particular stage of the conversation. But if he asks for clarification he will probably find his addressee somehow taking his own words as a 'slip of the tongue' as well, and not as something containing a degree of reality for him.

Rochester (1977) emphasizes that the 'listener's task' in a conversation with a schizophrenic participant is a very difficult one. This conclusion, however, is derived from the analysis of the utterances of the schizophrenic speakers, as described in their later study (1979): they asked judges who did not participate in the conversation to point out the most disrupted parts of the typed-out transcript, which were then analysed. Since they used judges who were no participants to point out the most disrupted parts of a typed-out interview, their study is not really an analysis of interaction. Also, they concentrate on the schizophrenic speaker, and in their case the 'difficult task' of the listener refers especially to the non-schizophrenic participant. That listener's task may well be an interesting point, but in a conversation all participants are both speakers and listeners, of course.

Therefore an analysis of what happens in a conversation with a schizophrenic and a non-schizophrenic participant should not be restricted to an analysis of the utterances of the schizophrenic speaker.

1.3. Data

Two types of conversations were collected. The first one was a 'free' conversation: participants having coffee together and no instruction about a set topic that could serve as an agenda.

The second type, however, did have an agenda: the non-schizophrenic participant was asked to try to stick to the topic as much as possible. This topic was something of concern involving the daily life of the schizophrenic participants of which the non-schizophrenic participants did not know very much. The schizophrenic participants were all familiar with it, and therefore the information they could give was 'real' information for the non-schizophrenic partner.

It is a serious problem in the research of language and schizophrenia that results are difficult to compare, schizophrenia being rarely defined (Wykes 1980). Therefore in this study all schizophrenic participants were selected on the basis of their diagnosis according the criteria of Diagnostic Statistical Manual III (1980). The schizophrenic participants had been living in the hospital for at least 7 years. The non-schizophrenic participants were a psychiatrist and a 'layman'. Each of the latter two had a conversation with each of the schizophrenic participants twice, once without and once with an agenda.

However, since a diagnosis does not give information on the intensity of the symptoms, nor on the precise nature of the individual symptoms, there was an interview and a Brief Psychiatryc Rating Scale was completed by two psychiatrists after each conversation.

All participants were invited for the conversations. This

implies that the conversations were organised, and not collected via participant observation for instance. This method evades the methodological problem that speech should be collected in a natural setting, if a study of natural speech is to be made. On the other hand there were good reasons for deciding against the method of participant observation: none of the schizophrenic participants as very talkative in the ward. Most of them could not be expected to take the initiative. Moreover, the most natural setting of conversations for the schizophrenic participants was via appointments. As a matter of fact I found that it was very unusual to invite them to 'drop in for some coffee'. The only one who accepted my invitation was rather disturbed to find that I did not have any other reason for the invitation than to chat with him, that there was no special purpose, and that I had no intention of switching on the tape. The invitation 'to have a conversation' was acceptable for an appointment, and making an appointment was the natural thing to do.

For the non-schizophrenic participants it was less natural, at least at first. I always asked some questions afterwards, e.g. whether the tape-recorder had bothered or distracted them. Uninvited by me they always told me whether they had experienced the conversations as 'difficult' or 'easy'; never once when they reported that the conversation had been 'difficult' did they say that they had noticed the tape-recorder.

2. On privacy

2.1. The notion 'privacy'

There is a common sense meaning of privacy, there are things people do not want to discuss with everyone or maybe even with no one. Respect for, i.e. the need for privacy may appear in conversations.

This, however, is problematic, as privacy concerns things that are not 'mentionable', whereas the conversation is the display ground for such non-mentionable matter.

Toshow the need for privacy explicitly, to say something like "I don't want to discuss this" (or even mitigate the directness of it), involves the interactional risk of refusal and therefore it has to be made acceptable on a level of interaction. On the other hand implied in the notion of privacy is that it should be revealed as little as possible.

So apparently we are dealing with some kind of tension here which makes privacy a delicate kind of refusal.

Depending on how eager a participant is to continue the conversation these interactional activities will be more or less attended to. Motives to indicate a speaker's need for privacy can be given, but are not necessarily the 'real' personal motives, like for instance a fear to mention something, because it is painful, uninteresting, embarrassing, etc. Should these motives be mentionable, the privacy would again be partly revealed.

Because a participant has various options to guard his privacy without having to explain that he wants to do so or why, 'privacy' is an umbrella for motives that might be private. Consequently, if one wants to discuss 'privacy' as a problem for a conversation, the discussion cannot concentrate on these motives; I do not want to discuss the underlying motives but the way in which 'privacy' can be operationalised in a conversation.

Inherent in the notion is that it is something that does not come out into the open. At a topical level there are topics that are always mentionable, like for instance the weather, in other words topics that will never be considered as 'private'. But of course there are also topics that are always 'private'. It is not easy to list them, as privacy is something personal as well. Among friends there may be less privacy than among speakers who hardly know each other. So inherent in the notion is relativity as well, in the sense that 'privacy' depends on the situation and that it is personal. 'Privacy' then is the private ground participants in a conversation have apart from their shared -common- ground. Conversations are partly about the boundaries of the common and private ground[1].

Visualized and oversimplified there is the following scheme of topics concerning 'privacy' of any participant X in a conversation:

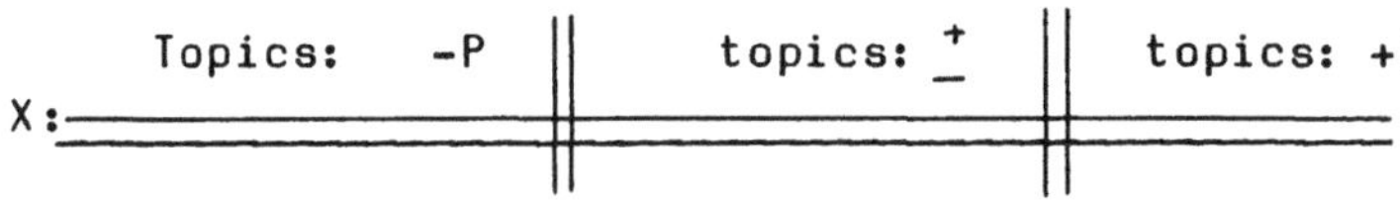

In the scheme there are 2 sets of vertical lines referring to the boundaries; one of them indicating the personal aspects, the other indicating the situation. The exact place of these sets of boundaries depends on the identity of the participants in the conversation.

Defining i.e. creating those boundaries involves attempts to get access to a partner's private ground, which can be experienced as such only if 'guarding privacy' is a conversational problem; in other words, if those boudaries are not congruent[2] for participants.

Elsewhere I described techniques the non-schizophrenic participants can use to get access. Accessibility is something speakers have to deal with; at a topical level the propositions with which speakers compose their topic will have to be accessible in order to constitute the topic at all. Accessibility may become a problem as soon as getting access becomes the main activity of the participant. Access involves a matter of degree. A conversation which is evaluated as 'good' (or 'not difficult') is a conversation in which participants experienced accessibility to a satisfying degree: accessibility involves -as is the case with privacy-relativity. Inaccessibility does not necessarily imply privacy, because a proposition might also be unintelligible and therefore inaccessible, for instance.

Privacy, however, certainly involves inaccessibility; as I shall try to show in the next paragraph the conversational activity of 'guarding privacy' involves diminished attempts at access.

2.2. The complexity of a privacy sequence

In the fragments to be discussed A is the non-schizophrenic, and B the schizophrenic participant. All fragments are excerpts from different conversations. The first fragment was transcribed using 'play-notation'; in the others 'partiture-notation' is used because overlaps and pauses are crucial there. (For the symbols used in the transcription, see appendix I)

Consider the next fragment; A and B are talking about drawing, which B used to do a lot, and which as a therapy is part of daily life in the hospital:[3]

I.

1. B: I don't do that anymore
2. A: why not?
3. B: you wear away here, don't you, you wear away here
4. A: you feel less and less like doing things,
5. B: yes.
6. A: awful

7. (6)

'Drawing', the topic discussed, was initiated by B. This implies, that apparently the topic as such was not 'private' for B, and consequently in principle accessible for A. A's question in line 2 'why not' can be seen as an attempt to get access to B's remark that he does not draw anymore. B's answer to the question reveals the reason: 'you wear away here'. In line 4 A tries again to get access to B's remark:

3. B: you wear away here, don't you, you wear away here
4. A: you feel less and less like doing things

A offers B a tentative interpretation is his former utterance, thereby inviting B to continue and at the same time diminishing the attempt to get access via the cautious formulation[4].

B indeed continues, but minimally and with a downward intonation:

4. A: you feel less and less like doing things
5. B: yes.
6. A: awful
(6)

A's comment 'awful' is an equally short reaction. In fact it is a very delicate one on A's behalf, as the reaction is explicitly an empathic interpretation of the emotional 'colour' of B's former utterance. Nevertheless it leaves the possibility for B to continue open; so it is a very 'light' attempt to get access. B however does not opt for continuing, and the long silence of 6 seconds can then be the respect for privacy which was built up in the previous reactions. After the silence there is a change of topic.

Silences are very difficult to understand. Apart from the fact that a noticeable silence is a turn that is not taken, which is a structural aspect of turntaking systematics, it is often not at all clear whose silence it is or how long a silence must be before it is a shared silence. The strain of long silences is well-known; psychotherapists have to learn to tolerate silences, and nevertheless conversations with long silences are rarely experienced as 'smooth' or 'good'. What I intend to say here is not that a silence can be interpreted as a straightforward privacy-marker. But rather that it seems plausible that to initiate a topic shift and certainly a topic change without a previous silence would seem a rude thing to do.

The remarkable aspect is that though usually it is not at all easy to point out one turn as the turn of a topic shift, as this is rather a shared activity of all participants, it is not difficult to point out that turn in this sequence; the participants do not return to this later on in the conversations.

This long silence does not imply that there always has to be such a long silence in a privacy sequence, but it certainly must be a noticeable one.

Guarding B's privacy is a shared activity in this fragment. The sequence of that shared activity then is:

> Topic B--► attempt at access A--► attempt at privacy B--► diminished attempt at access A--► silence--► topic change

The scheme of this sequence can be longer, depending on the number of attempts by A. As a matter of fact in the material I have it very rarely happens that the sequence is so simple. More often the sequence is part of a longer sequence, or it is disconnected by other sequences: the overall sequence of all turns of the conversation consists of sequences which can overlap and be part of other sequences as well, as far as the transparency of the overall sequence goes.

2.3. Can locatives locate privacy?

The next question is which part of the topic initiated by B, and consequently in principle accessible for A, can generate the activity of guarding privacy?

In the fragment above it can be seen that A's first diminished attempt to get access is a reaction to:

> B: you wear away here, don't you, you wear away

B's description of what happens 'here', namely 'wear away', has two components: a locative 'here' and his personal experience 'wear away', both referring to his life in hospital, of which A, being a 'layman' has a common sense knowledge. Hearing this description and consequently the reference of the locative 'here', A may have been prepared for this privacy-sequence. Now it is well-known that locatives are often more than a geographical reference. Discussing therapy-talk in group sessions, Turner (1976) mentions for instance, that the question 'why are you coming here?' is a problematic one for members of the group. To quote Turner: "coming to terms with 'here' in therapy sessions requires some sense of what it is that is taken to be going on; and this will be as much a matter of the questioner and the questioned as of geography"; he implies that 'here' in therapy sessions has to do with the expectations of the participants in relation to the therapy. In the conversations that form my material 'here' always refers to life in the hospital, as do the various other locatives like 'the ward', 'the building', 'the room', or the names of the buildings. For all participants the geographical meaning is that these are all places which can be visited, should participants want to do so; they also refer to the environment of the conversation.

A second type of locatives refers -geographically- to places that belong to the biography of the speaker, and consequently are not necessarily 'known' to all participants. When used by the schizophrenic participants this second type refers to the location of events which happened before they lived in the hospital. In that respect they are connected with the 'here'. I shall not discuss the second type of locatives in this paper, however.

In the fragment above, I tried to describe the activity of guarding privacy as a **shared** activity: both partners indicated at that stage of the conversation that 'wear away' was a possible private topic. Apparently this belonged to the collection of topics that may be private, as I mentioned at the beginning of this paper.

There I spoke also of topics that are always mentionable, which are never connected with privacy, and those which always are, cf. the following scheme:

topics: -P	‖	topics: $\pm$P	‖	topics: +P
	I		II	

I shall illustrate in the next paragraph that a topic considered to be devoid of the risk of being private, was indeed considered as such by the schizophrenic participant, and a topic which was considered private by the non-schizophrenic participant, was apparently not judged as such by the schizophrenic speaker. In other words in both cases there is an incongruence in the participant's experience of a topic as private.

The first fragment illustrates the incongruence around the schematic boundaries, the second fragment shows the incongruence around the schematic boundaries II.

2.4. Incongruence of privacy

In the next fragment the topic, again initiated by the schizophrenic participant, is the study he used to pursue at the university a long time ago and the question as to whether he still kept up with the subject:

II.

```
[1.  B: you've got to keep up with everything (.) once you've left the university
[2.  A:
[3.  B: you keep up with everything (.)  otherwise your year|s are quite fruitless
[4.  A:                              yeah                 y|eah
[5.  B:                                                              |yeah      |yeah
[6.  A: yes that (.) yes 'cause you go on when you study you always |go on studyi|ng,
[7.  B:        |yeah   yeah                                                    I read
[8.  A: don't  |you,          and do you read something from time to time? or ehm,
[9.  B: something from time to time=      ye|ah
[10. A:                              =l see(.) |yes (.) you also get some magazines
[11. B:             |magazines                  but we keep it rather  lig|ht
[12. A: or things li|ke that       hm.(l) yes (l)                         |sure that's
[13. B:          |we're tired most people here are tired      is one of the greatest
[14. A: fine we  |keep                                  yes (.)
[15. B: ailments that is, is |n't it                     tireoness yes
[16. A:                      |yes tiredness isn't it (.)               yes that is
[17. B:                                                       yes wrong use yes wrong
[18. A: certainly true (1 1/2) wrong use of energy or something?
```

Of course A knows that his condition is imcompatible with studying; in line 6 A generalizes 'studying', offering a tentative interpretation of B's former remark, and in line 8 this interpretation of A in line 6 appeared to be a preface to shifting the topic to 'reading'. B's minimal reactions (lines 5 and 7) apparently lead A to another attempt to get access to the topic 'reading' (line 10). B's minimal answers in line 9 seem to induce A to guard his privacy according to the equally minimal reactions and the short silences. Then (line 11) B mentions in 11 'but we keep it rather light', which apparently is interpreted as a topic shift by A: 'Sure that's fine we keep/'; A agrees with B to keep the conversation light (or else the 'we' would have been an insincere 'we'). B, however, continues in line 13 with an explanation of 'keeping it light', referring to 'light' reading, because people are tired. So at that point B did not change the topic after all. In fact the complexity is, that there is an incongruence in topic (reading magazines is according to A not a possible private topic) and in the place where A and B are engaged in guarding privacy. Again it is the locative 'here' that generates the diminished attempt of A, and only after the repeated remarks about 'tiredness' of B (lines 13 and 15) does A initiate a question about that.

In the following fragment the non-schizophrenic participant takes the utterances of the schizophrenic partner as 'private'.

Initially the talk was about the new ward B had moved into, then B starts to mention complaints about the doctors in the ward: they forgot to give him his medication, namely, hashish; he needs this as a counterbalance for the ammonia in his body. He complains about the doctor's lack of knowledge on the subject. (In fact the story is too complicated and too long to present here.) Then A generalizes:

III.

[1. A: uhuh and such is daily life there, I sEE
[2. B: yes (1)but I never really dIEd
[3. A: nO no no tnere is (.) well (.) strong (.) from counterbalance dcn't they
[4. B: yes.
[5. A: ($1^1/_2$) yes. (.) but those things (.) well you talk about them (.) but
[6. B:
[7. A: you're not occupied with them constantly now are you,
[8. B: no
[9. A: no you're not are you=
[10.B: =the beginning is horrible one gets an Acid a degree
[11.A: uhuh uhuh
[12.B: of acIdity all over the body and if one still stays alive then
[13.A: sUre I should think so
[14.B: one could say it turned out wEll

a privacy sequence. Note that this time it is A who uses the locative (line 1) and who after the silence in line 5 initiates a topic shift, hedging the story to 'those things' which might occupy B's mind constantly. A is concerned about this matter and explicitly states that the story does not belong to the topics mentionable for A: 'well you talk about them', expressing a feeling of reservation with respect to this topic. So here we can see an incongruence in privacy of topic in the sense that the topic is not private for the schizophrenic speaker while it is so for the non-schizophrenic partner. Note that in line 8 B answers 'no', immediately demonstrating that at least during the conversation 'those things' are indeed occupying his mind.

3. Concluding remarks

The notion 'privacy' was not meant to be connected with the common sense notion directly. Of course a lot could be said about the 'privacy' people who live in a hospital have, and their need for privacy (or their lack of this need), which is sometimes discussed in the conversations.

I wanted to show how privacy was operationalized and what generates privacy in this conversation-technical sense. I chose one locative 'here' and its variations. This does not imply that only locatives generate privacy-sequences, however. The fragments selected must be considered as illustrations of the last paragraph, in which I tried to show that some topics are more 'private' for a schizophrenic speaker than usual, whereas some are less. In other words incongruence of private topics of the participants is one of the problems to be solved in these conversations, and it is certainly a problem for both participants.

As the schizophrenic participants had been living in the clinic for a long time, hospitalisation may play an important role in the incongruence of private topics; this incongruence may be less obvious in conversations with schizophrenic people who do not live in a hospital, as they can manage a greater variety of social situations than life in a hospital can offer.

Also, the conversations were organised, so it might be argued that in a situation like this a greater number of topics will be private. The point is, however, that apparently there are topics which are not private and that there can be an incongruence of the participants on that matter.

Of course I did not mean to argue that these two instances prove that schizophrenic people have different boundaries for privacy. The idea is rather, that apparently it is sometimes difficult to strike a balance between 'privacy' and 'accessibility'. For if everything is private there is hardly any reason to talk at all; whereas should no topic at all be private, there would be no reason to talk either. This idea can be connected with the theory that in psychosis 'ego-boundaries' are weak: that at least for some experiences all thoughts are accessible for everyone. In the conversations I collected this never occurred so extremely, and certainly not the fragments selected for this paper. The reason seems very simple: the schizophrenic participants all decided to have those conversations, at least they had the notion of 'privacy'.

NOTES

1 Compared with A-events and B-events (Labov and Fanshel 1977): if A and B are talking about an A-event, for instance, then B gets access to the degree of A's privacy that is, if the A-event belongs to the topics that are not necessarily private.

2 Following Goodwin (1984) I use the term 'congruent' rather than 'shared': (conscious or unconscious) knowledge cannot be shared, but is congruent; an activity is shared.

3 The translation of original fragments is always a delicate and problematic matter, and always imprecise. The specific problems of the fragments discussed in this paper are the translation of 'yeah' and 'yes'. In fragment III the problem lies in the moments when the non-schizophrenic participant is searching for words in line 3; this line has been translated literally.

4 Heritage (1983) calls this type of reaction a 'formulation'. In interviews for a third audience the interviewer often uses such a formulation to elicit more information from the interviewee. The interviewer does not make a 'real' contribution to the topic, and can change the topic in the direction that the audience, for whom he is an intermediary, might be interested in. Heritage mentions that this formulation is rarely seen in conversations, and when it occurs

this formulation always has a component of 'caution'. In the conversations with schizophrenic participants, however, this type of 'formulation with caution' can be found in massive quantities.

5. This research is supported by the Foundation for Linguistic Research, which is funded by the Netherland Organisation for the Advancement of Pure Research ZWO. I want to thank Doro Franck, Erica Huls, Martha Komter, S.C. Dik and H.G.M. Rooymans for their comments on an earlier draft of this paper.

Appendix I:

Symbols used in the transcription of conversational fragments

(These symbols are adapted from those which are commonly in use for Conversational Analysis)

1. B: otherwise your ye[ars are quite fruitless
   A: [yeah

The **extended straight brackets** indicate the point at which a current speaker's talk is overlapped by that of his partner.

2. B: I read something form time to time=
   A: =I see

The **equals signs** at the end of one speaker's utterance, and at the begining of that of the next speaker's indicates that there is no discernable interval between the first speaker finishing, and the next starting.

3. a. A: yes that's certainly true ($1^1/_2$) wrong use of energy or something?
   b. A: I see(.) yes(.) you also get some magazines,

Single brackets are used for silences; a short gap between turns or a gap within a single speaker's turn (i.e. less than 1 second) is indicated by a **dot inside brackets.**

4. **Intonation patterns** are indicated as follows: a **question remark** indicates upward intonation on the whole word

after which it is placed. Commas indicated upward intonation at the end of the word. A dot indicates a downward intonation. Capitals are used to indicate stress on (part of) a word.

Appendix II

Original fragments

(I.)

1.B: dat doe ik niet meer
2.A: waarom niet?
3.B: je slijt hier weg he, je slijt hier weg
4.A: u hebt steeds minder zin in dingen
5.B: ja.
6.A: akelig
7.(6)

(II.)

1.B: je moet alles bijhouden (.) als je eenmaal van de academie komt hou je
2.A:
3.B: alles bij (.) anders brengen je jaren niet veel zoveel vrucht
4.A: ja ja nee dat
5.B: ja ja
6.A: (.) nee want je blijft als je studeert blijf je altijd studeren
7.B: ja ja ik lees nog wel eens
8.A: eigenlijk he, en leest u nog wel eens wat of eh,
9.B: wat= ja tijdschriften
10.A: = jaja (.) ja (.) krijgt ook nog wel tijdschriften of zo
11.B: maar we houden 't aan de luchtige kant een beetje
12.A: hm. (1) ja, jA da's prima
13.B: we zijn moe he, de meeste mensen zijn moe hier is een van de
14.A: we houden ja(.)
15.B: grootste kwalen is dat he, moeheid ja
16.A: ja moeheid he, ja dat is inderdaad waar
17.B: ja verkeerd gebruik ja verkeerd ja
18.A: $(1^{1}/_{2})$ verkeerd gebruik van energie of zo?

(III)

1.A: jaja en zo is 't hele dagelijkse leven daar, jA
2.B: ja [1] maar ik ben nooit
3.A: nEE nee nee d'r zit (.) ja (.) sterk (.) tegenwicht vormen
4.B: dOOd gegaan
5.A: he ja.(.) maar met die dingen (.) ja u vertelt er nou over (.)
6.B: ja
7.A: maar met die dingen houdt u zich toch niet dagelijks bezig he,
8.B: nee.
9.A: nee he,=
10.B: = 't begin is verschrikkelijk men krijgt een zUUr een zUUrgraad
11.A: mja mja,
12.B: over het hEle lichaam en als men dan nog blijft leven dan mag
13.A: jA. dat lijkt mij ook
14.B: men van gelUk spreken

COMMENTS ON DIEK VAN BIJSTERVELD

Arrie van Berkel

In this discussion paper I will argue, after some general remarks, that the transcription analysis can be refined by using some notions from textual coherence theories. This will lead to the support of some observations made by Diek van Bijsterveld (henceforth: DvB), but also to the modification of some conclusions. Before doing so, I must emphasize that I am not familiar with mental illness and its specific manifestations. I may well overlook certain aspects in the transcriptions that are relevant in this special field.

In a previous paper (Van Bijsterveld: to appear) DvB pointed out that the means of getting access to conversations is coherence. This explains why her paper begins with a short survey about the "immediacy hypothesis": schizophrenic patients are not able to produce coherent texts of any length. In my opinion there are at least two reasons to regard this hypothesis with suspicion. First, coherence has been weakly defined, and second, little is known about coherence that "normal" people maintain in texts produced under the same situational circumstances. A dangerous consequence might be that this hypothesis, which is based on nonsystematic observations, will lead to stigmatization of schizophrenic language producers.

According to DvB the notions access and privacy are strongly connected. Privacy, if I understand it correctly, is evasive behaviour in conversations. I will elaborate this under the aspect of intention, which may be important to describe schizophrenic behaviour. Evasive behaviour may be intentional (avoiding) or unintentional (failing). Evasive behaviour in action patterns has been studied by Rehbein (1977: 233ff.) who emphasizes that evasions, or the experience of evasive acts, are highly dependent on the actors' expectations of each other. Evasive behaviour, when it is experienced by an actor, is always connected with feelings of disappointment about the co-actor(s) or the interaction.

These feelings may be caused by strong expectations of getting access. When the expectations are low the disappointment will be low too. Though DvB's paper mentions that the nonschizophrenic participant was disappointed, it does not give us any detail about the reason why the expectations of getting access could be so high. Hospitalized schizophrenic patients may have perfectly "normal" reasons for evasive behaviour. According to DvB's description of the situation in which the conversations between a schizophrenic and a nonschizophrenic participant took place, the discourse type can be defined as informal, despite the institutional pressure that cannot be neglected in mental hospitals. Basically, the conversations are symmetric ones. The latter notion means that the involved participants have no specific (institutional) goals other than to keep the conversation going in order to kill the time. Participants have no conversational obligations or rights and even their participation as much is not obliged (Springorum 1982). Other examples of symmetric conversations can be found in waiting-rooms. Considering the fact that expectations of getting access in such conversations under moral conditions cannnot be high, it follows that under the conditions as described by DvB they must be even lower. Conversely, the need for protecting one's privacy will also be relatively high. Now I shall look at the first transcription in DvB's paper:

1. B: I don't do that anymore
2. A: why not
3. B: you're wearing away here eh you're wearing away here (fragment, new translation)

DvB argues **inter alia** that the use of the locative 'here' generates a privacy sequence. I shall extend this observation to the use of pronouns in this fragment with respect to coherence as a stronger indication of a privacy sequence. I shall restrict myself to this fragment. All transcriptions in DvB's paper have similar phenomena so that my remarks also apply to them.

B's utterances show a remarkable shift from the pronoun 'I' to 'you', whereas the syntactic position (topic and subject) is unchanged (syntactic parallellism). Further, there is a conceptual shift from AGENT ('I') to AFFECTED ENTITY ('you') under indentical syntactic position. Perfect coherence can only be processed if (textual) co-referentiality occurs, which is here between 'you' and 'I'. Less perfect coherence can be processed if co-referentiality can be inferred. This may happen under the principle of sense **constancy** which means that meanings will be kept constant under certain conditions, unless there are signals to change them (Hörmann 1976). Both according to coherence principles and the nature of syntactic parallellism the relation between 'you' and 'I' is co-referential, which implies that the meaning of 'you' is at least 'I'.

In Dutch, just as in English, it is not incorrect to speak about oneself using the pronoun 'you' ('je') or 'one' ('men'), even when the topic is a personal experience. The use of these indefinite pronouns shows that a private topic can be uttered in a non-private form. In this case B's attempt at privacy is not as strong as DvB suggest. On the other hand we have to realize that the utterance under discussion is an answer to the question 'why (did you stop reading)?'. This leads to the plausible fact that B did in fact change the topic from 'I' to 'you' in the sense of 'we all'. A third possibility which cannot be excluded, is that we have to take 'you' literally as a reference to the adressee. The utterance thus becomes a sort of counterfactual: 'if you would be here then you would be wearing away'. In this case a real topic change has been carried out, which means a strong attempt at privacy.

I already mentioned that at the conceptual level the shift from 'I' to 'you' is a shift from AGENT (or actually: NON-AGENT) to AFFECTED ENTITY. The intentional behaviour that has been expressed is transformed into a non-intentional being affected, just after A's question about the backgrounds of B's intentions. This may be interpreted in such a way that undesired non-acting cannot be changed because of the undesired process that victimizes B. In this respect B's utterance can be interpreted as a complaint, i.e. an assertion about a deficient or undesired state that B cannot change into a sufficient or a desired one. The vagueness of the complaints is rather common in medical settings where it is often connected with an equally vague notion like "mental weakness". Bremer (1980) pointed out that complaining often slows down the other's aggression because it expresses weakness. The complainer may even become a martyr who saddles the hearer with feelings of guilt. This may coincide with the third interpretation of B's utterance: the counterfactual one.

If all this is correct, then B's utterance may be considered an attempt at privacy, a depersonalization or limited generalization, an expression of weakness, of victimization and martyrship and even an attempt at provoking the hearer at the same time. Textual coherence decreases proportionally along this sequence.

7

The evaluation of discourse structures with a probabilistic sequential approach

The case of the psychosomatic ward round

D. Fehlenberg

Introduction: Discourse analysis as an evaluative tool

One of the many interests in using communication data within studies of social situations is the **evaluation** of practical change accomplished by professional intervention, which may be of an organizational or a personal nature. With respect to doctor-patient interaction there are several medical approaches which lay stress on an intensification of communication between doctors and their patients for humanistic as well as for inner professional reasons. These are, for example, the approaches in 'Behavioural Medicine', in so-called 'Humanistic Medicine' and in the traditional 'Psychosomatic Approach'. I shall here report on a study of ward-round discourses where the ward's organisation in general and the daily round in particular was organized in accordance with a psychosomatic view of illness and its treatment.

The ward round's discourse within the traditional clinical setting

In Germany the clinical ward round is a comparably well-studied field of medical interactions (cf. Fehlenberg, 1983a). The results of extensive empirical investigations within the last ten years may be summarized in 3 major ways:

1. The round's discourse cannot be characterized as being solely doctor-patient communication. As a matter of fact, clinical and organizational functions, which have to be performed in doctor-doctor or doctor-staff communication clearly structure the round's discourse of the traditional kind. Most typically there is a predominance of topics in medical consultations, i.e. the discussion of the 'case' by the different physicians participating in the round, or in the exchange of information between the physicians and the nursing staff and in the assignment of diagnostic and therapeutic tasks. Put in terms of interaction, the patients

are excluded from participation in these parts of the discourse by several interactional characteristics of the staff's communication (Nothdurft, 1983, Gück et al., 1983).

2. When patients participate (or are allowed to participate), it is typically the case that their turns are required for ongoing staff inter-communication, i.e. they help with information concerning their complaints, their pains and the like. If patients take the initiative, for example, by requesting information, or by making attempts to tell a story on some occasions, the staff's typical reaction is that of nullifying the initiative in one way or another; or at least, the patient's initiatives are re-defined so that their purposes better conform to a professional medical context (Bliesener and Siegrist, 1981).

3. This disregard of the patients' own interest seems to be particularly marked where a patient with an unfavourable prognosis is concerned. It seems almost as if physicians when dealing with terminally ill patients follow a medical routine and do so in an extremely formal and aloof manner (Siegrist, 1978).

The patient centered programme of the psychosomatic approach

With respect to this situation encountered within the traditional clinical setting the psychosomatic clinicians have 4 major goals for the daily round:

1. **The deconcentration of clinical functions:** the tasks relating to the organizational functions should be carried out in principle outside the door of the patients' rooms. The time at the bedside should be reserved exclusively for doctor-patient interaction.

2. The **'communicative symmetry'**: by this term physicians mean a conversational behaviour that should encourage the patients to talk about their interests. The patients should have the same chances of influencing the topics of discourse as the physicians.

3. There should be **no disadvantage for terminally ill patients** with respect to these goals.

4. **Psychotherapeutic help:** relying on the basic assumption of the psychosomatic approach that psychical factors are of some importance in the course of **every** disease (cf. Weiss and English, 1944) it is a special goal of the round's discourse to open up new ways of resolving (psychical) conflicts by means of psychotherapeutic verbal interventions.

The goal of psychotherapeutic help has been described in several case-based analyses, which served the function of exploring typical problems of interaction associated with leading a round's discourse therapeutically (cf. Fehlenberg, 1983b, Bliesener, 1982, Fehlenberg and Köhle, 1984). I will disregard this aspect here. Instead I will concentrate on the first three aspects of intended changes, the 'deconcentration of clininal functions', the 'symmetry or influence' and the 'avoidance of disadvantage for terminally ill patients'. In doing so I would like to discuss the possibility of a representative and concept-oriented or criteria-oriented evaluationof goal attainment using communication data.

The evaluation of discourse structures by a probabilistic approach

There are some strong advantages in using a quantitative, probabilistic approach in situations where the problems of interest are essentially known in advance and where there are clear-cut criteria which can be checked. A probabilistic approach, then,

- o gives information with respect to representativity and generalizability;
- o gives information about the degree of confirmation regarding the evaluation hypothesis;
- o allows for the integration of non-communicative features with those of the communicative process, thereby linking micro- and macro-sociological perspectives;
- o and it lays the foundations for making cross-situational comparisons.

But some conditions must be fulfilled. Models for analyses should take into account the processual and interactive nature of the data under investigation. So an adequate model of analyses has to consist of two structural parts:

(1) A **processual part**, i.e. a structural model for the **sequential qualities** of the data. This part should include statements with respect to the local length of dependence and their structural components.

(2) A **co-processual part** incorporating assumptions regarding the **influence of non-communicative factors** and their relation to the communicative process.

Another essential condition is that the communication phenomena under study are classified in an exhaustive way, i.e. the interaction process should be described as a sequence of consecutive actions, giving a full picture of all activities relevant to the evaluative questions. Clearly the two preconditions are interdependent. Only an exhaustive categorization allows for the formulation of probabilistic models.

A coding system for the sequential description for participants' controlling behaviour

With respect to our evaluation hypothesis for reaching symmetry and deconcentration of clinical functions, we used a coding system to describe the participants' behaviour for controlling the topics of the discourse. The first stage of the analytical process changed the transcription into a formal sequential description of the participants' steering behaviour. The second stage, then, is the formulation and testing of a model on pragmatic structures expected under the hypothesis that the intended goals had been reached. The theoretical framework for the coding system is given by the pragmatic theory of dialogue control and steering as outlined by J. Schwitalla (1979). I made some modifications with respect to the definition of the categories, which I will not discuss in detail. Fig. 1, 2, 3 and 4 give a rough outline of the different sets of categories used in the system. Essentially, the result of the coding is a pragmatic description of two interactional layers: the local thematic innovation and the type of degree of pragmatic coherence, as achieved by any of the participants' continuations. Where the first aspect may be seen as a quality of sequences of single moves, the second aspect is conceptualised as a property of a speaker's whole turn.

Controlling the discourse progression by:

initiating ('forward control')	reacting ('backward control')
unit of description: move	unit of description: turn
o speaker o (first addressee o speaker's intention (cf. fig. 2) o topic/ thematic domain (cf. fig. 3)	o speaker o speaker of the turn the present speaker is relating to o type of continuation (cf. fig. 4) o argumentational function o treatment of obligations

fig. 1: Dimensions of the coding system for the description of participants' local controlling behaviour

As indicated by fig.1 each move is described under 4 headings:

(a) Who speaks?
(b) Who is the (first) addressee?
(c) What is the speaker's intention, with respect to the addressee's subsequent behaviour? (cf. fig. 2)
(d) What is the topic? (cf. fig. 3)

A move is an intentionally and thematically coherent activity; a turn may be built up of one or more different moves.

Each speaker's turn is classified according to 5 properties:

(a) Who speaks?
(b) Who is the speaker s/he is relating to?
(c) What is the type of the speaker's continuation? (cf. fig. 4)
(d) What is the argumentational function of the continuation?
(e) If there are any obligations resulting from previous speakers' turns, how are they treated?

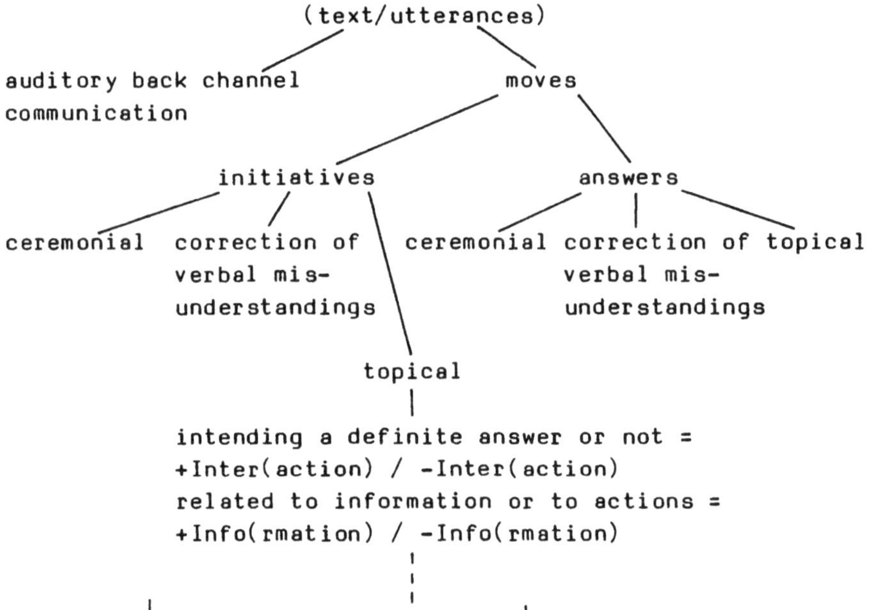

	+Info	-Info
	The present speaker requests:	
+Inter	o descriptions and other non-evaluative information o explanations o qualifying info. o reasons	o intentions o proposals o advice o decisions
	The present speaker gives/makes:	
-Inter	o descriptions and other non-evaluative information o explanations o qualifying info. o reasons/motivations	o intentions o proposals o advice o decisions

fig. 2: Categories describing the speaker's intention

'doctors' topics':
o (results of) examinations
o treatment
o prognosis
'patients' topics':
o patient's condition (complaints)
o subjective ideas about illness
o history of illness
o pt.'s life outside the hospital
'topics of shared knowledge / disputable topics':
o round's interaction / metacommunication
o hospital life
o general topics

fig. 3 Categories describing the round's topics and thematic domains

As it can be seen from fig. 2 and 4, some coding categories are complex hierarchical distinctions. All in all the system differentiates 375 possible constellations with respect to the intention and topic of any speaker's move, and it differentiates 36 constellations with respect to the speakers' continuations.

Sample

The analysis is based on 296 tape-recorded and transcribed ward round discourses with 74 patients, using the first 4 discourses during their stay in the hospital. The recording was done during a span of 3,5 years (1975-1978) in a ward of the Department of Internal Medicine/University of Ulm (FRG) where an attempt was made to re-organize the daily round according to the principles outlined above.

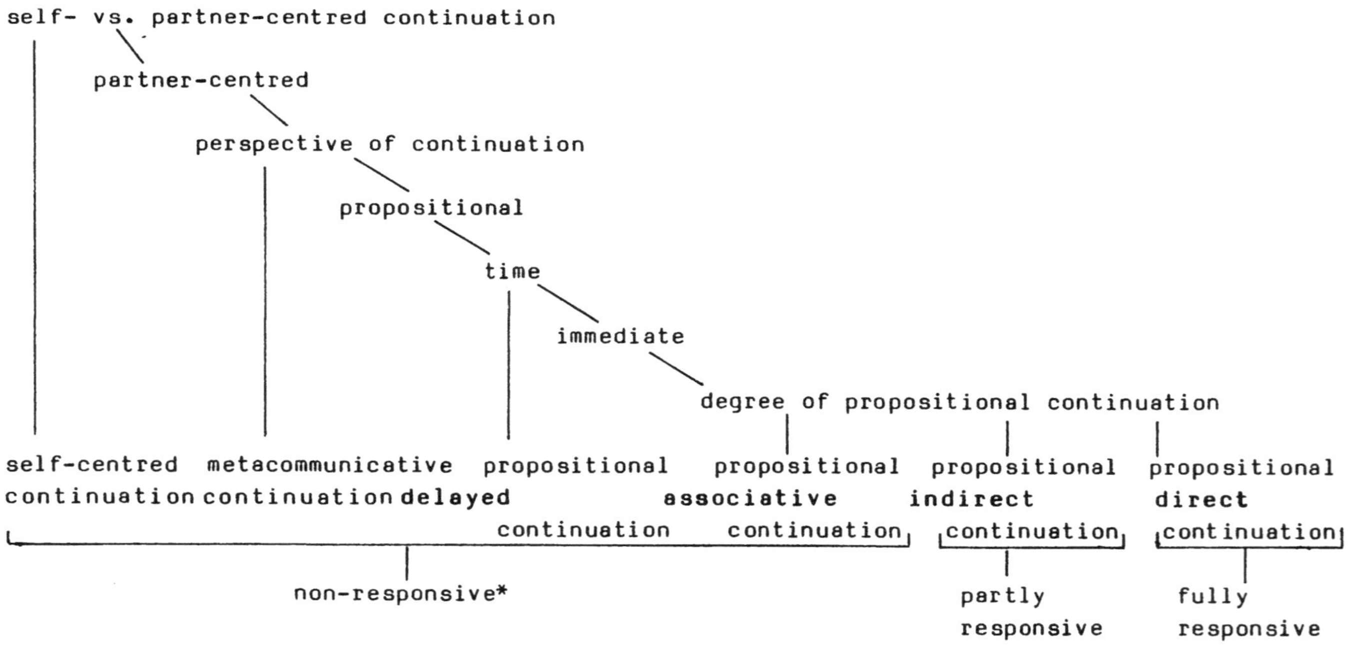

fig. 4. **Categories describing the type of continuation**

* category of the later analysis (contraction of the distinctions above)

The sample consisted of two groups of patients - 37 who were terminally ill and 37 who were not terminally ill. (Terminally ill was defined as having a diagnosis associated with a 30% risk of dying within the span of 3 months, or with an average span of expected survival less than two years according to medical literature.)

The groups and the discourse were matched with respect to 3 factors: patients' age and gender and the physicians leading the discourse. The discourses were gained from rounds with 7 physicians.

Coding procedure

The 296 discourses were transcribed and coded using the outlined system. The coding was done by 3 different coders. An extensive investigation of the coding procedure revealed that the categorization was highly generalizable with regard to coders and the time of coding.

The coding transformed the transcription into sequences of 23,329 moves (auditory back channel communications not included) and 10,794 turns respectively. These data are the basis for all the following probabilistic analyses.

The hierarchical structure of the system allows for an easy and theoretical-grounded grouping of the categories, dependent on the concrete interest of evaluation. This feature is useful in the data analysis.

3 examples for the formulation and testing of probabilistic models incorporating aspects of (macro-) social and sequential structure

The evaluation of the deconcentration of clinical functions

The first example for the formulation and testing of probabilistic sequential models is very simplistic with respect to the categorization it uses. It tests the attainment of the deconcentration of clinical functions. This is accomplished by looking at the sequences of different groups of speaker. The unit of analysis is the move and the observed variable in this analysis 'who is making the move'. The evaluation hypothesis to be tested can be stated as follows:

Given that the deconcentration of clinical functions has been attained, the participation of persons other than the physician leading the round and the patient (i.e. the second physician and the nursing staff) should be reduced to a minimum and should not hinder the coherent transaction of the doctor-patient dialogue. This kind of interactive organization should be found in discourses with non-terminally ill patients as well as in discourse with terminally ill patients.

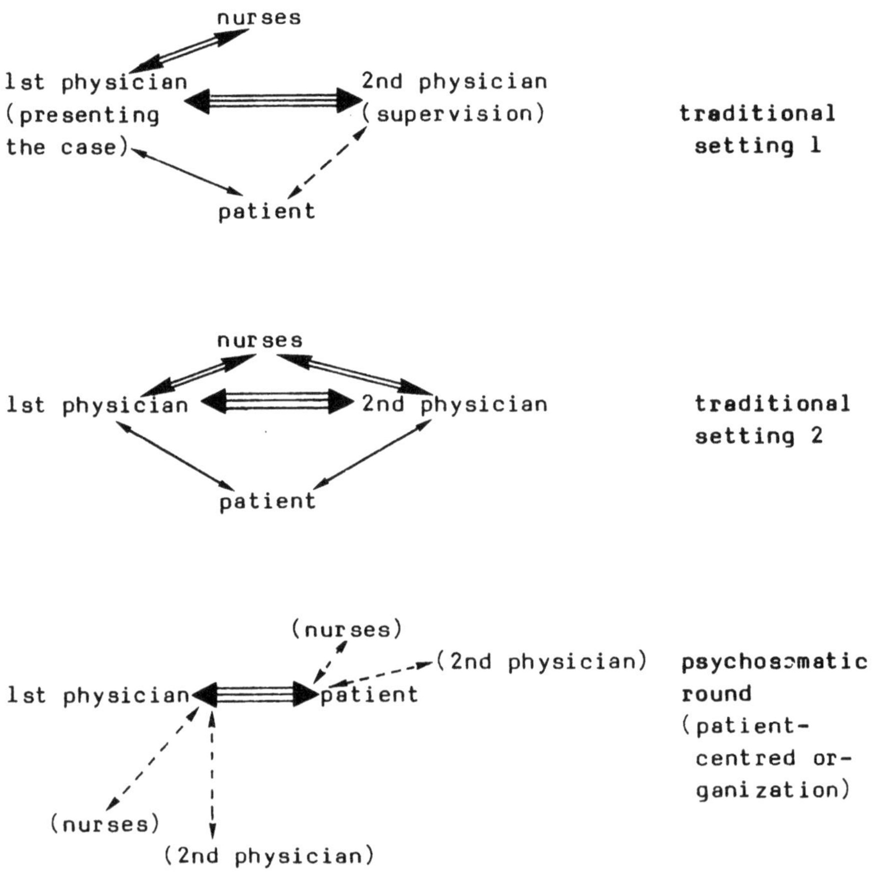

fig. 5: Dialogical relationships expected within the ward round's communication in different clinical settings

Fig. 5 gives three schemes for the dialogical relationship characterizing three different settings. Whereas the overall pragmatic structure of the traditional setting is characterized by a prominent and stable dialogical line between the 1st and the 2nd physician and an involvement of the patient only in an unstable and minor line of communication with the 1st, or with the 1st **and** the 2nd physician, the patient-centredness of the psychosomatic discourse is reflected by a stable and dominating relationship involving the 1st physician and the patient. All other participants are expected to be involved only in unstable and minor dialogical lines centred around the 1st physician or around the patient. A probabilistic equivalent of communicational lines between two or more speakers is the higher frequency of sequences with one speaker immediately followed by the other than could be expected from the overall participation of each speaker.

The first step in assessing the hypothesized structure of speaker sequences is to determine the length of the local stochastic dependence. Statistically speaking: Is the dependence of 1st order (i.e. whoever makes the next move is sequentially influenced only by whoever has made the previous move)? Or is it of a higher order (i.e. whoever makes the next move is sequentially influenced by a whole sequence of speakers who have previously made moves). This is the Markov question of predictability of a process from its own past. One way of answering this question is given by an analysis of the percentual reduction of uncertainty, that could be computed by using formulas derived from information theory as developed by Shannon and Weaver.

Fig. 6 shows the results of this analysis for sequences of speakers' moves. The graph gives the percentual reduction in uncertainty with respect to the question 'who makes the next move?', given the knowledge of who has made the previous move (S1), the previous two moves (S2), and so on. The analysis was performed separately for the two groups of patients. In both groups the essential dependence is that of a 2nd order process. This can be seen from the marked drop of the graphs' increments between the positions S2 and S3. (This conclusion is further confirmed by a series of LR-Chi^2 tests as described in Bishop et al., 1980).

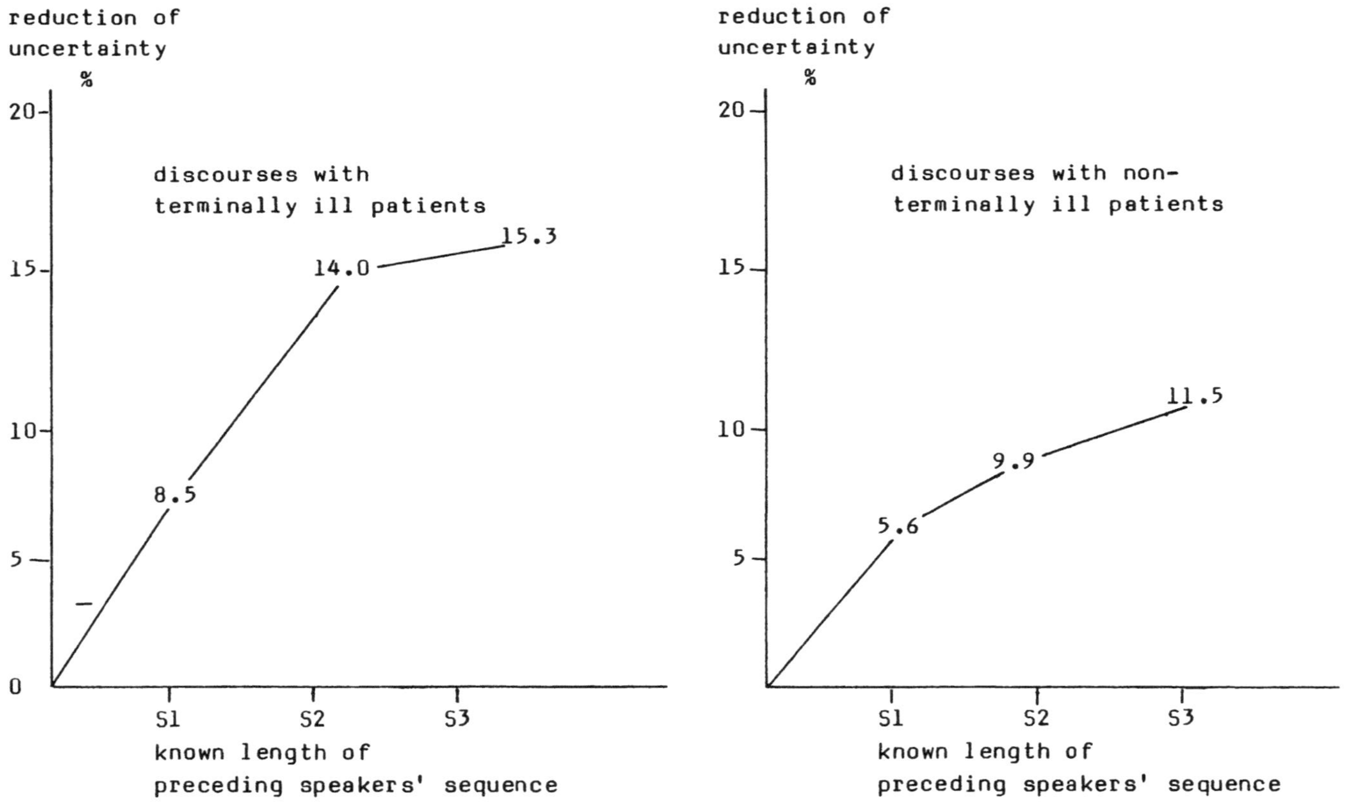

fig. 6: Information analysis: sequence of speakers

The next step in testing for the hypothesized form of sequential organization is the assessment of the relevant structural components underlying the process of speakers' sequencing. Since we have determined the process as being one of 2nd order, we have to look at a 3-dimensional contingency table, or transitional matrix where the relative serial positions are the dimensions and may be indicated as TØ, T-1, T-2. There are 4 possible structural models of dependence as given schematically in fig. 7.

(1) 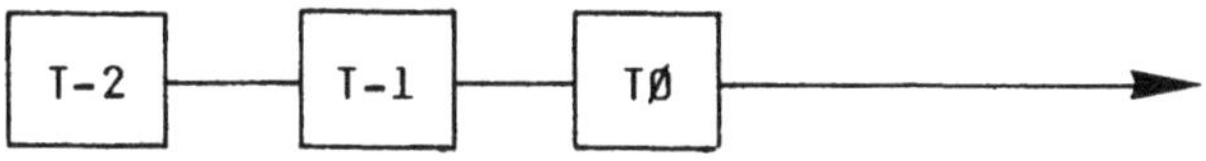

model of sequential independence

(2) 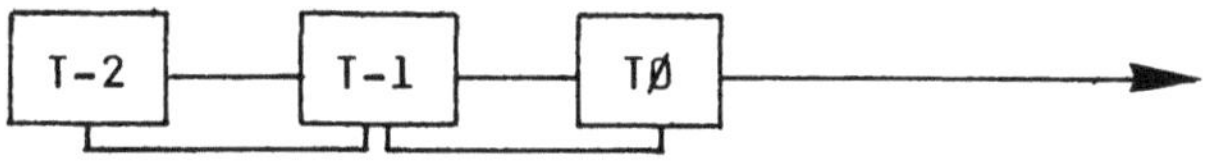

dependence of neighbouring positions
(1st order Markov chain)

(3) 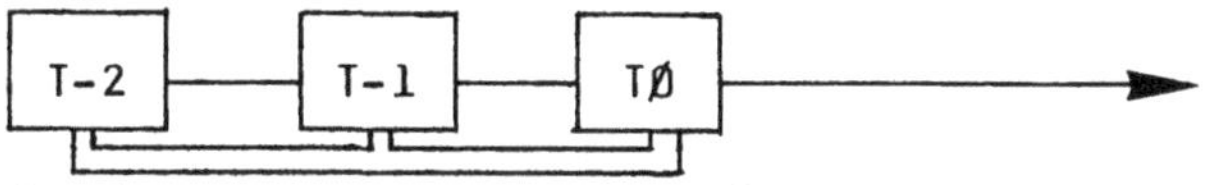

simple dependence across two lags

(4) 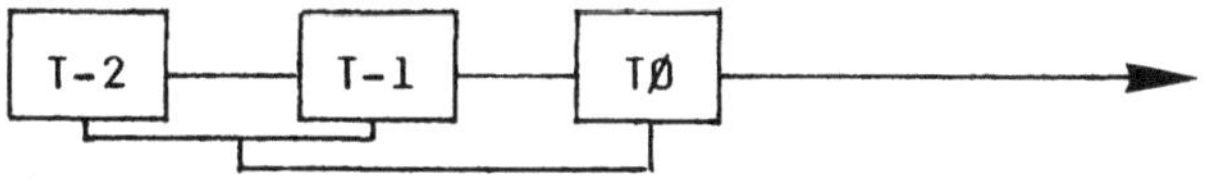

complex dependence: the specific constellation of T-2 with T-1 influences TØ (2nd order Markov chain)

fig. 7: Models of sequential dependence (processual part of a probabilistic model of analysis)

Model (2) is that of a first order dependence which we have already discarded. Model (4) is that of a full 2nd order dependence, i.e. who makes the next move depends on the specific sequence of speakers at the previous two positions. Model (3) lies somewhere in between. TØ is influenced by who was making a move at T-1 and at T-2, but the specific constellation of who was speaking at T-2 and T-1 is not essential. These models can be tested with a generalized factorial chisquare analysis as is given by the log-linear model conceptualized by L. Goodman and associates (cf. Bishop et. al., 1980). Fig. 8 gives the results of the tests computed separately for the groups of the terminally ill and the non-terminally ill patients.(fig.8, pag.178)

(N = 11310 moves)

model	DF	LR CHi^2	P	Q (%)
1. T-2, T-1, TØ (baseline model)	54	4 897.93	0.0	———
2. T-2, T-1, T-1 TØ	36	1 161.77	0.0	76.28
3. T-2 T-1, T-1 TØ, T-2 TØ	27	211.36	0.0	95.68

Discourses with terminally ill patients

(N = 10984 moves)

model	DF	LR CHi^2	P	Q (%)
1. T-2, T-1, TØ (baseline model)	54	2 999.20	0.0	———
2. T-2 T-1, T-1 TØ	36	800.10	0.0	73.32
3. T-2 T-1, T-1 TØ, T-2 TØ	27	229.78	0.0	92.34

Discourses with non-terminally ill patients

fig. 8: Sequence of speakers according to moves (1st physician, 2nd physician, patient, nursing staff)

As the N of the analysis is quite large the most adequate measure for judging whether the models fit is the proportion of explained variation as compared with a baseline model (this analogon of R^2 from multiple regression was proposed by Knorke and Burke, 1980). According to this criterion, the model (3) fits the data very well with respect to the discourses of the terminally ill patients (residuals of LR Chi^2 5%). With respect to the discourses of the non-terminally ill patients, model (3) still fits reasonably (residuals 10%), but its explanation of the sequential structure of the data is clearly worse.

Co-processual determinants, as for example the fact whether a patient is terminally ill or not, may be integrated with the sequential analysis by conceptualizing the transitional matrices of the sub-groups as marginal sub-tables of a higher order contingency table. The additional dimensions are the integrated co-processual determinants. The log-linear approach then allows for testing their actual relevance.(fig.9, pag. 180)

Given the sequential structure, it is possible to determine whether there is a difference only with respect to the frequences of categories, or whether there are differences with respect to the transitional structure. Fig. 9 gives 8 possible models incorporating processual and co-processual parts in different combinations. Fig. 10 shows the results for testing these 8 models for speaker-sequences and the mortality of the patients as a co-processual determinant.
(fig.10, pag.181)
Model (6), which is that of a full 2nd-order dependence in its sequential part and which incorporates an influence of the patients' mortality on the frequency of the different speakers occurring in the discourse fits best, although there is no difference in the sequential organization for the two groups. Having accepted this model as the best description of the observed data, it becomes possible to test the substantial implications of the hypothesized dialogical structure by comparing expected probable and improbable transitions and the parameters of these transitions under model (6). (fig.11 en 12, pag. 182 en 183)

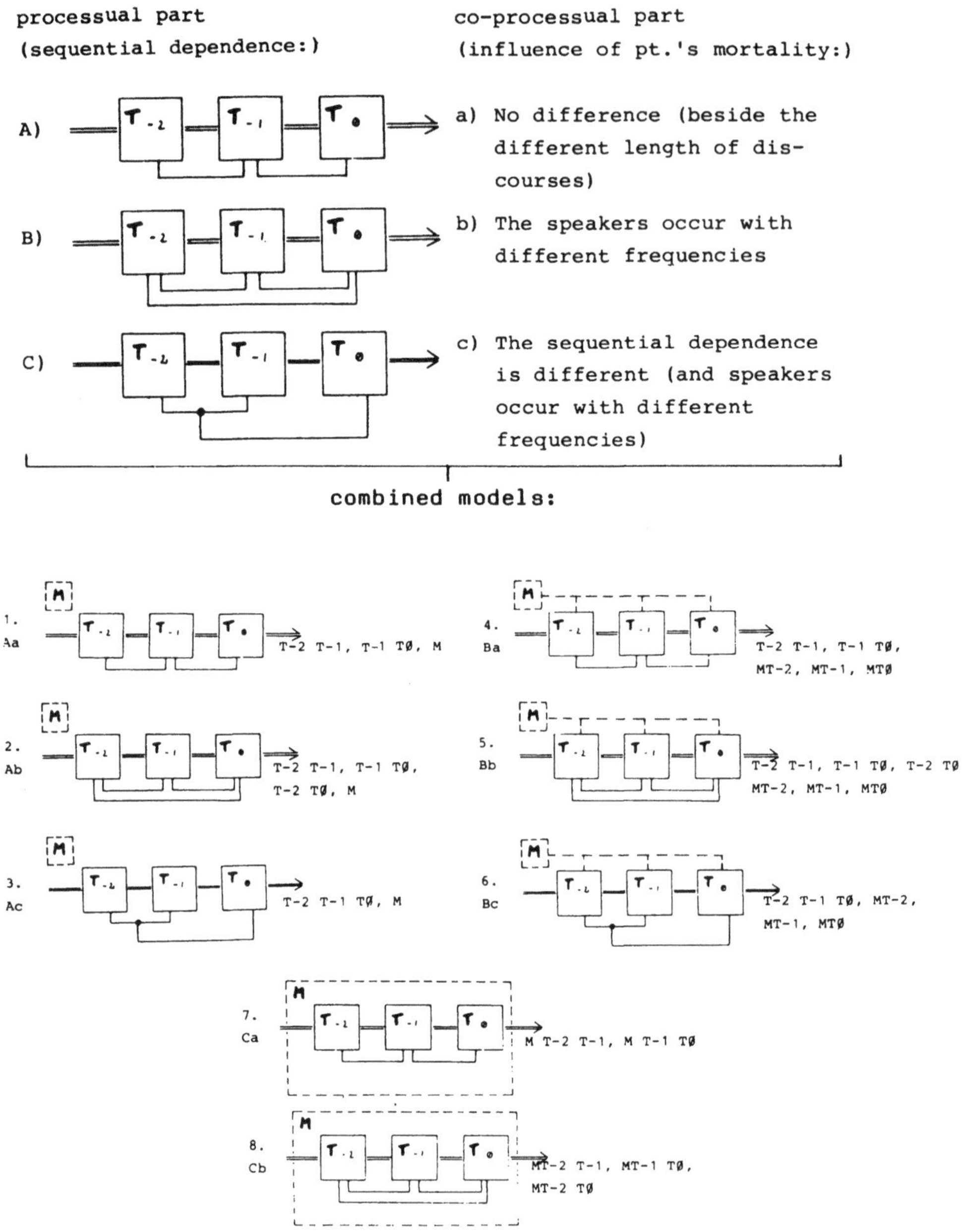

Fig. 9: Structural models combining different kinds of sequential dependence and influence of a co-processual determinant (M= mortality of the patient)

model	DF	LR Chi^2	P	Q (%)
0. T-2, T-1, TØ, M (baseline)	117	8 220.70	0.0	———
1. T-2 T-1, T-1 TØ, M	99	2 502.58	0.0	69.56
2. T-2 T-1, T-1 TØ, T-2 TØ, M	90	936.79	0.0	88.60
3. T-2 T-1 TØ, M	63	541.39	0.0	93.41
4. T-2 T-1, T-1 TØ, M T-2, M T-1, M TØ	90	2 183.86	0.0	73.43
5. T-2 T-1, T-1 TØ, T-2 TØ,M T-2, M T-1, M TØ	81	655.65	0.0	92.02
6. T-2 T-1 TØ, M T-2, M T-1, M TØ	54	260.92	0.0	96.83
7. M T-2 T-1, M T-1 TØ	72	1 961.88	0.0	76.13
8. M T-2 T-1, M T-1 TØ, M T-2 TØ	54	441.14	0.0	94.63

fig. 10: **The sequence of speakers and the influence of patients' mortality (N = 22,294 moves). Model (6) is accepted as the best description of the data according to Q%**

	Substantial implications with respect to the speakers' sequential relationships	number of predictions	confirmed (/z/1.96)	expected dir. (/z/ 1.96)	not exp. dir. (/z/ 1.96)
Hl.1:	all posible constellations of the 1st physician and the patient:+	6	6	-	-
Hl.2:	if y speaks after x, x speaks after y: +	10	8	2	-
Hl.3:	constellation with more than 2 different speakers: -	24	18	6	-
Hl.4:	no stable or substantial dialogue between 1st physician/patient and 2nd physician/nursing staff: -	12	8	6	2
Hl.5:	if the 2nd physic/nurs. staff makes a substantial turn it is following a 1st physic/pt turn: +	4	4	-	-
Hl.6:	no stable dialogue between 2nd physic/nurs. staff: -	4	2	-	2
Hl.7:	complex turns for all speakers: +	4	4	-	-
	overall structure	64	50	10	4

fig.11: hypothesized dialogical relationships of the psychomatic round (The z-scores are the standardized lambdas of the log-linear model (T-2 T2) TØ, M (T-2 T-1),M TØ which is identical to the accepted model (6) in its sequential part but allows for an easier assessment of sequential parameters because all possible combinations of T-2 and T-1 are treated as 1 variable.
+ = above chance expectation
- = below chance expectation)

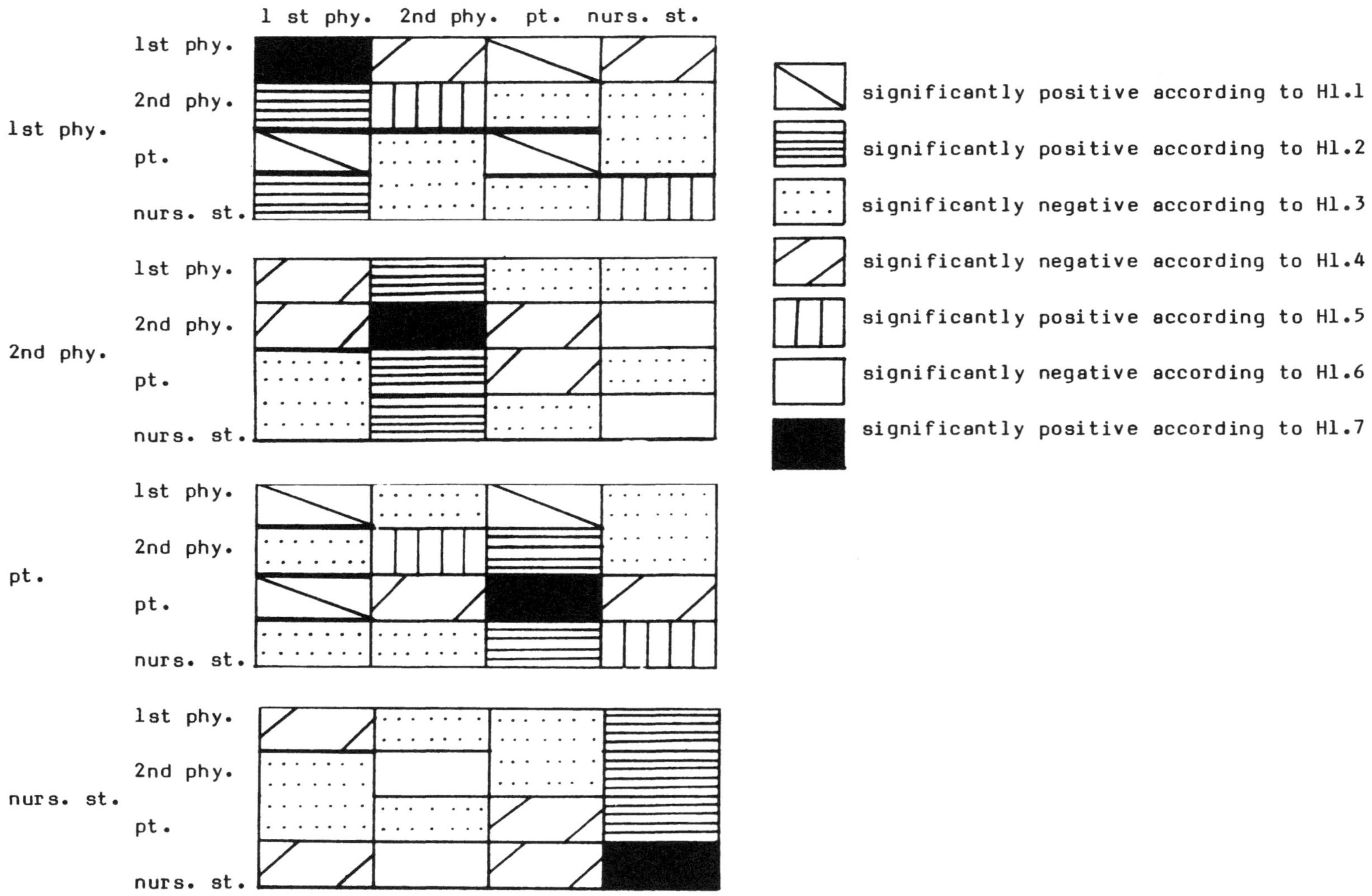

fig. 12: Summary display of dialogical relationships

Fig. 11 and 12 summarize 7 substantial hypotheses derived from the notion of functional deconcentration (cf. fig. 5c) with respect to the sequential parameters corresponding to the 64 possible sequences of speakers found in the 2nd order transitional matrix. As can be seen from fig. 11, 50 expectations are confirmed substantially, another 10 parameters are non-significant but in the expected direction, where only 4 parameters are not in the expected direction but still non-significant. So the dialogical relationship between the different speakers' groups that were postulated as implications of the deconcentration of clinical functions can be seen as very tenable. There is no difference between the discourses of terminally-ill patients and non-terminally-ill patients with respect to these dialogical relationships. But there is a marked difference between these groups with regard to the frequency of participation: there is a more frequent participation of the 2nd physician and of the nurses in the group of the terminally-ill patients. So a bad prognosis for the patient leads to a more substantial participation of the staff, but it leaves the dialogical relationship among the participants unchanged.

Testing for the attainment of symmetry

Social psychologists have given different definitions with respect to the notion of symmetry or dominance within social interactions. Dominance may be related to the frequency of special indicators, as for example interruptions, questions, etc., or it may be defined formally. A widely used definition is given by Gottman (1980) who defines dominance as differences in predictability. The participant whose behaviour is more predictable from the behaviour of another participant than vice versa is being dominated by the other. Gottman's approach characterizes asymmetry as differences in the influences people exert on each other, instead of by what they are doing. Both definitions, the one based on frequencies of speech acts and the formal one based on the sequential organization of participants' speech acts are applicable. The former may be seen as reflecting primarily the (pre-established) **situational** components of asymmetry, attributable to the professional and institutional constraints on action, whereas the latter reflects the **interactive** components of asymmetry that are the object of participants' bargaining. So it is a question of situational asymmetry whether a doctor is requesting more information, or is more frequently chosing indirect continuations. But it is clearly a feature of interactive asymmetry, if a request for information that has to be answered by the physician, given it was made by the patient, is answered in another way and to a different extent as a request for information made by the physician in the reversed situation.

A general evaluation of this point has to be quite complex, because it was to include all possible layers of participants' controlling behaviour. I will give two examples from the results of our study. The first deals with the sequencing of different moves, made by the physicians and the patients, the second is an analysis integrating the type of continuation.
The statistics are of the same kind as those introduced with the analysis of speakers' sequencing. All the sub-sections of the discourses were removed from the analysis, where the 2nd physician and/or the nurses participate (thereby retaining 9,154 moves from discourses with terminally ill patients - 1st physicians: 4,660; patients: 4,494 - and 8,620 moves from discourses with non-terminally ill patients - 1st physician: 4,688; patients: 3,932).

The local length of organization with respect to the sequencing of moves turns out to be of 1st order, i.e. who is making what kind of move is sequentially dependent only on which speaker made what kind of move just before. So the data can be organized as a two-dimensional contingency table (cf. fig. 13), containing 4 sections:

(A) the within-turn transitions of the physician,
(B) the transition from moves of the patient to moves of the physician,
(C) the transition from moves of the physicians to moves of the patient,
(D) and the within-turn transitions of the patient.

fig. 13 (pag.186)

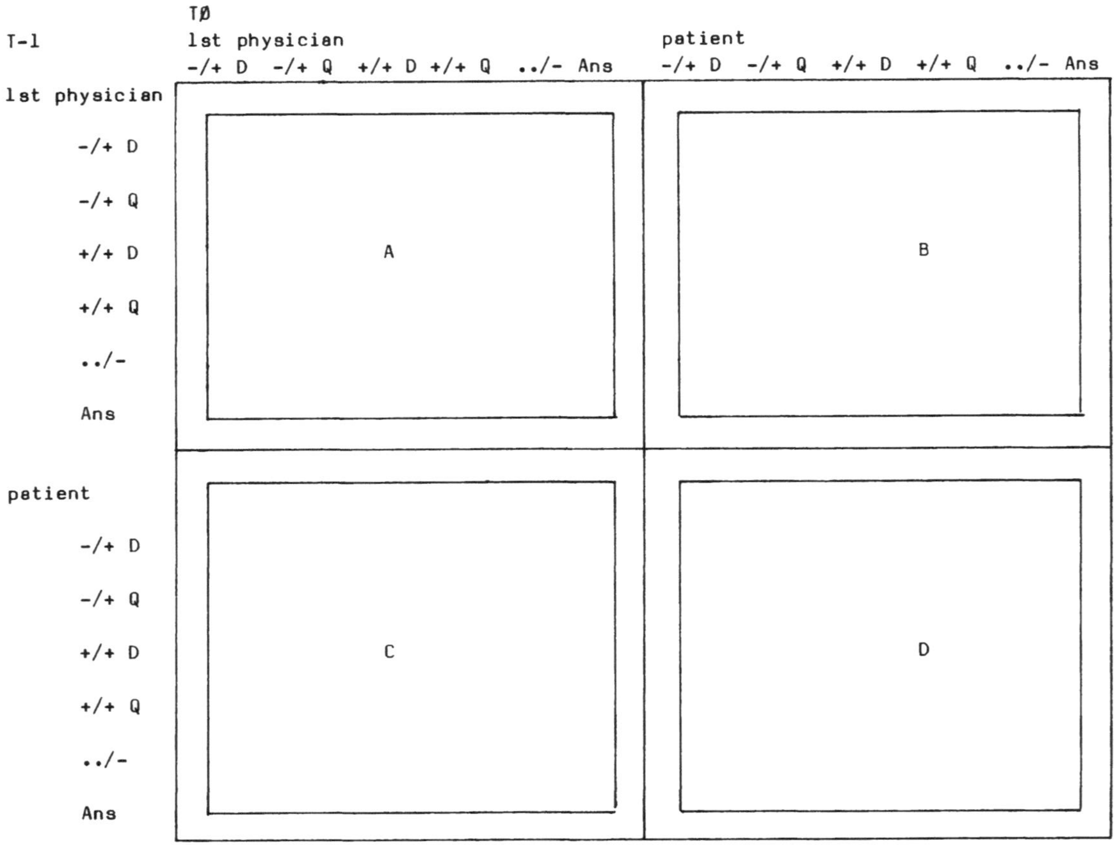

fig. 13: 1st order transition matrix of thematic moves made by the 1st physician and the patient

-/+ = D speaker is giving descriptive information
+/+ = Q speaker is giving a qualification
+/+ = D speaker is requesting descriptive information
+/+ = Q speaker is requesting a qualification
../- = any speaker's move related to actions
Ans = speaker is answering

Different log-linear models incorporating firstly no components of asymmetry, secondly only situational components of asymmetry, or thirdly situational and interactive components of asymmetry may be used to explain the structure of the observed transition matrix. The results, computed separately for the discourse of the terminally ill patients and the non-terminally ill patients and controlled for the subject domain are given in fig. 13 and 14. (pag. 186 and 188)

One can summarize these results as follows:

(1) In all thematic domains the psychosomatic round's discourse is asymmetric with regard to the first, the situational notion of asymmetry (cf. the significant LR-Chi^2 of model (2) in fig. 14). All differences between model (2) and models (3), (4) and (5) incorporating differences in the frequencies of move types between physicians and patients are highly significant.

(2) on the whole there is no need to introduce components of sequential, interactive asymmetry in order to arrive at a good explanation of the observed transitions. This is shown by the fact that model (5) fits almost perfectly with respect to 5 out of 6 instances (cf. fig. 14). With respect to the terminally ill patients and the topics of shared knowledge, the saturated model containing all possible components of interactive asymmetries is the only model consistent with the observed transitional structure (according to the significant LR-Chi^2 as well as to the criterion of explained variance, Q % 5).

(3) The log-linear approach allows for a further differentiation of interactive asymmetries:

o One can ask, whether there are differences between the physicians and the patients with respect to the possibility of using moves depending on whether there has been a speakerchange or not ('interactive asymmetry type I').

o One can ask, whether there are differences between the physicians and the patients with respect to the sequencing of moves given the fact that a certain move has been made at a certain interactional position ('interactive asymmetry type III').

	models		DF doctor's topics		patient topics		top. of sh. knowl.	
terminally ill patients	(1) TØT-1, X, S, F	105	2.103.82*	(Q%)	3.938.84*	(Q%)	1.096.82*	(Q%)
	(2) TØT-1X, S, F	70	911.21*	56,7	2.723.63*	30.9	511.49*	53.4
	(3) TØT-1X, S, T-1F	65	285.69*	86.4	428.19*	89.1	245.44*	77.6
	(4) TØT-1X, TØS, F	65	476.21*	77.4	573.06*	85.5	205.21*	81.3
	(5) TØT-1X, TØS, T-1F	60	68.98	96.7	64.91	98.4	88.60**	91.9
	(6) TØT-1X, TØS, T-1FX	55	56.25	97.3	56.96	98.6	85.35**	92.2
	(7) TØT-1X, TØSX, T-1F	55	63.34	97.0	55.33	98.6	86.67**	92.1
	(8) TØT-1X, TØSX, T-1FX	50	50.93	97.6	47.01	98.8	83.43**	92.4
non-terminally ill patients	(1) TØT-1, X, S, F	105	1.906.24*	(Q%)	4.224.75*	(Q%)	1.473.70*	(Q%)
	(2) TØT-1X, S, F	70	907.17*	52.4	2.689.83*	36.3	825.27*	44.0
	(3) TØT-1X, S, T-1F	65	376.39*	80.3	570.01*	86.5	265.89*	82.0
	(4) TØT-1X, TØS, F	65	443.23*	76.7	483.36*	88.6	337.89*	77.1
	(5) TØT-1X, TØS, T-1F	60	50.10	96.9	64.00	98.5	65.53	95.6
	(6) TØT-1X, TØS, T-1FX	55	55.01	97.1	62.92	98.5	53.09	96.4
	(7) TØT-1X, TØSX, T-1F	55	55.61	97.1	51.75	98.8	51.37	96.5
	(8) TØT-1X, TØSX, T-1FX	50	51.57	97.3	50.36	98.8	39.85	97.3

fig. 14: Models containing different components of situational and interactive asymmetry physician/patient: thematic moves (1st order transition matrix), LR-Chi^2 and Q% with respect to baseline model (1)
TØ = type of move at TØ (consequent position)
T-1 = type of move at T-1 (antecedent position)
X = speaker-change vs. within-turn transition
F = first speaker: physician or patient
S = second speaker: physician or patient
$*p \leq .0001$
$**p \leq .01$

The importance of asymmetrical components of type I may be assessed by the differences between model (5) and models (6), (7), and (8) (cf. fig. 15 pag.192).

4 differences proved to be significant as indicated by the asterisks in fig. 15.
The interactive meaning of these structural differences may be judged by looking at the standardized parameters of the significant effects. As all the effects are of minor importance (according to their low LR-Chi^2 values and the nevertheless perfect explanation of model (5)) their parameters tend to be insignificant, indicating that the observed differences are diffuse in most instances. There is only one marked asymmetry with respect to the terminally ill patients: when talking about doctor's topics, more of their within-turn transitions start with answers than could be expected from a model containing no interactive asymmetries of type I. Terminally ill patients have to wait for an interactive opportunity, such as responding to a physician's initiative, to put forward initiatives of their own.

With respect to the terminally ill patients and the topics of shared knowledge, no interactive asymmetry of type I could be found, whereas this is the only instance where type II asymmetries turned out to be of importance. The pattern of residual components (standardized residuals of model (8) in fig. 14) indicates two main differences with respect to the sequential effects of a given move. Physicians' requests for (non-qualifying) informations are more likely to be followed by patients' requests for (non-qualifying) informations than vice versa. And physicians' answers are more likely to be followed by patients' answers than vice versa. The whole pattern might be seen as 'question-to-a-question' sequences, where the 1st speaker is more likely to be the physician.

Not tested but assumed (implicitly conformed to by all models tested above) has been the differences between physicians and patients in making simple (1 move only) or complex turns (more than 1 move), which might be seen as an additional aspect of interactive asymmetry. Fig. 16 shows the analysis of this aspect. The results do not differ essen-

			doctor's topics		patient's topics		top. of sh. knowl.	
	effects	DF	LRChi^2	p	LR Chi^2	p	LR Chi^2	p
terminally ill patients	'T-1 FX'	5	12.73*	.026	7.95	.159	3.25	.662
	'TØ SX'	5	5.64	.343	9.58	.088	1.93	.859
	'T-1 FX, TØ SX'	10	18.05	.054	17.9	.057	5.17	.880
non-terminally ill patients	'T-1 FX'	5	4.09	.537	1.08	.956	12.44*	.029
	'TØ SX	5	3.49	.625	12.25*	.032	14.16*	.015
	'T-1 FX, TØ SX'	10	7.53	.675	13.64	.190	25.68*	.004

fig. 15: Relative importance of effects 'T-1 FX', TØ SX' and 'T-1 FX, TØ SX' (= interactive asymmetry type I) judged as improvement of model T-1 TØ X, TØ S, T-1 F

The entries are the differences between models from fig. 14:

(5) - (6) = 'T-1 F X' speaker- related differences in using move types in first (antecedent) position (T-1)

(5) - (7) = 'TØ S X' speaker- related differences in using move types in second (consequent) position (TØ)

(5) - (8) = 'T-1 F X' + 'TØ S X'

* significant differences ($p \leqslant .05$)

	F, X	doctor's topic	patient's topic	top. of sh. knowl.
terminally ill patients	LR Chi^2 (1) Phy.: Pt	213.51 (0.0) 1.32	51.31 (0.0) .87	8.89 (.00029) 1.08
non-terminally ill patients	LR Chi^2 (1) Phy.: Pt.	119.75 (0.0) 1.22	183.15 (0.0) .78	2.77 (.0961) .96

fig. 16: LR-Chi^2, (p) **and odds ratio of the cross-tabulation of first speaker (F: physician/patient) and** X **(speaker change /within turn transition)**

tially from one group to another. The physicians make more complex moves within their subject domain, whereas the patients do the same within their thematic domain. With respect to the topics of shared knowledge the discourses are almost perfectly symmetrical. The whole picture can be best characterized as a topic related asymmetry with an overall balanced structure between physicians and patients.

fig. 16 (pag.191)

The above analysis is an assessment of the asymmetry found in the layer of thematic innovation. Asymmetry of steering by continuations with different degrees of coherence may be analyzed by asking which features of a preceding turn influence the next speaker's type of continuation. The analysis uses 4 dimensions of the coding system: the kind of continuation (non-responsive, partly responsive, fully responsive), the type of the preceding speaker's last move (categories as above), the thematic domain of that move, and the complexity of the preceding turn, i.e.: is the turn built up of more than 1 move?

There is no need to assess the local length of dependence, because the type of continuation is related per se to the preceding turn. There are 5,662 transitions from a physician's turn to a patient's turn (2,886 with terminally ill and 2,776 with non-terminally ill patients) and 5,796 transitions from a patient's turn to a physician's turn (2,888 and 2,908).

fig. 17 (a b c) (pag.193)

Fig. 17 gives the best confirming structural models for these two types of transition. The type of continuation made by the physician is essentially only dependent on the complexity and the type of move of the patient's last turn. The structural model for the dependence of the patient's continuation is more complex. Beside the factors found to be relevant for the patient-doctor transitions, the patients' continuation is influenced by the thematic domain. And with respect to the terminally ill patients there is a higher order effect, the specific constellation of the physician's last move and thematic domain influencing the patient's type of reaction.

The pragmatic social substance of these structural differen-

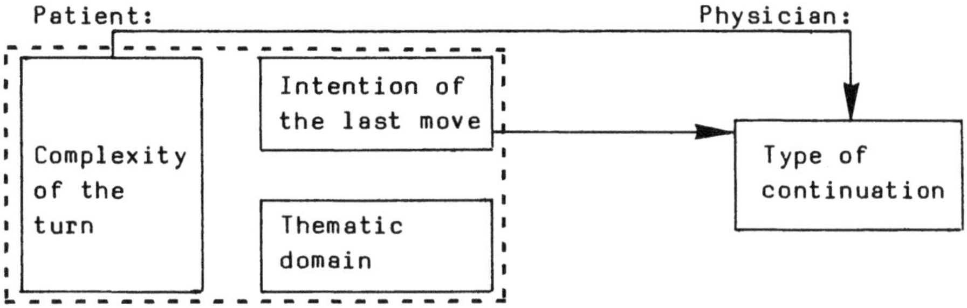

fig. 17a: A structural model of the physician's continuation following a patient's turn (no difference as to whether the patient is terminally ill or not)

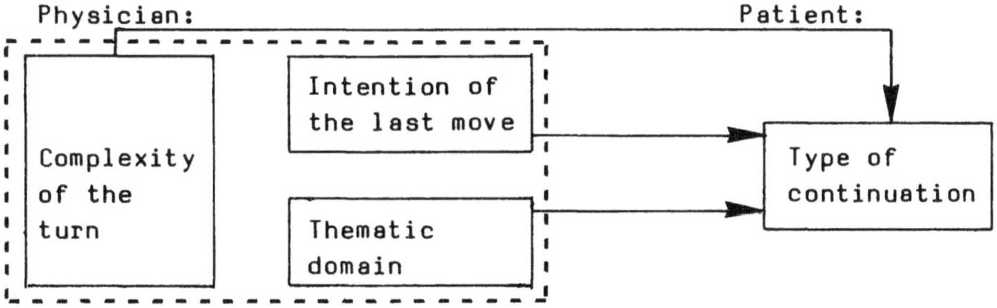

fig. 17b: A structural model of the patient's continuation following a physician's turn (non-terminally ill patients)

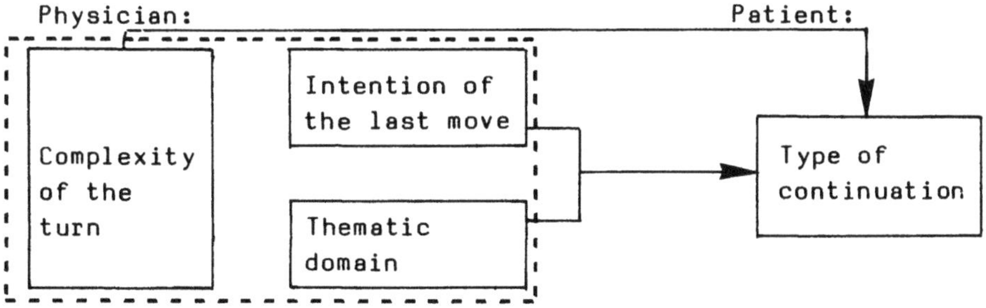

fig. 17c: A structural model of the patient's continuation following a physician's turn (terminally ill patients)

ces has to be interpreted by examining the significant parameters found in these models. I cannot do this here, because the least complex model is associated with 50 and the most complex model with 74 independent parameters. Yet the structural analysis reveals that the evaluative hypothesis of symmetry is not tenable with respect to the dialogical control as achieved by the type of continuation. Patients show a more complex consideration for what was done by the physician before. This asymmetry seems particularly marked for the discourses with terminally ill patients. With respect to the results reported, the dominating role of the physicians may be described as an extra freedom of steering the discourse by continuations of their own choice.

COMMENTS ON DIRK FEHLENBERG.

Paul ten Have.

The paper by Dirk Fehlenberg reports of an evaluation study of an effort to change the structure and contents of bedside communication. This effort had several objectives. On the one hand, the aim was to focus on the communication between the main doctor and the patient and to have the professionals discuss the case among themselves at another time and in a different place. On the other hand, the aim was to give both parties, physician and patient, an equal chance to influence communication. Furthermore, the 'disadvantage' that existed for 'terminal' patients in these matters had to be avoided. Fehlenberg tries to evaluate these efforts by using a probabilistic quantitative research design. A large sample of bedside discourse was coded, using a theoretically relevant coding system, and this data-set was then used to test how it would best fit a series of theoretical models, developed on the basis of the professed aims of the changing program. In this way, it is hoped that one can specify the extent to which the goals of the program have been reached. Roughly summarizing his results, one may say that the effort to focus the bedside conversation on the pair of main doctor and patient has been largely successful, but that the effort to equalize the influence of both parties on the communication - the creation of 'symmetry' - has produced only mixed results.

Fehlenberg's paper represents a highly technical exercisein probabilistic analysis. In fact, though it has 'discourse' as its object, there is not a single quote to be found in the paper from the discourses studied. Theoretically and methodologically sound efforts are made to adapt the methods of coding and analysis to the particularities of oral multiparty discourse, but the imagination of the non-technical reader is never assisted by illustrative examples of the phenomena under discussion. As to the technical intricacies,

I am not qualified to discuss them fully, so I will restrict my remarks to some substantial issues.

A general problem concerning attempts at planned change of social organization is that certain aspects of this organization differ in changeability. A further problem is that attempts at change may have unplanned effects. Fehlenberg's research design precludes the production of findings on this latter problem, since he has analyzed his data from the perspective of the program goals. As to this first problem, his research does produce some interesting results. The efforts to change the bedside meetings in such a way that the pair of main physician and patient is the focus of communication have been largely successful. The interprofessional discussion of the case has been separated from communication with the patient and the bedside meeting is mainly devoted to the latter. This is so even with the terminally ill, although there is a larger participation of the other professionals in those cases. So from this part of the research we may conclude that it is, in fact possibe to change communicative patterns - in the sense of who-speaks-to-whom.

The second major aim of the program was to have greater 'equality' among the communicative partners, that is less 'asymmetry'. Evaluation in the light of this particular aim has produced mixed results. We may speculate about the reasons for this lower level of success. The question of who speaks constitutes a more controllable aspect of organizational interaction than that what will be said and how people will react to each other's contributions. It should be noted that Fehlenberg uses a very specific notion of 'symmetry'. He focuses on a symmetry of pragmatic effectiveness and will call a communicative situation 'symmetrical' when the same kinds of speech acts have the same kinds of communicative effect, when they are followed by the same kinds of complementary acts, regardless of the parties involved. There are, of course, other concepts of (a-)symmetry to be encountered in the literature, such as those regarding topics or the distribution of kinds of speech acts over the participants. In Fehlenberg's conception an asymmetrical distribution of, for instance, 'request for information', does not count as a case of 'asymmetry', for, as he puts it, "these differences may be attributable to the situational logic and constraints of action". He seems to think that these kinds of asymmetry are somehow inessential and are not connected with the asymmetry of effectiveness that he wants to focus on. Without a theoretical argumentation and an empirical demonstration I am not convinced that these assumptions are valid.

It may be that we can find some indications of other aspects of asymmetrical organization from the findings reported by Fehlenberg. One difference between patients and physicians that he found is that the former tend to produce various initiatives (questions, decisions, etc.) immediately following a speaker change, while the latter tend to do that in the second part of their utterances. In other words, patients tend to attach their initiatives to doctors' preceding speech, while physicians attach theirs to their own previous talking. This result, which is not explained by Fehlenberg, can be easily understood by reference to the three-part sequence that is so pervasive in provider-client interaction - as I have shown in my other contribution to this volume. Since in this sequence the provider has a general right to both first and third positions, while the client takes up the second, it is very likely that doctors tend to produce two-move utterances, while patients are restricted to single-move utterances. More concretely, doctors' utterances will often contain an acknowledgement plus a question, while patients will only provide answers. Such an answer may, on occasion, be coded as an initiative in Fehlenberg's system. Another possibility for patients is to use their second position to ask a question, for instance a request for clarification referring to the preceding doctor's question (a Next Turn Initiator in conversation-analytic jargon). In Fehlenberg's analysis this would count as an initiative following a speaker change. So one usually has: doctor's question, possibly preceded by an acknowledgement of the preceding answer, followed by a patient's answer, and so on, or in some instances: doctor's question, doctor's clarification, followed by the patient's answer to the clarified question. This would be compatible with some of Fehlenberg's other findings. In general, he notes, there is almost no difference between parties as to the other person's moves that follow theirs. But there are some exceptions:

Physicians' request for (non-qualifying) information is more likely to be followed by patients' request for (non-qualifying) information than vice versa. And physicians' answers are more likely to be followed by patients' answers than vice versa.

That doctors would initiate less repair on patients' questions than the other way around comes as no surprise if one bears in mind that doctors' questions tend to have their origin in the medical frame of knowledge, which is not widely shared with patients.

These observations are tentative, of course. I have no access to Fehlenberg's data to check my account of his quantitative findings. But I do think that my suggestions are compatible with most analyses of doctor-patient interactions that have been published to date. I also think that physicians and patients usually take up different positions in both regular questioning sequences and in incidential repair sequences, in other words, that they display a sequential asymmetry. It seems clear to me that this kind of asymmetry is functionnally connected with some basic aspects of professional-client encounters, and that the former has expertise to deal with the other person's problems. So, contrary to Fehlenberg's assumption I am inclined to think that the various aspects of 'asymmetry' are functionally interdependent. And contrary to the aims of the ambitious program he evaluates I would think that a certain measure of 'asymmetry' is unavoidable. Striving for an absolute equalization of interactional influence may well lead to either a weakening of professional responsibility or to some form of hypocritical glossing over of an unavoidable asymmetry.

8

Summarizing in doctor-patient interaction

H. Houtkoop-Steenstra

1. Introduction

Dutch medical students are taught to communicate with their future patients effectively, as appears from Schouten (1982) and other coursebooks. Since patients are supposed to need encouragement to tell what they want from their general practitioner and what their complaints are, medical students are taught to summarize [1] the patients' utterances frequently. And when one listens to taped medical interactions, one does indeed find doctors using this Rogerian technique very frequently.

In this paper I will demonstrate how this summarizing technique may have an unintended and negative effect, if not applied very carefully. It will be made clear that summarizing may lead the patient's talk into a certain direction, whereas it is meant to give the patient the opportunity to express her or his thoughts freely (Schouten, 1982).

2. Mrs. Van Veen

The interaction to be discussed here [2], is one between an elderly male general practitioner and a woman of about 55 years of age. It becomes clear from the interaction that she has been seeing this doctor for at least some years. Doctor and patient are sitting in low comfortable chairs, next to each other, which gives the interaction a friendly character. The tape starts off with the presentation of the medical complaints. Last week the patient had a sore throat, and it hurt especially when she took hot food. After a few days these symptoms disappeared, but now she has a headache, and suffers from dizziness and nausea. After having reported this, the woman indicates that she had thought of blood-pressure problems [3]:

(1) lines 25-51 (see Appendix for transcript). key, and for the original Dutch fragment).

25 P. I thought at first it might be my blood-pressure,
26 (.)
27 but we:ll, that can't have to do/
28 D. (you thought so. Did you yourself have ideas about that?
29 (0.7)
30 P. Well yes because I/
31 D. (That your blood-pressure might not be alright?=
32 P. (Be/
33 P. =Because I had it then as well, y'know? Heada:che, and thi-thi-this
34.D. (Yes.
35 P. dizziness and also sickness;
36 D. (Yes.
37 (.)
38 P. I got then.
39 (0.7)
40 But we:ll, that was a long time ago. Y'know.
41 D. It was a long time ago, ya:h.=
42 P. =It was a long time ago now.
43 (0.3)
44 D. But you remembered that after all when you u:h (.) all of a
45 P. (Yes (. Yes. and then
46 D. sudden u:h/
47 P. (I also had balance-problems, but that nevertheless was something else.
48 Wasn't it.
49 D. °It was.°
50 (1.9)
51 P. But I don't know. I just don't feel we:ll

In line 25 the patient seems to offer a candidate diagnosis. By 'candidate diagnosis' I refer to the fact that patients produce a diagnosis which might, but need not, be the correct one. The candidate diagnosis is formulated in a careful way and the utterance usually contains modal verbs and particles. Patients may also present a "non-diagnosis" such as "I don't know what it is".

I would like to highlight this diagnosis-utterance in order to demonstrate that the patient is not offering a candidate diagnosis, although it may look like one on the face of it, and although the doctor seems to take it for one.

This utterance starts off with an "I thought at first". Jefferson (n.d.) investigated reports by people who had been in an earthquake, and who presented their experiences as 'At First I Thought X, Then I Realized Y'. Jefferson (page 6) summarizes Sacks (1968, pages 1-2) who writes about such "contrast classes" as follows: "So what we have is something like: 'Realized' stands in opposition to 'thought' by reference to the fact that 'thought' is used when it turns out to be wrong. (....) Thus, particulary with respect to reports of past events, one wants to look which verb is being used, to see whether the verb is doing things besides, say, reporting a reaction, a feeling, etcetera, i.e. that the verb is saying about that thing it was true or false". She furthermore states that "Asserting the wrong "first thought" reaffirms, in the fact of the actuality, the **in principle-correctness** of the ordinary alternative. In effect, it is proposing that **it should have been right.**" (page 11).

This patient may be seen to use this device when she states that at first she thought it might be her blood-pressure. Later on in the interaction, we will see that she will also give evidence for the in-principle correctness and the plausibility of this 'at first thought' candidate diagnosis: she has had the same symptoms before and it then turned out to be blood pressure as well. On the basis of Jefferson's and Sacks' observations of this device, the patient's first turn component may be looked upon as projecting that this blood-pressure is not her candidate diagnosis, although this seems plausible at first sight.

The patient follows up this utterance by "but we:ll, that can't have to do/". As Sacks (1967; 1973) points out, "well" very frequently precedes a disagreement with the prior assertion of the prior speaker (cf. also Pomerantz 1984). I suppose one may claim that in that case, 'well' can also be used to preface disagreement with or distancing from one's own prior assertion. The patient may then be seen to be prefacing disagreement with her 'at first thought' candidate diagnosis: She had it "Then as <u>well</u>". She carries on this explanation by saying "But we:ll, that was a long <u>time</u> ago, y'know.", which makes her diagnosis a doubtful one.

This may be seen as a further indication that the blood pressure should not be taken as a serious candidate diagnosis. Nevertheless, the doctor continues to talk about this diagnosis: "But you remembered that after all when you u:h (.) all of a sudden u:h/".

In line 51 she provides a new general presentation of her complaints: "But I don't know. I just don't feel we:ll.". The diagnosis presented in line 25 and implicitly rejected again, is now replaced by this non-diagnosis and general complaint. Furthermore, the patient initiates this second turn-component with the adversative "but".

Having heard the patient using an "at first I thought", a "but" and a disagreement preface-item "we:ll", one may expect her to be in the process of rejecting her initially stated candidate diagnosis. Moreover, in overlap with the doctor's utterance, she even produces a fourth item in this series: "that can't have to do/".

So there are several indications that this blood pressure is in the process of being rejected as a candidate diagnosis. Asked by the doctor why she thinks of blood pressure, she will argue that she has had it before.

In line 82, the patient offers a new possible diagnosis:

(2) lines 82-94

(2.6)

82 P. But we:ll, it may also be nervousness perhaps, y'know.=
83 D. =Do you think it also might be nervousness?
84 P. I don't know of course, because I u:h (.) well, have troubles with my
85 parents. Y'know? So, very tense actually;
86 (1.0)
87 And well, you're trying to find a solution to it yourself all the time
88 and you're thinking it will blow o:ver again;
89 (0.7)
90 D. Could you tell me something about that? What it's all
91 about u:h with your parents?=
92 P. (Well
93 =My father (...) ((Patient tells about her parents))

After the first candidate diagnosis has been implicitly rejected by the patient herself as an implausible one, she now provides a second possibility: nervousness. As an explanation of why it might be nervousness, she provides a vaguely formulated problem: "troubles with my parents." (85). What the troubles are is not revealed, and they are pronominalized later on as "it" (88). Following Terasaki (1976)[4)], we may look upon this utterance as a Pre-Announcement about troubles. And after the doctor has produced his elicitation to tell him about them, the patient talks about her troubles at great length ($4^{1}/_{2}$ pages of transcript).

The troubles are, in short, the following. Her father has had a stroke and is now in a nursing-home, which he likes very much. Although he is not able to do much, he is a very contented kind man. This talk about the father is not the trouble itself, but only leads to the troublesome point, which is the mother, who also lives in this nursing-home. This "got a disa:ster" however. The mother has a "painless cancer" of the gullet, and is demented. She is behaving very badly towards the doctor and nurses and everybody who is nice to her. Very threatening for the patient is her mother's wish to go back home again, about which the doctors have said that nobody can stop her from doing so, "but in that case the children will get saddled with it." So she is in a permanent fear of what will happen. "And u:h well this doctor said it's already impossible for one nurse, so let alone for me, Y'know?".

This talk of the patient's is treated by the doctor as Troubles Talk.

Jefferson & Lee (1981) distinguish between an Advice Giving Sequence, in which one party seeks, and the other party gives advice, and a Troubles Talk Sequence, in which the troubles talk is responded to by all kinds of affiliation responses by the troubles recipient. In this part of the interaction under discussion, the doctor gives responses such as "°yes yes°", "Isn't that something" or "°I can understand that very well.°". This troubles talk was presented as the explanation for the new possible diagnosis, the nervousness. In line 347 the patient returns to this diagnosis itself:

(3)lines 347 356

347 P. And my husband says well "o:h you're <u>all</u> nerves," but we:ll. May be that's
348 <u>so</u>, but on the other hand I figured/
349 D. (That's your husband's opinion of your

troubles;=
350 P. =O:f my troubles. Yes.
351 D. (Yes.
352 And what do you think yourself?
353 You mentioned as a matter of fact/
354 P. (I (Well,
355 that too, Y'know. But I find this really a little strange because
356 D. (Yes.
357 P. I've had it more often.

So the woman claims to consider nervousness as a possible diagnosis in fragment 2, a diagnosis for which causes are explained in the troubles talk. Now she returns to this candidate diagnosis in order to say that, although she is very nervous indeed, this might not be the correct diagnosis after all. Notice that in this section, the patient again makes use of a contrast-class: her husband thinks X, but she herself thinks differently.

"Maybe that's so, but on the other hand I figured/" (in Dutch: "Misschien is het ook wel zo;, maar aan de andere ka:nt dacht ik/") is a type of utterance which is characterized as a concessive-adversative construction" in Houtkoop-Steenstra (1980). It is a construction containing the contrast-class 'wel-maar', or 'that may be right, but'. The first concessive 'wel'-part projects on the second 'adversative 'maar'-part.

While the patient is still producing this 'wel-maar' utterance, the doctor interrupts her in order to unravel this double construction into its separate parts. He summarizes the "maybe that's so" as "That's your husband's opinion of your troubles.", with which the patient agrees. Then the doctor summarizes the patient's unfinished "but on the other hand I figured/" as "And what do you think yourself?". This summarizing by means of interruption becomes interesting when the doctor, by saying "You mentioned as a matter of fact/", leads her back to the subject of blood pressure.

While the patient is in the process of establishing a contrast between nervousness and something else, the doctor directs her into a contrast between nervousness and blood pressure. And since the woman has expressed her doubts with respect to the blood-pressure diagnosis on several occasions, one may assume that the contrast she is establishing was not that of nervousness versus blood pressure. Hence this instance of the doctor's summarizing is clearly a way to direct the patient's talk into the direction he thinks she should go.

When earlier on the patient mentioned the blood pressure, she claimed to have thought of it because she had it "then as well". Now she uses this argument in the opposite way: "But I find this a little strange, because I've had it more often" (notice also the difference between "then" and "more often").

Having returned to the blood pressure again as the diagnosis, the doctor will propose having that checked:

(4) **lines 354-376** (continuation of fragment 3)

354 P. But I find this really a little strange, because I've
had it often.
355 D. (Yes.
356 (0.6)
357 P. And then I was/
358 D. (You would still like to have this blood-pressure
checked.=
359 P. =Ye:s. That certainly yes.
360 D. That certainly.
361 P. (Yes certainly. Yes.
362 D. (Yes.
363 P. But I had it then as we:ll, and I saw you too, but in
364 those days I weighed hundred and seventy pounds.
365 (0.5)
366 And you said "we:ll that might be it." Y'know? The
fat around here. •hh And
367 I reduced it till a hundred and fifty-five, remember?
And (.) it indeed got
368 better. Really. Finally.
369 (0.8)
370 And now I got it agai:n.
371 (0.9)
372 Last week.
373 (.)
374 I'd say well now I'm not that heavy anymore.=
375 D. =No:
376 (3.0)

Although the patient expresses doubts with respect to the blood pressure diagnosis again in line 354, the doctor proposes having that checked. The patient accepts this proposal, although her utterance "That certainly yes." might be heard as 'that', (the blood-pressure) plus something else, not mentioned now, or 'at least that, among other things'. When the doctor and patient have come to an agreement about this blood-pressure check, the patient explains that, whatever may be wrong, it cannot be the overweight it was the last time. This explanation may also be heard as a new signalling of doubt with respect to this blood pressure being the only problem.

The doctor recognizes this 'more than just blood pressure':

(5) lines 381-400 (continuation of fragment 4)

381 D. Would you like to have one and another checked?
382 (0.8)
383 P. Ye:s. ((sighing deeply; doubting tone?))
384 (0.3)
385 D. Except for the blood pressure,
386 P. (Ye:s.
387 D. also uh
388 P. (Ye:s. I guess so.
389 (0.6)
390 D. having it checked physically?=
391 P. =Yes.=
392 D. =Yes?=
393 P. =Yes sure. That's alright with me.
394 (1.5)
395 The:/ I guess that would be a reassurance.=
396 D. =That would be a reassurance for you, I suppose.
397 P. (Yes. (Yes.
398 D. That is what you really want from me?
399 P. That. And honestly speaking ye:s indeed.=
400 D. =Yes.

So they come to an agreement [5] about an extensive physical examination, for reasons of reassuring the patient [6].

What is it that the patient thinks she might have, when it is not (only) blood pressure problems? This finally becomes clear in the next part of the transcript. I will continue the preceding fragment.

(6) lines 401-430

401 P. =One cannot/ I was so: involved. A:ll these years

with my mother. I walked
402 in and out of the hospital. (operette) I was involved with her.
403 ˙hh And when you (.) then get (.) something yourself, you come to
404 think "Oh Go:d, Surely I haven't got it as well, have I?"=
405 D. =°°Yes.°°=
406 P. =You know?=
407 D. °°Yes. °°
408 P. But we:ll, they say it is not contagious right? Something like that.
409 D. No, a malignant affection of the gullet, you mean?=
410 P. =Ye:s.
411 D. Yes.=
412 P. =Ye:s. That isn't/
413 D. (Is not contagious, no.=
414 P. =Isn't it can't be contagious can it?=
415 D. =That's not contagious (.) but I can understand very well now that you
416 yourself are feeling something like/ that one may think (.) you put it
417 P. (°°a little lump. °°
418 D. into your head, that you say "We:ll I hope I haven't got it as well,
419 right?"=
420 P. =Yes.
421 (.)
422 Because I had it more often uh in the past really.=
423 D. =Yes.
424 (.)
425 It's not something of uh (.) a few days:
426 P. (no. It's not only once, or so.
427 D. We'll check that as well.

Now that the fear of cancer has been expressed, other parts of the interaction come into a new perspective. In the very first lines of the transcript, the woman reports throat-problems: it ached when she took hot food.

Furthermore she said that her mother had cancer of the gullet. However, both assertions were made in such a way that they are difficult to recognize as important remarks. Her throat problems had already disappeared in a few days, and therefore her throat is painless now. Her mother's painless cancer is mentioned as a minor detail of the entire story about the mother. And in the lines there are indications that the doctor has not understood the following utterance as signalling a fear of cancer:

(7) lines 403-404
P. And when you (.) then get (.) something yourself, you come to think "Oh Go:d, Surely I haven't got it as well, have I?"

Except for the Troubles-Talk Sequences earlier in the interaction, this is the only other context where the doctor produces his soft "yes"-es. The misunderstanding of the gist of the patient's utterance may be caused by the patient's apparently resuming to talk about complaints and worries, especially because it follows talk which belongs to a different part of the interaction, the identification of the patient's reason for seeing the doctor:

(8) lines 398-404 (preceeds fragment 7)
398 D. Is that what you really want from me?
399 P. That. And honestly speaking ye:s indeed.=
400 D. =Yes.=
401 P. =One cannot / I was so: involved. A:ll these years with my mother. I walked
402 in and out of the hospital. (operette) I was involved with her. •hh
403 And when you (.) then get (.) something yourself, you come to
404 think "Oh Go:d, surely I haven't got it as well, have I?"

Notice also, that the woman does not mention the word cancer, but instead talks about "it", which later will be referred to by the doctor as "a malignant affection of the gullet, you mean?" (cf. Cicourel 1984). But since the interactants have previously come to the conclusion that the woman wants a general examination, this "it" might have been heard as 'some unknown disease'. It is only after the woman talks about "it" perhaps being contagious, that the doctor indicates that he understands she might be referring to cancer.

Whether or not the fear of cancer was the main reason for

the woman to come to see the doctor, the doctor treats it as a different worry of hers, which also needs assuaging by physical examination. ("We'll check that as well.") And apparently he does not treat this as her main worry, because he now proposes having the blood pressure checked today, and doing the rest of the check-up on a later occasion.

(9) **lines 438-451**

438 D. May I propose that I'll check your blood-pressure
now? So we'll
439 P. (Ye:s.
440 D. know that now. That we'll make another appointment
for the examination,
441 because that's a little difficult now
442 P. (Yes. (Yes. (Yes. (Yes. (Yes. And also
another pap-smear
443 please. That's been almost two years now.=
444 D. (And a pa:p-smear (as well)?
445 =Fine.
446 P. Yes?
447 D. We'll make another appointment for that. If that's
alright
448 P. (Yes.
449 D. with you.
450 Shall I check the blood pressure now then?
451 P. (Yes.=
452 D. =Yes?=
453 P. =Yes.

Conclusion

Although summarizings are meant to encourage the patient to go on talking, it may have become clear that it may do more than that. Doctors make choices when they summarize; in summarizing a certain utterance, they indicate that this is important information. It highlights information to the effect that it may become topicalized. And once it has been topicalized, this information becomes more prominent and may have an effect on how additional information will be received and consequently be dealt with again. So, instead of being a device to encourage the patient to go on in the direction she wants to go, it may turn out to become a device for leading the interview into an other direction.

We have seen how the patient mentions the blood pressure as a possible-diagnosis-to-be-rejected, and the doctor inquires about her reasons for having thought so. The woman then finds herself in a position to present an explanation which strengthens the logic of this blood pressure diagnosis, and which makes it more difficult for her to drop this diagnosis again.

In the second instance of this summarizing practice, the doctor unravels an ongoing concessive-adversative construction, in order to steer the patient in the direction of the blood pressure diagnosis again, although she has rejected this diagnosis several times.

That summarizings may have this unintended effect has to do with the unequality of the relationship between doctors and patients (cf. Fisher, 1984 on this 'institutional authority'). In several places in this interaction, the patient will claim to agree with the doctor's talk, although she demonstrates that she does not agree (cf. Sacks, Spring 1970, on the distinction between claiming and showing agreement). For example, the doctor may propose something, or may initiate a new topic or perspective, and the woman will claim agreement but give an example which shows disagreement, or she will return to the prior topic. See for example line 401 in which she returns to the talk about her mother, when it has just been decided to have a general check-up. In returning to this prior topic, she also returns to a prior phase (the presentation of the complaint) in the interaction.

Taking this (virtual) 'obligation to agree' as a feature of doctor-patient interaction into account, one will see that summarizing presupposes very good listening skills on the part of the doctor, first of all because it may highlight and topicalize information which had better not be topicalized, and secondly because it may trigger disagreeing talk which is formated as agreeing talk.

I should emphasize here that I do not mean to say that summarizing is a bad device as such. I only meant to demonstrate that it may be counterproductive when it is not applied very carefully.

It seems important to me that the effects of summarizings be investigated in detail. While I have demonstrated how summarizings may lead the patient's talk in the wrong direction, there are many other instances of summarizings which seem to obstruct the patient's talk rather than encourage it. I will give only two examples of this:

(10)
P. I just don't feel we:ll.
D. You don't feel well.=
P. =No::.
(1.1)

(11)
P. (...) it started to get sore again here,=
D. You got pain there.=
P. I got pain.=
D. Hm mm.
P. And it hurt also with hot food.

Instead of continuing her talk, the patient will acknowledge the doctor's summarizing utterances first. This may then lead to sequences which stagnate fluent further talking by the patient. Although this is not as dramatic as the two examples I have discussed before, one may say at least that it does not encourage the patient to go on freely.

It may very well be that summarizings become more effective when they are produced in a questioning way. For example, when the woman states that the fact that her mother went into the nursing-home turned out "a disa:ster", the doctor responds with "Did it turn out a disaster?" and the patient starts to explain all the problems her mother is causing.

So, if medical students are to be taught to summarize, it is important to have more knowledge about the effects the different types of summarizings may have. And Conversation Analysis may assist in the acquisition of this knowledge.

Notes

1. Although "formulating" (cf. Heritage & Watson, 1979; Davis 1984) is a more adequate term to refer to rephrasing the patient's words in one way or other, I will nevertheless use "summarizing" since that is how general practitioners refer to it themselves.

2. I thank Dr. Leendert Krol for giving me this tape so generously and for being willing to discuss my analysis of it.

3. The original Dutch transcripts have been translated into English in such a way that the most important information of the original conversation is captured in the translation, as far as possible. This implies that the underlinings, indicating some form of stress, may not correspond with the Dutch versions, since stress is strongly related to the word-order and syntactic structure of languages. It is also related to pragmatic features; whereas Dutch expresses modality mainly by means of modal particles and modal verbs, English in that case prefers paralinguistic means. Therefore, the English version of the fragments may contain underlining, where Dutch does not.

4. Terasaki (1976) elegantly describes sequences consisting of:
   1. Pre-announcement sequence First Pair-Part,
   2. Pre-announcement sequence Second Pair-Part, functioning as a solicit for:
   3. Announcement (of new information)

   She points out that in the pre-announcement the speaker may make use of nominal forms such as 'things' or 'something' which function as a generic noun projecting new information to be given in the next-next turn, after the recipient has solicited the speaker to do so.

5. In my Ph. D. work in progress, I am studying proposals of different sorts which set up five-sequences:
   1. speaker : proposal (request, invitation, promise etc.)
   2. recipient : acceptance (e.g. "Yes, that's fine.")
   3. speaker : request for confirmation (mostly a "ja?"/"Yes?")
   4. recipient : confirmation of acceptance
   5. speaker : sequence closing item (mostly an "okay.")

   In Houtkoop-Steenstra (1985) I have demonstrated that, when the proposal has been responded to by a single "Yes.", this response will not be treated by the initial speaker as an acceptance of the proposal. After the occurrence of such a "yes.", the speaker will continue producing talk to the initial proposal, instead of producing the third-positioned request for confirmation.

   In fragment (6) it may be noticed that the doctor is

reluctant when producing his request for confirmation, which signals that the patient's prior responses to the proposal are not treated by him as whole-hearted acceptance.

6. Krol (1979:867) claims that patients often come to see their doctor, not because they are primarily interested in the cause of their medical problems, but in order to have certain causes excluded. In this way it is not the trouble as such which induces the patient to see the doctor, but the worries caused by the trouble.

Appendix

(1) 25 Ik dacht eerst misschien m'n bloeddruk,
26 (.)
27 Maar ja : dat heb 'tan hier weer/
28 A. Dat dacht u. U had daar zelf uw vermoedens over?
29 (0.7)
30 P. Nou ja omdat ik/=
31 A. =Dat mogelijk de bloeddruk niet in orde zou kunnen zijn?=
32 P. (Om/
33 =Omdat ik dat toen ook gehad hebt, he. Hoofdpijn, en da-da-dat
34 A. (Ja.
35 P. duizeligheid en ook wel misselijk;
36 A. (Ja.
37 (.)
38 P. was ik toen.
39 (0.7)
40 Maar ja:, 't is wel lang geleden he.
41 A. 'T is lang geleden ja:.=
42 P. ='T is nou wel lang geleden.
43 (0.3)
44 A. Maar dat herinnerde zich toen toch weer toen U e:h (.) ineens e:h/
45 P. (Ja! En ik heb
46 toen ook e:venwichtsstoornissen gehad, maar dat was toch
47 weer iets anders. He.
48 A. °Ja.°
49 (1.9)

50 P. Maar ik weet het niet. 'K voel me alleen niet pre:ttig.

(2) 82 P. Maar ja, het kan ook missschien wel nerveusiteit zijn he?=
83 A. =Dacht u dat ook nerveusiteit zou kunnen zijn?
84 P. Dat wee:t ik dus nie:t, omdat ik e:h (.) ja, erg sukkel
85 met m'n ouders du:s. he. Dus erg gespannen eigenlijk;
86 (1.0)
87 En ja, je zoekt het zelf eigenlijk iedere keer maar een beetje
88 en dat je denkt van het zal wel o:ver gaan;
89 (0.7)
90 A. Kunt u daar iets van vertellen? Hoe dat u e:h is met uw ouders?=
91 P. (Nou ja/
92 =Mijn vader heb ik dus in Mei: (.) ben 'k hier ook al bij u
93 geweest voor pilletjes, ee:n hersenbloeding gehad, =

(3) 346 Jah.°En daarom hoo:r. en m'n man zegt wel "jij stikt van
347 de zenuwen,", maar ja:. Misschien is het ook wel zo:, maar
348 aan de andere ka:nt dacht ik/
349 A. (Dat is uws ma:n's (oordeel over uw klachten;=
350 P. =o:ver mijn klachten. Ja.
351 A. (Ja.
352 En wat vind u d'r zelf van? u noemde 't zelf eigenlijk ook al e:h,
353 P. (Ik/
(ach
354 dat ook wel maar ik vind dit wel een beetje vree:md, omdat ik dit
355 A. (Ja. (ja:.
356 P. wel es meer gehad heb.

(4) 354 dat ook wel maar ik vind dit wel een beetje vree:md, omdat ik dit
355 A. (Ja. (Ja:.

356 P. wel es meer gehad heb.
357 (0.6)
358 En toen ben ik/
359 A. U zou toch wel prettig vinden om e:ven die bloed-
druk te
360 kontroleren.=
361 P. =Ja: dat ze:ker wel.
362 A. Dat °zeker wel.°
363 P. (Zeker wel. Ja.
364 A. (Ja.
365 (0.8)
366 P. Maar ik heb het toen ook geha:d, en ben 'k ook
bij u geweest,
367 maar toen woog ik honderdzeventig pond.
368 (0.5)
369 En toen zegt u nou: dat kon het wel es we:zen he,
't vet
370 wat hier omheen °hhh En toen ben'k toch terug
gegaan tot
371 honderdvijfenvijftig, en (.) is 't ook o:ver
gegaan. hoor. op
372 den duur.
373 (0.8)
374 En nu had ik het wee:r.
375 (0.9)
376 Vleden week.
377 (.)
378 'K denk ja nou ben ik toch niet zo: zwaar meer.=
379 =Nee:.
380 (3.0)

(5) 381 Zou u 't prettig vinden om toch nog es een en
ander na
382 te kijken?
383 (0.8)
384 P. Ja:. ((twijfelende toon?, wat zuchtend))
385 (0.3)
386 A. Behalve de bloeddruk,
387 P. (Ja:.
388 A. Ook nog eh
389 P. (Ja:. Dacht ik wel.
390 (0.6)
391 A. Licha:melijk es bekijken?=
392 P. =Ja.=

393 A. =Ja?=
394 P. =Ja hoor. Daar heb ik niks op tegen.
395 A. (1.5)
396 De:/'K geloof dat dat een gerustställing is.=
397 A. =Dat zou toch wel een geruststelling voor u zijn denk ik.
398 P. (Ja. (Ja.
399 A. Dat is eigenlijk wat u van me wi:lt?
400 P. Dat. En eerlijk gezegd we:l.=
401 A. =Ja.=

(6) 402 P. =Dat kan je niet/ 'k ben zo: betrokken geweest. A::l die jaren
403 met me moeder. Ik heb zie :kenhuis uitgelopen.
404 (operette) heb ik met d'r meegemaakt. ·hh En
405 als je dan nou (op 't ogenblik zelf ook iets hebt, dan denk je "Go:d, ik
406 zal toch ook niet hebben."
407 A. = °°ja. °°=
408 P. =he?=
409 A. = °°ja. °°
410 P. Maar ja:, ze zeggen besmettelijk is het niet he. zoiets.
411 A. Nee een kwaadaardige aandoening van de slokdarm, bedoelt u?=
412 P. =Ja:a.
413 A. Ja.=
414 P. =ja:. Dat is toch
415 A. (Is niet besmettelijk (hoor).=
416 P. =Is toch dat kan niet besmettelijk wezen?=
417 A. =Dat is niet besmettelijk. (.) maar ik kan me heel goed
418 voorstellen dat u nou u zelf hier ook iets voelt van
419 P. (°bobbeltje°
420 A. Dat je dat toch toch voor de gee:st komt, dat je zegt nou:
421 P. nou omdat ik het al/
422 A. a-als ik dat maar niet ook heb. he?=
423 P. =Ja.
424 (.)
425 Omdat ik het al eh de laatste tijd al meer gehad heb hoor.=

426 A. =Ja.
427 (.)
428 'T is niet iets van eh paar dagen;
429 P. (Nee. 'T is niet maar een
keer, of zo.
430 A. Gaan we dat ook bekijken.

•hh En
(7) 405 Als je dan nou (op 't ogenblik zelf ook iets
hebt, dan denk je "Go:d, ik
406 zal toch ook niet hebben."

(8) 399 A. Dat is eigenlijk wat u van me wi:lt?
400 P. Dat. En eerlijk gezegd we:l.=
401 A. =Ja.=
402 P. =Dat kan niet/ 'k ben zo: betrokken geweest. A::l
die jaren
403 met me moeder. Ik heb zie :kenhuis in ziekenhuis
uitgelopen.
404 (operette) heb ik met d'r mee-
gemaakt. •hh En
405 als je dan nou (op 't ogenblik zelf ook iets
hebt, dan denk je "Go:d, ik
406 zal toch ook niet hebben."

(9) 447 A. Mag ik u voorstellen dat ik dan: nu eventjes uw
bloeddruk
448 opmeet? dan weten we dat vast. Dat we voor het
onderzoek een
449 P. (ja:.
450 A. andere afspraak maken, want dat gaat nou: 'n
beetje moeilijk.
451 P. Ja (Ja.
(Ja.En
452 oo:k weer een uitstrijkje graag. Da's bijna: twee
jaar geleden.=
453 A. (En 'n
uitstrij:kje:(erbij)?
454 A. =Prima:.
455 P. Ja?=
456 A. =Dan maken we daar een aparte afspraak voor. As
dat goed is.=
457 P. (Ja.
458 A. =Zal'k nu even de bloeddruk meten.

459 P. (Ja.=
460 A. =Ja?=
461 P. =Ja.

Transcription symbols

Apart from some minor changes, I use the transcript symbols as developed by Jefferson.

(	Indicates the starting point of speaker's overlapping talk
= =	Equal signs, one at the end of one line and one at the beginning of the next, indicate no 'gap' between the two lines
(0.6)	A pause of e.g. 0.6 of a second
(.)	A pause of less than 0.3 of a second
word	Underscoring indicates some form of stress, via pitch and/or amplitude
::	Colons indicate prolongation of the immediately preceding sound. The length of the colon row indicates the length of the prolongation.
word	Arrows indicate shifts into higher resp. lower word pitch than would be expected from the sentence structure ten language
°°	The part between the two degree signs is produced in a relatively low voice
ho/	Cut-off
⟨word⟩ ⟨word⟩	The utterance (part) is speeded up resp. slowed down.
°hh	Audible intake of breath
( )	Part of the speech was not understood by the transcriber

(word) Dubious hearing of the word

(( )) Double parentheses contain trancriber's descriptions.

Comments on Houtkoop

M. Fahrenfort

This paper takes a closer look at a conversational device that has always been taken for granted as a useful device in doctor-patient conversations, namely summarizing. The paper attempts to show some of the drawbacks that can be involved in this conversational activity - a fresh outlook that in itself makes it worth reading.

Being a medical sociologist and psychologist with a micro-sociological outlook, I naturally looked at it from this point of view. Seen from that angle, the remarks on goals and procedures in doctor-patient conversations look a little naive. To me, the most striking feature of this naïveté, is that the writer does not look at a doctor-patient conversation with the ethnomethodological openmindedness that would leave to be determined "what it is about". Instead, she starts out from the culturally tacit assumption that a medical encounter is a "problem-solving" encounter. In this way, she does exactly what a conversational analyst should not do, i.e. start out from a preconceived notion about the conversation.

To make matters worse, the preconceptions she starts with are highly dubious in themselves, taken as they are from the literature on medicine and medical psychology and reflecting the bias of practitioners in these fields.

Contrary to this, I would propose a doctor-patient conversation to be a joint endeavour in which conversational work is being done to construct the problem in terms that both parties can go along with. This view would allow us to lay aside theoretically dubious notions like "first and second diagnosis", "hidden information", or the distinction of medical and/or psychosocial problems. Following this line of reasoning, there is no reason whatsoever to assume a difference between psychotherapeutic interviews and doctor-patient consultations.

This would allow us to treat summarizings in this conversation for what they are, i.e. formulations. As one formulation follows another in a mutual searching process, indicating one or another interpretation of these formulations as the "correct" one, and providing explanations why one or the other interpretation would be more valid, is equivalent to constructing yet another (observer's) reality of which the validity will always remain to be proved. Is there really a way for the observer/analyst to determine with any certainty which matters should and should not be topicalized, or are productive and counterproductive? Whose point of view, if any, should prevail here? If we would really like to say something about these matters, which is, of course, not impossible, more sophistication on the matter in question is necessary: it is not sufficient to state "it is not clear what empirical basis the assumed function of summarizing has and to what extent it is successful", as Houtkoop does.

If we do this, however, we do not look at the process of pattern-construction. We stop being conversational analysts and become partners in the construction of the social reality in question.

9

Public discourse and the problem of social order

W. Labov and T. Labov

Much recent research on language in its social context has focussed on verbal interaction in everyday life, where little conscious attention is given to the forms of speech. Both sociologists and linguists have found that everyday interaction is more highly structured than general impressions led us to believe.

In this paper we turn our attention to discourse in formal settings, where issues of considerable importance to society as a whole are discussed. In these public contexts, speakers give evidence of careful attention to their choice of words and manner of phrasing, and the relations of implications and entailment between propositions. Yet close examination of the discourse will show a number of inconsistencies, and a purely logical analysis of the propositional content will not account for many of the linguistic forms used. We will propose that the interpretation of this discourse requires the recognition of a set of **moral premises** that dominate the propositional content. More generally, we believe that an understanding of the development of language requires an understanding of principles of social order which control social behavior and govern what can be said in the public domain.

A great deal of public discourse is oriented towards persuasion, and moving an audience to action. The features of public discourse that we will examine here are typical of much that is heard in modern Western society. Facts and numbers are marshalled in a syntactic framework with logical and causal subordination. The overt appeal is to conviction through rational argument. Yet closer examination will show a number of puzzling inconsistencies and contradictions in the discourse. We will propose that these inconsistencies can be accounted for by the operation of a mechanism more fundamental to the discourse that we will call **moral predication**. Uses of linguistic forms that appear inconsistent or contradictory within a framework of logical propositions will be understood as the result of their subordination to such moral predications.

Behind the investigation of particular features of public discourse, there lies the general question of the relation of public to informal or private language. Because public discourse embodies many literary forms, and literature has been affected by prescriptive norms isolated from the main body of grammatical rules, it has been suggested that two different sets of grammatical rules are needed to account for public and private discourse. It will appear that public discourse is not fundamentally different from other forms of language in its orientation to moral premises and the subordination of logical argument to social and emotional expression. Certain relations are brought into sharper relief in public discourse, and the particular forms used are often different from that of every-day language, but the general mechanism is the same.

The principal texts that we will examine here are from public hearings on violence and vandalism in the schools of the United States, conducted by a Senate Committee headed by Senator Birch Bayh in 1975.

1. The use of quantifiers

In the informal uses of English, quantifiers are common currency. A good proportion of these are the universal quantifiers **all**, **every**, **each**, any and **ever**, along with their negative counterparts **no**, **none**, and **never**. These universal quantifiers are not always used with the strict interpretation that the logical calculus specifies. For the majority of the speakers studies so far, it is even more common to find them used with a loose interpretation in which 'all' and 'almost all' are not distinguished (Labov to appear).

Among the occurrences of these universal quantifiers in informal English, we find a number of **conventional** uses, where the strict or loose interpretation is automatic. These include "approximates", where the quantifier demands a loose interpretation:

(1) So I don't work or anything.

There are also conventional uses where the strict interpretation would be an obvious falsehood:

(2) He eats all the time and don't even get fat.

Besides these conventional uses, universal quantifiers are frequently used for subjective contexts where the truth or falsehood of a strict interpretation could not reasonably be established by observation:

(3) Her daddy got a goat one time, I never will forget this.

On the other hand, universal quantifiers are sometimes used in situations where the number of the set being quantified is easily determined, and where a strict interpretation is much more likely:

(4) He gets in on time for us all to go to wrestlin' on Friday night, and we go.

The loose interpretation of universal quantifiers is closely associated with their use as markers of intensification, comparable to adverbs like **really**, **very** and so **much**. A study of the distribution of other marks of intensity shows that they are heavily associated with the use of universal quantifiers with the loose interpretation or in the "unobservable" condition shown above. They are used much less often with universal quantifiers in denumerable and known contexts, where the strict interpretation is confirmable (Labov to appear). A typical pattern is shown by the speaker cited in (1-4), a working-class woman from Knoxville, Tennessee. Nineteen per cent of her sentences contained universal quantifiers. For a sample of 100 universal quantifiers, we have the following distribution:

		N	% intensified
conventional uses:	strict	5	20
	loose	28	46
unobservable:		39	72
observable:		28	18
		100	

A very different use of universal quantifiers appears in public discourse. As an example of public discourse, we will consider the first statement presented on April 16th by the first witness in the 1975 hearings, the President of the teachers' union in New York City. It is printed in the hearings as it was presented orally, and as a written statement.

The oral presentation uses most of the material of the written statement, with adaptations to spoken style, and elaborations of certain points. The substance of the statement can be summarized as follows:

a. The incidence of violent crime in the New York City schools has increased very much in recent years.

b. There are three causes for this:

(1) Victims of assault are reluctant to report the crimes and press charges.
(2) The current legal procedures protect the accused but make it difficult for the victims to present their case.
(3) The courts cannot act to remove dangerous students because there are no institutional facilities to place them in.

c. Congress should therefore take action to:

(1) Appropriate funds for alternative schools for children who cannot adjust to the regular schools.
(2) Appropriate more funds for early childhood education.
(3) Appropriate funds for more security personnel in the schools.
(4) Require schoolsystems to keep accurate records of crimes and vandalism.
(5) Provide additional funds for narcotics education, since drug addiction is one of the causes of violence.

d. We should not have negative publicity about the schools, reporting that they are failing or that children are unsafe in the schools.

e. Part of the responsibility for the present situation lies with those who have given ideological support for violence by viewing students as an oppressed minority.

In both style and content, this statement is characteristic

of the public discourse in the hearings as a whole. The following analysis is based on the oral presentation, with comparisons to the written statement specifically indicated.

There are a good many quantifiers in the 94 sentences of the statement: 65 altogether. Unlike the pattern of informal speech, universal quantifiers are a minority of the total: 15. Furthermore, the majority of these are in that part of the oral presentation that goes beyond the written text. Only two universal quantifiers appear in the written statement. The first of these is in the opening paragraph, a passage that will play an important role in our discussion:

(5) Many authorities on education have written books on the importance of producing an effective learning environment in the schools by introducing more effective methods of teaching. None of them, however, seem to understand the shocking fact that the learning environment in thousands upon thousands of schools is filled with violence and danger.

None of them refers to the set of "authorities" who have written on education. Though the whole set is not easily denumerable, the set of those who understand the issue is, and the quantifier must be taken in the strict sense here: if a single writer had seemed to understand the issue, it would have come to the speaker's attention.

The second universal quantifier in the written statement is found in a statement that there are "no special schools or facilities available" in New York City. This set of schools in New York is observable and denumerated, and the no is evidently to be taken in the strict sense.

The other universal quantifiers of the oral presentation occur in the speaker's elaboration of the written text: most of these are reconstructions of the thinking of students and teachers in the everyday life of the school:

(6) Or, if he says to the student who is carrying money, well maybe it was your fault, that is really a way of saying, "I'm a busy man. I've got an impossible job. I've got all these pressures on me. And, if I proceed with your case, it's ... going to take me away from all of my other duties and responsibilities here."

(7) ... the child each year has a greater and greater be-

lief that he will never learn these things.

(8) so they get skills before they develop negative feelings about themselves - feelings that they will never learn and that they are bound to fail.

One use of all occurs as the speaker characterizes the position of critics of the school system:

(9) ... viewing students as a kind of colonial minority who are oppressed by teachers and principals and school systems, who are subjected to all sorts of "torture", namely, to traditional learning.

Two universal quantifiers are used in a counter-factual:

(10) If with each and every instance of assault that has taken place the principal has to involve himself ...

In this public discourse, the universal quantifiers are severely restricted in their application to real-world situations. The speaker uses them primarily to evoke the discourse of everyday life, as approximants with loose interpretation or in imaginative, non-real contexts. In realworld contexts they are confined to the strict interpretation.

The fifty other quantifiers are distributed over four different types. Nineteen are numerals, defining periods of time or reporting statistics:

(11) For the first five months of school, 31 incidents involving handguns have occurred.

Seven of the quantifiers are cardinal or ordinal numbers, that enumerate points of the argument. Thus half of the quantifiers used are figures that are closely associated with factual evidence or logical precision. The remaining 24 are less precise terms that refer only generally to quantity. Eight of these give the impression of a large number without specifying it, as in the "thousands and thousands" of (6), or:

(12) I know that thousands of both teachers and students could come forward ...

(13) our public schools are doing an excellent job for the

overwhelming majority of our students.

The largest number of these residual quantifiers are partitives like "some", "many", "most", "a large proportion", which are used where everyday speech tends to use lessqualified statements (W. Labov to appear). The speaker frequently selects these partitives at the most polemic points of his argument:

(14) I submit to you that part of the responsibility for the increasing violence lies with some of these very books and writers themselves.

On the whole, the use of quantifiers gives an impression of precise, carefully reasoned argument, consistent with the logically connected substance of the statement. Quantifiers with loose interpretation are limited to the parts of the statement that evoke everyday situations, and the thought processes of others.

The conclusion is invited that this particular style of public discourse is based on logical argument and reasoning, and is governed by strict rules of evidence and inference. It seems clear that the president of the teachers' union, and the other witnesses at the hearings, are making strenuous efforts to present their arguments in such a form.

However, there are a number of inconsistencies in the use of quantifiers that might lead one to hesitate before drawing this conclusion. Let us examine the statistical evidence presented by the president of the teacher's union to support the initial point made in (5): that violent crime has entered the school house. He reports that there were 474 assaults in the schools in the first 5 months of 1974-75, and describes this as an increase of 95.6% over the same period a year earlier. He then introduces data from the New York City police department to show "comparable" increases for the city as a whole: arrests of youth under 16 increased 10% in the same period, and for those 16 to 20, 10%. In a scientific paper, one might expect the author to make some inference from the fact that the increase of arrests in the schools is nine times as great as the general increase in arrests of youth. A nine times greater incidence of arrests within the schools makes it seem likely that crime within the school was being prosecuted actively. However, this inference would not be consistent with the first "major reason" that the speaker gives for the increase in crime:

(15) First, the victims of assaults - both teachers and students - are reluctant to report them and to press charges because of the all-too-prevalent stratagem of shifting blame from the assailant to the victim himself.

He then lists a number of the causes that would lead victims not to prosecute their attackers. For example:

(16) The pupil-victim who has been mugged and had several dollars taken from him may be accused of having invited the attack by carrying too much money with him.

The chairman breaks in with an expression of amazement and moral indignation:

(17) Pardon me for interrupting, but are we so out of touch with reality that we regard a child's carrying too much money, as the major reason he or she is assaulted?

In (16), the speaker has used the auxiliary "may" in framing his statement. Because he is dealing with past events, and has reported an unexpected kind of event, he invites the inference that such an event has occurred at least once. His response to the chairman is consistent with this use of the auxiliary: "These are reasons that are given". He cannot be faulted for a failure to support the statements he has made with evidence. From such evidence he draws the general conclusion:

(18) the assailants soon learn that they can continue in their actions with virtual impunity because the innocent victims, instead of receiving official support, are themselves denounced when they ask for help.

This conclusion supports three of the proposals for congressional action made by the teachers' union. They propose that students rights to due process be curtailed, that students classified as dangerous be removed to special schools, and that more police be placed in the schools. The fact that the number of arrests within the schools has almost doubled in the past year does not support these proposals, and if the speaker had called attention to this aspect of the data, he would not have been supporting his own position.

It is commonly recognized that figures do not speak for themselves, and require evaluation to be placed within the framework of a logical or scientific argument. A figure of 25% can be characterized as "as much as 25%", or "only 25%", or "no more than a quarter", at the option of the speaker, without doing violence to the rules of evidence or thecanons of logic. The larger framework of the discourse can also provide an interpretation of numbers, without such adverbial modification.

The influence of the larger discourse on the interpretation numbers is illustrated in the statement of the Chancellor of the New York City Board of Education in the 1975 hearings.

(19) The big city school is an area in which many of the crushing social problems of the city itself intrude, and are acted out not only by the students themselves, but more often by forces that invade the schools, generating problems that have their genesis in the surrounding community.

(19) sets up an opposition of "students" to "forces" from outside the school. The immediate sequel shows that these forces are other people who enter the school for no good purpose.

(20) Of the 4,775 incidents, for example, reported in 1973-74 - the 1st complete school year - of the 4,775, 1,020 were by intruders who gained entry into the school building by a variety of means.

The same information might of course have been presented in formats that would suggest different interpretations of the significance of the same facts:

(20') Of the 4,775 incidents, only 1020 were by intruders who had to gain entry into the school building.

(20'') Of the 4,775 incidents ... 3,755 were by students within the school system, who did not have to use any special means to enter the building.

The actual form of (20) is consistent with the general framework provided by (19). (20) places the noun phrase "intruders ..." in a marked position where new and focussed information is usually found: an agent contained in a by phrase This reinforces the interpretation invited by (19) that the number of attacks committed by these outside agents is large compared to our previous expectations.

The chairman of the committee had a special interest in the proportion of incidents involving outsiders. He intervened to ask "That is about 25%? ... is that a consistent percentage ... When we say 25% intruders, are those intruders totally removed from the system?"

It is interesting to note that the chairman did not call attention to the fact that the figures of (20) contradict the Chancellor's general statement (19): incidents involving outsiders occur **less often** than those involving students in the school, not **more often**. The figures might well have been used to argue against appropriating federal money for police to keep people out of the schools, since so many incidents are caused by students in the schools. The ambiguity of the situation is shown by the multiple hedges in the Chancellor's final response to the chairman:

(21) We need them (school guards) very largely now to protect in part at least the pupils as well as the teachers against outsiders as well as of course against fellow students.

The public discourse examined here shows many features of logical discourse. Universal quantifiers are used with a strict interpretation; statements about groups are carefully qualified with partitive quantifiers; modal auxiliaries are used in a form consistent with the evidence; and numbers are used to indicate precise dates, times and amounts. At the same time, there are puzzling inconsistencies in this discourse that will be elucidated by the inquiries to follow.

2. Non-restrictive attributives.

One of the characteristic features of informal speech and conversation is that the great majority of sentences contain single logical propositions, which are directly asserted.

Narratives of personal experience preserve this feature in its most straightforward form: narrative syntax typically has simple subjects, auxiliaries with preterit or historical present, active verbs and right-branching verbal complements (Labov 1972: Ch. 9). Some of the most complex syntax occurs in the orientation of a highly skilled narrative, when detailed characterizations of the persons and the situation are supplied; these are typically given as separate predications. The following is the beginning of a narrative by Charles Triplett, an 72-year-old man born in Iowa who had worked much of his life in carnivals. He describes the three main characters in the following way:

(22) a. Well, in the business I was associated at that time - -
b. the Doc was an old man.
c. He had killed one man
d. or done time.
e. But he had a young wife,
f. and in those days I dressed well.
g. And seemingly, she was trying to make me.
h. I never noticed it.
i. Fact is, I didn't like her very well, because she had -
she was a nice-looking girl
until you saw her feet.
j. She had big feet.
k. Jesus, God, she had big feet!

Each characteristic of each person is introduced in predicate position. The complements contain attributive adjectives, which are in all cases restrictive: **old man, young wife, big feet.**

At the other extreme, the literary language of fiction writers makes free use of non-restrictive modifiers: relative clauses, appositives, and attributive adjectives. From the first chapter of a Conrad novel, a central character is introduced with many non-restrictive modifiers; non-restrictive attributive adjectives are bold-faced.

(23) Old Singleton, the oldest able seaman in the ship, set apart on the deck right under the lamps, stripped to the waist, tattooed like a cannibal chief all over his **powerful** chest and **enormous** biceps. Between the blue

and red patterns his **white** skin gleamed like satin; his **bare** back was propped against the heel of the bowsprit, and he held a book at arm's length before his **big, sunburnt** face.

Beginning writers also select non-restrictive attributives as legitimate literary tools to enhance their compositions, and use them freely to describe situations and characters. A talented student in a Michigan composition workshop began "Country Road PA" in this way:

(24) Irene was glad she had a Volkswagon. The **air-cooled** engine took the **August** heat and humidity well. As the **dark green** bus rolled down the **narrow** highway, Irene smiled to herself. The **thickly populated** pines adorning the mountain on either side of the road blocked out the **sizzling** sun; their shadows cooling the air.

Personal narrative and literary narration mark the two extremes of the use of non-restrictive modifiers. Most personal narrative is simpler than the example of (22), and identifies persons and objects with a single category device: **my mother, the doctor, the car,** just as we do in every-day conversation. The narrative, when it is effective, places the listener at the scene where he sees and reacts to the situation as the participants do. The literary devices illustrated above address readers as people who were not present, and know nothing of the scene: the non-restrictive modifiers fill in the details, much like a scene-painter does on the backdrop of the stage.

The public discourses that we are considering here are formal, but they are not literary in the sense illustrated above. Non-restrictive modifiers do appear, but far less often than in literary compositions. The modifiers that do occur are different from the literary types shown in (23) and (24). In the initial sentences of the hearing, cited above:

(5) ... None of them, however, seem to understand the **shocking** fact that the learning evironment in thousands upon thousands of schools is filled with violence and danger.

The adjective **shocking** does not inform the listeners of a characteristic of the head noun that they might not know about, as in **sunburnt face.** It provides no new information: instead, it evaluates the situation in a way that is already familiar to the listeners (and readers of the written statement). **Shocking** is not only an emotional or personal evaluation, but a social one. 'Shock' here refers to a feeling of moral indignation that the state of affairs should be so contrary to what one would expect in a good society.

The adjective **shocking** is one of a sizeable set of adjectives derived in a regular way from a corresponding set of transitive verbs. These verbs designate a subjective impression created on animate beings by an animate or inanimate object, or a state of affairs. We may refer to them as 'impression' verbs: **thrill, alarm, surprise, fascinate, frighten, terrify, interest, intrigue, disgust, revolt, touch,** and many others. Adjectives are formed from the verbs by the addition of the active participial suffix, **-ing.** These adjectives may be used freely in either predicate position or attributive position:

(25) a. The fact is certainly shocking.
b. A shocking fact was discovered.
c. The shocking fact is that ...

When such adjectives are used as predicates, they are of course asserted of the subject, and so restrict it. In attributive position, they may be restrictive, as in (25a), or non-restrictive, as in (25b), depending on the definiteness of the noun phrase and the larger context. As non-restrictive modifiers, their application to the noun they modify is presupposed, and not asserted.

The derivation of impression adjectives from verbs is regular but not entirely productive. For example, the verb **scare** is semantically parallel to **frighten** and **terrify,** but the adjective formed is **scary,** not ***scaring.** The verb attract is a legitimate member of this semantic class, but it forms the adjective **attractive,** not ***attracting.** No matter how the adjective is formed, the semantic interpretation of the effect involves some person or persons who are affected. The adjective cannot formally take an object complement. Instead, the object is expressed optionally by a prepositional phrase. This complement is appended directly to the predicate adjective. If it is added to a restrictive attributive modifier, the entire adjective phrase must be placed after the noun. In pre-nominal attributive position such a prepositional phrase is not normally found or easily accommodated. It has to be inserted, parenthetically, after the modified noun.

(26) a. The fact was certainly shocking to any reasonable person.
b. A fact shocking to any reasonable person was discovered.
c. The shocking fact - to any reasonable person - is that ...

These differences in the ways that object complements can be added reflect differences in the normal semantic interpretation of asserted predicate adjectives and presupposed non-restrictive adjectives. If no object is indicated it is understood that the impression registered is that of the speaker.

(27) a. That fact is shocking.
b. That fact is shocking to me.

If no particular stress is put on **me**, there is no clear semantic difference between (27a) and (27b), and the complement may be considered redundant. The situation is different with non-restrictive prenominal adjectives. The insertion of a to phrase is understood as explicitly controverting the interpretation that others are so affected.

(28) The shocking fact - to me - is that ...

One reason for this difference is that some stress must fall on the interjected prepositional phrase, but the fact that the phrase must be inserted as a parenthesis indicates in another way that the semantic interpretation of the presupposed adjective is different from that of the asserted predicate adjective.

Shocking is a prototypical evaluation in these hearings. Senator Bayh introduces each day of hearing with a statement which includes the phrase, "Shocking as these facts may be". We find other adjectives derived from impression verbs: "staggering amount" and "devastating effect". But we observe a number of other types of non-restrictive adjectives: **grim story, tragic circumstances, serious increase, outright defiance, eloquent testimony, utter contempt, lethargic**

courts. They all share with the impression verb derivatives a common semantic character: they provide a social evaluation of the events reported or testimony given in ways that are closely related to the theme of the hearing. One way of looking at these non-restrictive modifiers is to see them as intensifying the effect of the propositions on the listener, in ways that are parallel to the literary examples given above. But we believe that the non-restrictive attributives of public discourse are more than peripheral decoration or support for the propositional content. We regard them as markers of the fundamental premises of the discourse, which motivate the organization of discourse and account for much of its structure. Further, we believe that an understanding of these premises or underlying propositions is needed to account for the apparent inconsistencies and departure from strict logical form noted in the first section.

The particular discourse we are studying here concerns a social problem of great generality: violence and vandalism. It might be said that there is no more general problem, since the moral premises involved here are the fundamental social responses to the problem of social order. That problem, as first formulated by Hobbes, can be put simply as: how is social control possible? that is, how can an organization of human beings be created that will control the brute self-interest of individuals in their competition for scarce resources? One essential element of social control, in the societies that we know, is a set of **moral premises** which include the following:

I. In a good society, people ought to be protected from violence and danger to life or health.

II. In a good society, property ought to be protected from destruction or appropriation by others.

The hearings are concerned with establishing whether or not these fundamental principles have been violated and what action, if any, should be taken if this is the case. The determination involves features of human behavior that are specific to social and moral issues. Moral premises contain predicates of obligation and evaluation - **good** and **ought** - which call for an all-or-none mode of response (T. Labov 1980). Responses to violations of these premises are not cognitive responses based on rational calculation, but social and emotional responses such as **moral indignation.**

In this case, the response of the Congress may be no action at all even if violations of social order are established. Means to maintain social order and correct violations already exist: the disciplinary resources of the schools, of the local police, and the state authorities. Congress is empowered to act only when these methods of control are clearly proved to be ineffective. The witnesses who advocate Congressional intervention must therefore do more than show that violations of social order exist. They must show that a **crisis** exists: that the extent of these violations threatens the fundamental social order, a problem so serious that every informed and responsible person recognizes it. As in every act of social persuasion, this is accomplished by a mechanism of **moral predication**.

Moral predication is the process which relates the discourse to the set of moral premises which provide the broadest level of interpretation and motivation for the speech acts being performed. These moral premises are rarely asserted. Normally, as in the hearings, the moral premises are of such generality that they are always available and potentially relevant (T. Labov 1980). In the hearings on violence and vandalism in the schools, principles I and II are available in this way. Moral predication makes this potential relevance overt. The predication has three phases:

a) **Orientation**. The speaker indicates the polarity of the situation by a linguistic device that shows whether what **ought to be**, is so or is not so.

b) **Evaluation**. The speaker indicates the relative weight of the situation in terms of the need for action: for conditions that violate moral premises, how great the violation is; and for actions that restore conformity to moral premises, how difficult the achievement was.

c) **Alignment**. The speaker indicates the set of people who endorse the orientation and evaluation presented; this is the set of people that the speaker is (T. Labov 1983).

A moral predication does not usually involve an overt statement of orientation, evaluation and alignment, though this is possible. Most often the predication is signalled by a linguistic form that implies rather than asserts the orientation, and presupposes the evaluation. The act of presupposition then establishes the alignment.

The prototypical device of this type is the adjective derived from impression verbs; in the hearings, the phrase **shocking fact** operates in this way. **Shocking** implies the orientation that what is, ought not to be. The Webster's New International (2nd ed.) definition of this term is:

> pres. ptcp. & verbal noun of shock: hence, adj. causing to shake or tremble, as by a blow; esp., causing to recoil with horror or disgust; extremely offensive; also bad; abominable.

Shocking evaluates the situation described as far removed from any acceptable situation, and within the framework of the hearings designates the state of crisis that is the prerequisite for congressional action. Further, its use as a presupposition permits the broadest possible alignment. In presupposing that a fact is shocking, the speaker can be heard as speaking for the great majority of people.

The facts and figures introduced by witnesses are to be understood within this framework. The statistics of rates and percentages of increase provided by the speaker are not compared and interrelated in the manner of a scientific argument. They are presented as demonstrations of a fact already known to the speaker and by presupposition to a much wider audience. It is thus possible for the speaker to disregard interrelations between these figures and the theories put forward to explain the situation. Anyone who would disagree with the need for the actions proposed by the teachers' union is open to being shown as tolerating or approving the gross violation of the moral premises I and II that are demonstrated by these facts.

In the final part of the statement of the president of the teachers' union, he warns against negative publicity about the schools, saying:

(29) ... overall, in fact, our public schools are doing an excellent job for the overwhelming majority of our students.

and concludes:

(30) ... we should not create the impression that parents should not send their children to schools because they are unlikely to come home some day in one piece, because that is just not true.

Here moral predication takes the form of overt assertion. (29) establishes a positive orientation to the moral premises: teachers and administrators should be praised for accomplishing what ought to be done in the schools. There is the further implication that they should not be blamed for the problem outlined earlier, and this fits in with preceding statements that assign "part of the responsibility" to writers who produce negative material about the schools and "glorify lawlessness and disorder in the name of some sort of revolutionary gains". (30) follows with the overt evaluation that the present situation is not dangerous enough for parents to worry about. Yet in his presentation of the basic problem, the head of the teachers' union concluded:

(31) While major cities and school systems, under pressure from teachers and parents, have taken steps to protect both school employees and students, their efforts on the whole have not been effective.

The inconsistency of (30) and (31) can be understood in the light of the different moral predications they subserve. (31) is subordinated to the moral predication that all reasonable persons recognize that the violations of personal safety in the schools have reached an unacceptable level. (30) is subordinated to a different predication, and the arguments for it are viewed from a different aspect. It is not inevitable that the statements used to support the two different moral predications should be inconsistent, but there are no guarantees that they will not be.
In the first section, we considered inconsistencies in the presentation of the Chancellor of the New York City schools to the congressional hearings. His statement also provides examples of moral predications through the use of non-restrictive attributives.

(31) The big city school is an arena in which many of the **crushing** social problems of the city itself intrude ...

The Chancellor refers to the "catalogue of criminal activities that impact on the school" and characterizes them as

(32) ... **grim** statistics of a social pathology that has characterized city living increasingly in the last decade.

The moral predication here orients listeners to violations of social order, and evaluates the scale of these violations as surpassing any capacity of the schools to deal with them. The fact that 25% of the crimes are committed by outsiders is then used to argue for more police to keep people out of the schools. As noted above, it might have been argued that since 75% of the crimes are committed by students in the schools, the major problem does not come from outside. But someone who pointed out the inconsistency in the Chancellor's statement would be open to the charge of not taking seriously the 1,020 crimes committed by outsiders. In the light of the moral predications that govern the discourse, such a search for logical consistency might itself be characterized as a violation of moral principles.

3. Overview

We conclude that the language in these examples of public discourse is not different in its fundamental organization from discourse used in less formal settings. There are many differences from informal speech in the surface forms, in the lexicon, and possibly in grammatical rules. We have noted the restriction of the use of the universal quantifiers to strict interpretation, the free use of non-restrictive attributives, and the frequent use of numbers and percentages. We also observe logical inconsistencies that indicate that the use of these quantifiers is not comparable to their use in the calculations of business or engineering. We have proposed that public discourse is regulated at the broadest level by moral predications, in this case related to the fundamental principles of social order.

The arguments and quantifications of the discourse are best understood as subordinate to the moral predications. These predications are accepted by speakers at the outset of their discourse, and attributed to the widest possible speech community. Moral predications are advanced as a basis for community action, and opposition to the arguments of the discourse can be portrayed as oppositions to the moral predictions endorsed by the community as a whole.

PUZZLED OR SHOCKED? THE RHETORICS OF PRECISION IN PUBLIC AND SCIENTIFIC DISCOURSE.
COMMENTS ON W. AND T. LABOV

Dorothea Franck

While I agree with most of what the authors assert, I do not agree with several of their implicit premises, i.e. with what I think the authors must presuppose. In particular I agree with the main conclusion of W. and T. Labov's paper:

(1) ... that public discourse is not fundamentally different from other forms of language in its orientation to moral premises and the subordination of logical argument to social and emotional expression.

Since the paper deserves a more thorough discussion than flat agreement I should like to apply a reflexive analysis to it: i.e. to examine it in a similar way as the paper itself examines its object of study: a particular public discourse (henceforth the former is called meta-text and the latter object-text; MT and OT). I will focus particularly, just as MT does with respect to OT, on some general premises underlying the argumentation and a very general rhetorical device or principle which both MT and OT have in common.
Let me start with a general remark or rather an attempt to categorize the linguistic activity and orientation of the paper. It marks a transition in (socio-)linguistic theory from linguistic analysis in the narrower sense to rhetorical analysis:

(2) A great deal of public discourse is oriented toward persuasion and moving an audience to action.

With this statement the core of the situation is defined, which is the classical domain of rhetorics. To my amazement, the notion of rhetorics is not mentioned once throughout the paper. This would not be worth mentioning were it only a terminological matter. That it is more, I should like to make plausible with the ensuing notes.

Let me first quote the sentence on which I want to focus attention. Like the preceding sentences they give the upshot of the analysis in a nutshell. They immediately follow the sentence in (2).

(3) The features of public discourse that we will examine here are typical of much that is heard in modern Western society. Facts and numbers are marshalled in a syntactic framework with logical and causal subordination.

(4) The overt appeal is to conviction through rational argument.

(5) Yet closer examination will show a number of puzzling inconsistencies and contradictions in the discourse.

And later in the article they conclude:

(7) We have noted the restrictions of the use of universal quantifiers to strict interpretation, the free use of non-restrictive attributives, and the frequent use of numbers and percentages. We also observe logical inconsistencies that indicate that the use of these quantifiers is not comparable to their use in the calculations of business or engineering.

(8) We have proposed that public discourse is regulated at the broadest level by moral predications, in this case related to the fundamental principles of social order.

What makes these assertions "tellable"? In other words, which are the silent assumptions which account for the fact that they appear as non-trivial assertions in general and as relevant statements at the present stage of sociolinguistic discussion?

According to the authors the use of quantifiers, numbers and facts in OT makes us expect 'rational argumentation'. "Us" referring both to the adressees of the discourse and to us, the analyzers. "Rational" is understood -throughout the article- in an unnecessarily (as I will argue) narrow sense of logical calculation "as used in e.g. engineering and business". On closer inspection the discourse in question does not fulfil these expectations: the authors express their puzzlement about some inconsistencies and contradictions which depart from strict logical form.

How rational is it to expect the mentioned sort of rationality in a public discourse like the public hearing in question? Are we fooled by (dubious? manipulative?) rhetorical devices of the speakers and/or by our own expectations about what 'rational' discourse (including our own) is supposed to look like?

The use of 'puzzling' in MT is somewhat comparable to the use of "shocking" in OT. "Puzzling" presupposes the silent assumption that the academic community to which the paper is addressed, subscribes to a particular model of rational discourse which makes the signalled "inconsistencies" unexpected, if not in some sense "illegal".

From a rhetorical point of view, however, they are all but puzzling in a public discourse of the given sort (and countless others). From this perspective one can also see further parallels between MT and OT. Both texts make use of facts and numbers in a way that is "typical of much that is heard in modern Western society". I should like to call this device (or rather: style of argumentation) 'rhetorics of precision': Facts and numbers are given abundantly (e.g. about the use of quantifiers and non-restrictive adjectives in different discourse genres), but the most important conclusions are not reached by strict logical inference from these data but through a 'qualitative jump', no matter how plausible the inference, once stated, seems. 'Plausibility' is a rhetorical, not a logical category.

Now I should like to make it clear that from my perspective this is not a piece of criticism - on the contrary: it accounts for the fact that the given statement is not trivial. (If critical questions are to be asked: then here is one: are the numbers/the given details necessary?)

The rhetorics of precision is an extremely frequent device in academic/scientific and political discourse: The use of numbers c.q. facts of a quantifiable sort creates a climate of precision and expectations of impartial exactitude from which a high degree of credibility derives. This effect operates to some extent independently of the actual stringency of the argumentation, and imparts itself to other parts of the same discourse which are not strictly related to the "exact" parts.

Now let us take a quick look at the two major cases of "puzzling contradictions and inconsistensies". How contradictory and inconsistent are they in fact? If we look at the contradiction between the examples (19) and (20) of the paper

(19) The big city school is an area in which many of the crushing social problems of the city intrude, and are acted out not only by the students themselves, but more often by forces that invade the schools, generating problems that have their genesis in the surrounding community.

(20) Of the 4,775 incidents, for example, reported in 1973-74 - the first complete schools year - of the 4,775, 1,020 were by intruders who gained entry into the school building by a variety of means.

the question arises: is it possible to give a reading of the two sentences without ensuing contradiction? I think it is. If we try to be cooperative recipients (in the sense of the Gricean Cooperation Principles), and give (19) a benevolent interpretation, taking into account its position as precedent to (20) and, moreover the previous context and general setting of the speech, we could "dissolve" the contradictions by the assumption that (19) is meant as a more general statement about the genesis of the specific problems inside the school from wider social problems outside the school. Then the "**forces that invade**", said after "**the crushing social problems itself intrude**", do not have to be understood as coextensive with the "**1,020 intruders**" from sentence (20), representing "only" 25% of the cases. If we give the speaker a good portion of the Gricean goodwill-principle: why should we assume that a speaker would construct blatant contradictions between two consecutive sentences? The "benevolent" reading is exploiting the vagueness of the formulation; the result being not a contradiction but an eloquent rhetorical arrangement of facts which interprets and evaluates these facts in a partial but logically not impossible way. For the calculation of this implicature (namely that the "forces" in (19) have a more general meaning, such that they would affect both delinquent students and 'intruders') we do not strictly need to recur to the moral principles laid out by the authors. But that does not mean that I should like to deny the relevance of these principles. Their function is not primarily to fill, in some way, the logical gaps of reasoning. Rather, they function as a motive for the displayed or implied evaluation of the facts and justify the choice of the recommended actions.

Since the moral predication and the Gricean Cooperation Principle play a comparable role (or could even be combined) in reconstructing and repairing seemingly deficient chains of reasoning, my interpretation could be seen as a paraphrase of W. and T. Labov's analysis. The difference of approach might get clearer in the next case: the inconsistency ascribed to (29), (30) and (31). I would like to argue that the 'inconsistencies' are not (or not in the first place) inconsistencies on the level of discourse but rather represent the "ordinary" case where a speaker tries to discern between wanted and unwanted practical consequences of a presentation of the situation. The given discourse is designed to move the audience to action. The formulations are representative of the problem-solving nature of discourse: competing preferences, risks and goods have to be weighted and balanced continuously. In the given case the interests of students and teachers are deeply interdependent but not identical. The leader of the teachers' union has to care about both but in case of conflict cannot be expected to be impartial. Here he manages to safeguard the position of the teachers by introducing certain distinctions which are not obvious but logically not impossible: e.g. between the moment where the teachers and politicians have to worry about the safety of the students and the moment where parents should start to worry to a point as to keeping their children at home. He states that it is not yet unlikely that the children "come home in one piece". Implicit in this presenttation of course is a comparison of advantages and disadvantages (risks) for the children of going to school, where the advantages are assumed to prevail.

Similarly he draws a line between effort and result when speaking about the teachers and employees' attempts to protect the students. They have tried but without sufficient result: this is exactly why help from outside is called in. Here the speaker is in fact making a tightrope walk, balancing the fear of being blamed for failure with the desire to describe the situation in the schools as so critical that the adressees cannot refuse to take measures within the scope of their competences.

This is a typical situation for human actors, inside and outside of discourse. The question for us analyzers is: where do we locate the contradictions? Can speakers be blamed for inconsistency when e.g. they try to fulfil the delicate task of criticizing somebody's actions without hurting the person? Or for prescribing or taking a medicine in spite of expectable negative side-effects? When do we consider the speaker as creating the contradictions, and when do we see the contradictions as given conditions, i.e. as a task and challenge for the speaker. When we think that the latter is the case, recurring to moral principles is indeed to be expected. But for deeper reasons than those indicated by T. and W. Labov.

In their analysis the given moral principles are considered only on the discourse level: in their function to fill the gap between a logical-rational model of discourse and the observed deviations from it. But how this is to be achieved is not quite clear. While there is no doubt that the speakers of the discourse under investigation certainly appeal to shared moral principles, there is no explanation offered as to how it is possible (linguistically/rhetorically), that a moral appeal all by itself would make up for (or overrule) the indicated logical inconsistencies. The 'internal' analysis of the "mechanism of moral predication" does not account for the way it manages to remedy the signalled inconsistencies. On the other hand it seems clear that even without these cases the speaker could be understood as appealing to these same moral principles.
By giving the device of moral predication the function to account for the departure from logical form, they construct a strict opposition between **moral** and **reason**, which - at least in this form - is neither desirable nor necessary.

Moral principles, although not derivable rational principles themselves (but from values), are not opposed to rational action or speech but rather a necessary foundation of it. But I am using 'rational' here in a wider sense than T. and W. Labov do. I call 'rational' any action (discourse) through which we pursue our aims, within the real or assumed limitations of our resources, in an expectably efficient way. Only in a very limited range of situations, 'rational' in this sense coincides with 'logical', viz. rational discourse with explicitly logically connected statements. It can be perfectly rational of speakers in certain contexts, to produce a non-logical or even 'irrational' discourse. This means that we should not only distinguish between 'logical' and 'rational', but also the levels on which we want to use predicates like 'rational': the discourse, the speaker, the context.

In rational action we need moral principles as guidelines which allow us to choose priorities for competing aims and interests and to rank values and relevances whenever they do not coincide. Of course this also pertains to our scientific activities. Since the (natural language) discourses we investigate will never be totally explicit and unambiguous, our analysis always relies on interpretation with a considerable speculative and subjective side to it. To a large extent our analysis will always reflect our own attitudes and expectations towards the text and/or the speaker. We can choose, for example, among degrees of benevolence of interpretation: do we prefer an 'exegetic' or a 'critical' reading? In the first (extreme) case, the speaker (text) is assumed to be always right (ratinal, meaningful, truthful...); only our interpretation could be insufficient. In the second extreme, we are out to catch our speakers/writers at any error or mistake, at attempts to mislead or manipulate the recipient or, at least at signs of in-sufficient or distorted competence.

Both procedures are of course equally susceptible to the interpreter's subjectivity. The choice of a particular inter-pretive attitude is, nevertheless, ultimately a moral choice.Of course neither of them is in itself morally superior or inferior, but the choice should be conscious, such that the dangers of arbitrariness and unreflected (hidden) subjectivity can be met each time in the appropri-ate way. In the first case the analyzer will stick as close-ly as possible to the perspective of the speakers and has to adopt for the moment all the tacit assumptions which allow him to reconstruct the discourse as meaningful and even in a sense as optimal under the given circumstances. In the second case, we have to make our own set of premises parti-cularly explicit and clear, in order to account for the dif-ferences in perspective between the speaker's and our own point of view. Naturally we can at most aproximate these methodological requirements.

In the given article any overt evaluation of the analyzed discourse is carefully avoided; this seems to point to the first perspective. But then the interpretation lacks the necessary cooperativeness of this perspective when it assigns 'contra-diction' and 'inconsistency' labels, derived from different norms than the speakers might adhere to. Here the authors seem to dissociate themselves from the speaker's point of view. This ambivalence, i.e. the abstinence from explicit critical evaluation of the rhetorical "tricks" in OT, combined with an - ever so slight - implicit bias towards certain discourse ideals from which OT deviates, may account for my vague feeling of confusion and of somehow having missed the point, while the explicit point of the paper seemed sufficiently clear.

But now notice the ironical parallel again, this time between my own discourse and MT. I could be blamed again for practically everything I noted critically about the article I discuss. Only by not giving an optimally cooperative interpretation, by not sharing some of the background assumptions and by coining a terminology that fits my own purpose and reflects my expectations and ideals concerning discourse, was I able to contrast my view with theirs. Also the use of 'rhetorics of precision' could be seen in the fact that I give a somewhat detailed analysis of two fragments, creating the impression of a thorough and careful reading from which my criticism would be derived, while in fact the differences of opinion cannot be derived from the different analysis of the examples. It is rather the other way round. The examples are illustration rather than proof. The difference in analysis stems from a more general difference in our philosophical and methodological outlook on discourse, including the fact, that I am more oriented towards rhetorics than grammar, phenomenological than 'mainstream' sociology, and last but not least, that I am developing a different model of discourse than the one on which the present analysis is based, a fact which of course compels me to look for flaws in every different approach.

Back to square one or to a non-committal relativism? I think not. Our discourse does not have to be logical in order to make sense, and our mutual understanding does not have to be perfect in order to further our insight into both our own position and the position of the other person and into our object of study: discourse.

10

Conversational analysis of political interviews

A diachronic survey

J. Schwitalla

1. Introduction and survey of research

The invitation to this meeting states: "The central issue of the workshop is: how can theories of language use be used for practical applications?" I interpret this sentence in a specific way by asking whether linguistic theories and definitions might have a beneficial or clarifying - in short, a useful - function in certain areas of language use. But it becomes apparent at once that the words "useful" and "to be used for" are endowed with several meanings, depending on the question: In what respect and, in particular, for which group of persons and interests are scientific findings "useful"?

Everyday life seldom calls upon us to encounter the situation of interviewing a politician, let alone of being exposed to an interview in the same way as a politician. Compare this with the more familiar interaction between doctor and patient. From this I conclude that our task of clarification (assuming that we were to give it practical effect) should primarily be for the benefit of passive listeners, so that they can see through the mechanisms which so often characterize political interviews.

As a second line of approach, the very fact that in interviews sequences of action and reaction may be shown to run according to fixed patterns should help journalists to check on their techniques in presenting questions and also on their subsequent linguistic treatment. How often do we gain the impression that politicians tend to evade certain types of questions, give a good account of themselves or portray the world in such a way that their own actions and decisions appear plausible. It is here that a journalist can profit by taking a more calculated attitude toward his practical linguistic action.

With these questions in mind I should like to deal briefly

with a few publications which have appeared in West Germany within the last few years. I should like to compare these investigations with the question: Which objectives did the authors of these surveys have in mind in the course of their research?

There is first the work of Franz Josef Berens (1975) "Analyse des Sprachverhaltens im Redekonstellationstyp 'Interview'". This term "Redekonstellationstyp" - "type of constellation of verbal interaction" - gives the clearest indication of the scientific aim of this study. The concept that spoken language is realised in different ways according to the type of text was at that time being examined in a variety of separate surveys. Berens compared the type of text "interview" with those of "narratives" and "conversations". In using the term "interview" he has in mind particularly the political television or radio interview. He finds differences in the allocation of the length of each speaker's contribution as well as in the way the subjects are dealt with (argument predominates over narrative or association). Moreover he observes the asymmetric distribution of dialogue which is so typical of interviews: The interviewer has the prerogative of putting questions, he starts and concludes the interview and introduces the topics to be discussed.

I presented my own findings on dialogue control in interviews a few years later than Berens did, namely in 1979. At that time various research groups in West Germany began their projects on dialogue research. In my work, I used interviews as a readily available source for demonstrating fundamental categories of dialogue activities, for instance, turn-taking, back-channel behaviour, initiating and responding acts, responsiveness, strategies continuing through several turns and methods of argument.

The study of these categories, conducted on types of interview with politicians, experts and stars, was then examined within the tradition of text analysis. The object was to bring to light differences between these types of texts.

Some special phenomena of communication for political interviews and with them hints to the listener are to be found in some passages where I deal with the type of question expecting agreement, or with the way in which politicians evade questions or, again, with the interviewer's persistence in dwelling upon a question and the politician's steadfastness in keeping to an answer already given so as to create a situation of talking at cross-purposes.

Heinz-Günter Hang, who wrote about "Signals for Questions in Spoken Language", also used interviews in evaluating frequently-used questions and phraseology. He hardly deals at all with the interactive qualities of interviews.

In 1977 a small volume entitled "Textform Interview" by Ecker, Landwehr, Settekorn and Walther was published. The authors are very sceptical vis-a-vis the journalistic genre "interview". They refer to the written text type "Spiegel-Gespräch" and contend that a combination of people and political circumstances tempts producers and audiences alike to adopt either an attitude of veneration or identification or else one of aggression. From these opposing interests they determine those strategies of the interviewer which they call strategies of affirmation or confrontation. Although it is not uncommon in radio and television interviews for the interviewer to display neither admiration nor aggression with regard to the politician, the question in the mind of a potential listener is: will the interviewer support or criticize the politician? Which may be useful in assessing important communicative aims of interviews.

In other respects, the authors also give clarifying indications concerning "tricks", strategies and techniques of those interviewing and those being interviewed; for instance, "answers" of politicians which are no answers, vague phraseology, change of subject, propagation of one's own policy - and, as regards the interviewer, patent and latent questions, trap questions, persistent questions, etc.

The first analyst of interviews in West Germany to stress the importance of institutional conditions for political interviews and the first to include them in his surveys was Rolf-Rüdiger Hoffmann with his thesis "Politische Fernsehinterviews" - political television interviews (1983).

Hoffmann points to the big difference between short interviews, consisting of few changes in speaker, and the long interviews found in "magazine" broadcasts. With the help of extensive material he establishes that, in putting questions, journalists are more often concerned to discover opinions and facts than with the formulation of critical and problematic questions. These critical questions asked by the interviewers are more frequently to be found in the larger scale "magazine" programmes of the broadcasting companies than, for instance, in the small interviews inserted into news broadcasts.

Hoffmann reaches various other interesting conclusions, of which only a few need to be mentioned here. In the political interviews, "leading politicians" from the parties and the executive branch of government tend to dominate. Topics concern "top-level" politics: foreign, domestic and economic policy. The interviewers work their way through a catalogue of questions, rarely persisting when their questions have been answered evasively, playing down reproaches and differences of opinion by, for example, failing to admit that they hold a different point of view, but hiding instead behind the criticism of other politicians or observers.

Hoffmann's results correspond to the intuitive perception of an alert though not scientifically-minded observer of interviews about political issues on television. (One might, however, have wished for more accuracy in the use of terms, such as "inferred problems" and "refusal" which are too broad and vague. Hoffmann does not create his own theory about linquistic behaviour which he checks against interviews. He employs sundry theoretical applications from conversational analysis to argument research with eclectic skill. This, however, means that his survey has the advantage of realistic density).

Yet, even after Hoffmann's survey, nobody in West Germany has so far attempted to examine how interviews originate, what fears and apprehensions journalists and politicians experience, what secondary aims they pursue and what effects they have on the public. The answers to all these questions would explain a lot about the social foundation and functions of interviews, and they would explain all this from different social and political positions and groupings.

We do have some surveys and results of conversations between researchers and journalists, but these do not address themselves to the problems mentioned above. In 1976, the sociologist Jürgen Friedrichs presented a few of the dilemmas inherent in political interviews:

- an interviewer adapts his position "to the interests of those whom he interviews, allows them to "carry on" without interrupting, reads off previously agreed questions, an so on. This happens particularly often in the course of political interviews and can be traced back, inter alia, to the interviewer's fear of not being accorded further interviews if his questioning is too uncompromising" (p. 173);

- in political interviews "it is often the case that the person to whom the question has been put is less interested in providing a self-exposure". And he adds: "It is, with respect, a big mistake on the part of broadcasting companies to carry such interviews or, indeed, to be obliged to broadcast them". (p. 174).

As far as I am aware, Friedrichs is the only person to have organized seminars and courses with journalists in which both sides discussed selected interviews. Amongst other things, some "hints" about successful interviewing were brought to light. The interviewer should, for example, ask first those questions aimed at eliciting information and only then those questions which seek to obtain an explanation. Conditions were discussed under which a journalist is required to ask an "open" question and those under which a "closed" question - i.e. one which foresees the answer - is called for. The journalist who receives an evasive answer should continue with a statement by way of interpretation so as to force the politician to take up a certain position.

(If, however, an interview is talked about as being an example of "exemplary planning", in which the journalist represents the same political standpoint as the politician and only uses more elegant phrases on his behalf (p. 181) then I should like to enquire whether the efficiency of the politician's non-evasive behaviour might not result in the absence of any critical component. Here I would prefer the journalist clearly to show evasive answers for what they are whilst insisting on "agreeing to differ" when a controversial subject is being discussed. I also think that the term "information" has a very wide range when used by Friedrichs; it includes information on political events, yet also on explanations, motives and justifications. It is, however, with exactly these distinctions that one directs people's attention to the vital communicative acts which surround the image in political interviews.)

We therefore find that in the various surveys terms and categories of conversational analysis are capable of giving a clearer account of the complexity of the happenings in interviews whilst, on the other hand, the vital aspects of appraisal (i.e. the question of how much room the journalist may give a politician to present his own policy in a propagandistic manner) are more dependent on political views of the social norm.

2. Supplementary documentation: some strategies used in conversation by interviewers and politicians, 1984.

In October and November 1984, I taped 23 political television interviews in the random order in which they were broadcast in news and "magazine" programmes in West Germany. I wanted to find out whether there had been major changes in comparison with interviews of the early 1970s.

The first important distinction to be noted when studying these dialogues is that between long and short interviews. Hoffmann (1982) rightly points out the relevance of this distinction and its significance for media integration in relation to other broadcasts. I am nonetheless unable to confirm his thesis that questions seeking information predominate in short, unprepared interviews. It is here, in particular, that matters of opinion are raised and also questions which presuppose specific value judgments on the part of the politicians:

Example 1: Interviewer (on the resignation of Rainer Barzel, Speaker of the Bundestag): "Do you consider that this resignation came too late" ("kommt dieser r̈cktritt nach ihrer meinung zu sp̈t?"
Biedenkopf (a party-colleague of Barzel): - after a pause - "I am unable to make any comment".
(dazu kann ich nichts sagen").

Politicians use no uncertain terms in expressing their refusal to answer a "snap" question.

A comparison of very short with very long interviews reveals the markedly artificial character of the latter. There is an inherent willingness to talk, and those being interviewed refuse to answer questions much more rarely.
In many respects, results of earlier studies are confirmed:
- Politicians speak for longer periods than their interviewers;
- The journalists ask the questions and lead deliberately into new subjects. These rules, which are fundamental to interviewing, remain valid. (An exception proves the rule in that politicians have been known to apologise for parrying a direct question with a counter-question):

Example 2: **Gatter:** "But was Herr von Brauchitsch with you on the fifteenth of August 1978?"
Matthöfer: "How do I know? Where were you on the fifteenth of august 1978?"
Gatter: "In poland" (laughter)
Matthöfer: "I really do apologise, but that is six years ago..."

- Looking at my little collection of interviews as a whole, there are considerably more questions seeking facts and evaluation than explanation and justification. I counted more questions demanding information (37, of which 8 implied slight criticism or inference) than those demanding opinion or evaluation (12).

Open criticism is rare. Critical or reproachful elements are usually cloaked by journalists in questions demanding information or evaluation. This procedure allows them to remain implicit. The politician is thus enabled to overlook the critical element.

Example 3: **Interviewer:** "But determining the course presumably means that the course must be newly-defined. Is there something wrong with the course?" ("stimmt denn etwas nicht am kurs?").

Where interviewers allow themselves a critical remark, they will often do so by means of a statement or an interrogative sentence, in which the deprecated behaviour appears to attach a label to the politician in question:

Example 4: **Interviewer:** (to a "green" MP in Hessen)
"Do you still want to engage in fundamental opposition?" ("wollen sie noch immer fundamental-opposition machen?").

Politicians either ignore criticism expressed in this way or contradict sharply when, in their opinion, such exaggerations are uttered (in Example 4: "We do not in any way engage in fundamental opposition; that would not be possible in any case." ("wir machen keine fundamental-opposition, das wäre gar nicht machbar".))

Decisive questions implying criticism or containing the risk of damage to the politician's image are countered with a flat denial.

When I compare these interviews with those from the early days of the Socialist-Liberal coalition, I find that, in 1984, Members of Parliament are more often confronted with critical opinions not from counter-proposals made by opposition parties but from politicians attacking from "even further to the right" and contending that the person in question had not gone far enough.

Two examples may prove helpful: The Federal Minister for Post and Telecommunications is attacked not on the grounds of pursuing a comprehensive and far-reaching programme to provide cable television to private homes so much as for refraining from using the latest and most expensive technical system (optic fibre versus copper cable). Again: The Federal Minister of Defence is reproached for lacking sufficient courage either to extend the basic period for national service still further or to accept women for service with the Federal Army. By this technique the interviewer gives the politician the change to stamp his policy with the hallmark of moderation. It seems to me that this is where a dilemma becomes apparent. The journalist must adopt a critical attitude towards politicians, come what may. He then draws upon the spectrum of public opinion in order to arm himself with critical arguments whereever he happens fo find them.

Journalists seldom insist once a question has not been answered. It is only in the critical magazine programmes that they interrupt politicians and insist on putting a divergent opinion after an answer has been given. This is especially so in the case of well-known journalists. Even here interviewers tend to hide behind the opinions of others ("some observers are under the impression that ...").

Openly critical questions tend to predominate in interviews forming part of political magazine broadcasts whose socio-critical bias is well-known, or else where interviewers themselves enjoy the status of "star" journalist.

Compared with the interviews of the early '70s I notice that journalists rarely ask so-called questions inviting confirmation. This type of question is one by means of which the interviewer anticipates confirmation of his views and to this end formulates the question with words of negation in expectation of an answer in the affirmative.

Example 5: Nowottny: "Should not the FDP have identified the source of the donation at once?"

("hätte die fdp nicht gleich ausweisen müssen, woher die spende kommt?).

Of the 85 conversational exchanges involving interviewers I can find only three such confirmatory questions. Whether we are being confronted with a new understanding of the interview situation which allows journalists to forego interrogative sentences when formulating their opinion is a matter requiring closer examination.

One particular interview makes it perfectly clear that journalists use opinions expressed by politicians in order to provide a counter-balance to contrary political opinions expressed earlier in the interview. The interview concerned deals with the introduction of computers into primary schools throughout Lower Saxony, a State ruled by the Christian Democrats. The Socialist Minister with responsibility for schools in the Hamburg area was interviewed immediately afterwards and he condemned these endeavours in strong terms. The female interviewer, who was confining herself in this case to questions seeking information and evaluation, supported the politician's viewpoint in this instance.

Finally, it should be noted that certain journalists, like some politicians, have their own style of conversing. The journalist Friedrich Nowottny, who has a predilection for injecting unexpected witty and ironic formulations even into political news magazines, likewise adopts this ironic tone in the interviews. When the Federal Chancellor once said that nobody had forced him to become a candidate for his own high office, Nowottny confirmed his finding with the ironic admission "quite so" ("es ist wohl so").

Let us now turn our attention to the replies favoured by politicians. Their most important counter-mechanism is to contradict opinions or critical evaluations and premises contained in questions. Compared with my earlier findings they do this just as frequently, if not slightly more often (in the case of replies by 200 persons in the 1970s 35 times; in the case of 85 contributions during 1984 18 times). As already indicated, an open **refusal to answer** is employed by politicians more frequently during an unprepared interview than in a previously arranged one.

Two general strategies emerge in relation to politicians' replies when confronted with disagreeable facts or opinions: First they contradict, then they either put themselves in a positive light or else attack (usually third parties, seldom

the interviewer). Occasionally they combine the latter two tactics.
Here is an example to illustrate the sequence of **contradiction + positive self-exposure:**

Example 6: **Interviewer:** Isn't that just a way of playing for time because you cannot be quite so sure of the Free Democrats at this juncture?"
Wörner (Minister of Defence): "No, not in the least. I wonder what else you want. This Government has stated that it will solve the personnel problems of the nineties. It will indeed be finding a solution during its present term of office ..."

Where journalists fail to confer praise on politicians, some of them respond by going beyond all limits in extolling their own virtues. If such personal statements were to be made during the course of a private conversation they would be embarrassing.

Example 7: **Wörner:** "and of course one looks to the Germans because the Germans are a corner-stone in the area of defence ... we're not just a pretty face, we are trendsetters." ("wir können uns nicht nur sehen lassen, wir haben ein zeichen gesetzt").

Example 8: **Kohl:** "Our policy is good, as everyone can see for himself at a glance by looking at ourforeign, security and essential parts of our domestic, economic and social policies. Our standing is high ... and I am not impressed ..." ("wir machen eine gute politik ... wir stehen gut da, und ich lass mich nicht beeindrucken ...").

The alternative to this strategy is to mount an **attack** on another politician after the **disagreement**. In reviewing political interviews I have come to be struck by the frequency with which politicians use interviews in order to address their points of view to those of other political persuasions. These are usually representatives of other parties, but most frequently they are other parties in general. They may also be "forces within this Federal Republic of Germany" (Kohl) or foreign governments. Occasionally politicians combine their reproach directed at third parties with an

appeal (as for instance where a representative of the SPD calls upon the "Greens" to participate in government). This approach to the outside world - in which the addressee is neither the interviewer nor the audience - points once again to the institutional peculiarity of political interviews. Politicians consider such an interview not only as a chance to reiterate their point of view and to canvass votes for their party but also as a direct means of implementing their policies. The content of such interviews, especially those on Saturdays and Sundays, is then repeated in news bulletins and newspapers as a statement of opinion. The parties at which it is aimed then make it their business to make counter-statements.

On some occasions politicians who are being interviewed direct their reproaches at journalists. This can take the form of general complaints with regard to specific practices - as favoured by the Minister President of Bavaria, Franz Josef Strauss ("in this connection I call for a greater degree of responsibility on the part of some sections of the media. This is not a matter of sensational headlines or of lavishing affection on our best-beloved prejudices"). Sometimes they utter a rebuttal of presentations of fact which might harm the politician:

Example 9: **Matthöfer** (former Finance-Minister): "... I can only marvel at the accuracy with which you produce quotations of Brauchitsch which have long since been gainsaid ..."

In many recently recorded interviews politicians know only too well how to use public broadcasts for their own purposes. In two interviews of medium length (4 and 6 exchanges only) they really repeat with new phrases what they have said already. They add a few reasons for the opinions which they have expressed, and sometimes make an appeal. However, such an opinion or appeal leaves the impression that each has been the main concern behind appearing for the interview.

In order to demonstrate typical strategies used by journalists and politicians in political interviews I have written down two interviews. (See Appendix).

The first interview deals with an inquiry discussed during the well-known socio-critical political broadcast entitled "Panorama" (20.11.84). The journalist asked the former

Federal Finance Minister Matthöfer to explain how the Flick-concern came by a tax rebate in spite of the fact that his Secretary of State had expressed his opposition.

I wish here to draw attention to the following details to show how a journalist can steer an interview:

- He interrupts the politician's flow of words on several occasions (turns numbered 3, 9, 13, 17, attempt to interrupt in no. 10) and once without a pause he virtually attaches his next comment to the speaker's last words (14-15).
- The interviewer repeatedly voices a difference of opinion over the subject-matter and thereby forces the politician to comment on facts which essentially contradict his own account (turn 3, 7, 9, 15, nascent contradiction in 18). Divergence of opinion is opnely shown through signals of dissent such as "but" ("aber"), "no" ("nee"), "still" ("doch") and need not be inferred. In one instance, where the politician tries to mitigate a set of circumstances through the model verb "should", the interviewer immediately steps in and insists on the fact of the decision in question.
- From the point of view of content the journalist constantly confronts the politician with information of a controversial nature. The audience is supposed to infer from this that the assertions made by the politician do not ring true, or at least not quite true (turns 3, 7, 9, 15). In putting forward such brief proposals regarding the subject-matter, the journalist aims in each case to blunt the edge of the politician's argument. Thus, in the initial question he implies that the decision on tax rebates was deliberately taken at a time when one of its opponents was on holiday.

We thus have here one example of the interviewer's strategy for dissent. It is only at the beginning that he puts an indirect question tinged with reproach. Thereafter he confines himself to an attack on the politician's defence.

Let us now turn to politician Matthöfer's strategy. It may be seen as the art of **minimization** (playing down relevance). He in turn picks up the indirect reproach concerning the **deliberate** choice of timing (turn 2) and describes it as coincidence. After a brief, positive selfportrayal he endeavours to play down the element of truth contained in the tabled fact.

The second strategy of minimization occurs in turn 6, when he not only plays down the conversation with Von Brauchitsch, the former chairman of the Flick-Concern, as one of many with a variety of persons but also makes light of the sum of money then involved.

The third playing down of relevance affects the decisions for or against Flick: their number is claimed to have been legion (turn 12).

At the beginning of these counter-proposals he also contradicts with undisguised indications of dissent the account put forward by the journalist (turns 8, 12, 16) so that the interview takes on the character of a battle of opinions.

This interview has been selected in order to give an example of "hard" and systematic steering of a conversation by the interviewer. It is also designed to show the politician's counter-strategy which is likewise advanced on a logically and pragmatically developed aura of plausibility. The commitment of both parties is great, at least that is how it appears to the audience. The impression is given of a spontaneous debate, be it through interrupting each other, through counter-questions put by the interviewer, exaggeration and consequent irritation (as in turns 3-6 and 9-11). It could equally well be that this spontaneity had in fact been skilfully staged, that the journalist had decided from the outset to appear as a "hard" interviewer. In this particular case, the visual image on television needs to be examined as follows: Are the verbal and paralinguistic facts on the one hand compatible with the pattern of non-verbal behaviour on the other? This was not the impression which I, for one, gained when watching this interview.

Let us now compare this interview with that given by the Federal Minister for Post and Telecommunications Schwarz-Schilling. Here the journalist takes up the argument raised by another journalist in the preceding programme: Multi-channel optic fibre cable is capable of transmitting many more and diverse channels of communication.

This time the interviewer leaves the politician totally free to present his views. He refrains from interrupting even when a catalogue of past achievements finds its conclusion in over-powering self-congratulation. The interviewer does not ask supplementary questions, nor does he put any critical questions (apart from his opening remarks). He confines himself instead to requesting information (turns 3, 5 and 7).

The interviewer's sole concern is the viewpoint that optic fibre cable is more suitable than copper cable. To this end he picks upon a date suggested by the interviewee in order to enquire whether that would be the right moment for switching from copper cable to optic fibre cable.

In general, the interviewer leaves aside the central topic of criticism levelled at the Minister for Post and Telecommunication's policy. (For years there has been open argument in the Federal Republic of Germany on the subject of whether it is sensible to install a costly and comprehensive cable network purely so that Federal citizens may in future be able to view, say, ten instead of three television programmes. Such programmes are broadcast for the greater part by private commercial television companies. The decision on this development is pregnant with grave consequences for the structure of radio and television companies, for individual leisure-time pursuits, for families and the character of public media).

The politician for his part has prepared himself for the critically slanted question at the start of the interview. Advance publicity had been given to this interview. Probably the comparative costs and the time factor involved in the two possible forms of cable television had been calculated in advance. The Minister speaks calmly, in measured tones and with many "filled" and "silent" pauses. His intonation conveys a sense of security and authority. He glances down diagonally from time to time, as if he were reading from a set of notes. In his subsequent statements the Minister only once reverts to the argument that copper cable would be cheaper. From this point onwards he concentrates exclusively on propaganda to illustrate his political objectives:

- he attacks his opponents, without mentioning either names nor parties ("this dogmatic polemic" - turn 4);
- he endeavours to conduct a "strategy of disclosure": the technical argument (i.e. that optic fibre is better than copper) is only a pretext for attacking the policy on cable television as a whole (turn 4);
- he speaks of his own political decisions in a manner which shows that the testing and introduction of optic cables are due entirely to the Federal Government's openness to new technologies and to the provision of Government contracts to industry. He enumerates the many projects and their operation in individual cities and thus substantiates the great activity of his Ministry in this area

(turn 6).

As a general pattern of pre-planned answers the politician uses the following sequences:

- Dissent and counter-argument
- Dissent and attack on third parties (turn 4)
- Unlimited positive self-exposure (turns 6-8).

In quoting from these two interviews it is my intention to present examples of contrasting sequences in the course of an interview. I consider them to be typical of the contemporary scene. Whilst controlled and strict steering of an interview by the journalist raises the suspicion of a stage battle, the unbridled manner in which a politician is permitted to revel in self-glorification is a matter of great disappointment to the politically-interested spectator.

3. Comparison with political interviews during the '50s

I should now like to indicate only one aspect of enquiry which appears to me to show promise in casting light upon the social significance of political interviews. With regard to the analysis of political interviews it would be desirable if forms of linguistic expression were to be examined historically. In order to gain a first impression I examined 10 political radio-interviews from the years 1954-1958. Almost all of those are long interviews from various radio stations with a total of 144 exchanges.

Even a cursory perusal of the interview texts is sufficient to reveal that the interviewers then adopted a very different, very much more friendly and polite, in part almost obsequious attitude toward politicians.

In the 10 interviews selected we find no strategy of confrontation whatsoever. The journalists do not contradict their partners in conversation or, if so, then very rarely. Instead both parties assure each other of their agreement. Politicians refrain from attacking other political institutions.

The text classified as "interview", displaying an undisputed prerogative on the part of the journalist to put certain types of questions, would seem at that time not to have been in the foreground of the participants' minds. Instead one gains the impression that the partners in conversation comply with the style of conversation used in public exchanges of political opinion. They treat each other with politeness. The journalists do not wish to be obtrusive, their tenor betokens the fact that they feel ill at ease where the occasion demands that they act otherwise. They do not persist in following up a point, even when a politician has confined himself to a vague statement. I wish, at this juncture, to illustrate these remarks by reference to certain observations:

- The journalists **respect the fact that politicians do not wish to disclose everything.** They accordingly go out of their way to formulate explanations to indicate their understanding for the politician's reluctance in disclosing his knowledge: "full understanding on our part for the German delegation's reserve" ("unsererseits volles verständnis für die zurückhaltung der deutschen delegation"); "... the evening of the third day of the conference is hardly the time for making major forecasts or allowing glimpses behind the scenes ..." ("am abend erst des dritten konferenztages kann es sicher keine grosse prognosen oder blicke hinter die kulissen geben"); "What were the main points of discussion? Would you be able to put them in a nutshell?" ("... ist das zu sagen?").
- **Journalists and politicians each speak as though belonging to the rank of the initiated.** (Interviewer: "anyone who knows the circumstances will at once realise that you are evidently thinking of socalled unwieldy massproduction ..."). The interviewers contribute their own thoughts in order to advance a politician's exposé and definitely not to contrive an argument against them. Politicians in turn take up the journalists' interpretation and ideas, agree with them and develop them further: Thus it is that from time to time interviews take on the complexion of joint deliberations. (Some politicians even put themselves in the place of their audience for the purpose of sharing worthwhile information or else shielding them from unpleasant events. "You know that we would have to implement this treaty with an act of Parliament dealing withnational service. It is certain that when the time comes there will be many interesting and worthwhile aspects to be discussed with you on the air for the benefit of your listeners." ("... über das dann bei gegebener zeit sicherlich auch für ihre hörer sehr interessantes und wissenswertes hier am mikrophon mit ihnen zu besprechen wäre). "Herr Albert, I could draw on concrete examples but I dare not

present them to our listeners. They are so pitiful as to end in general merriment ...")

- **Personal concern** is the order of the day. Politicians do not only address their interviewers by name ("dear Herr von Zahn" ("lieber herr von zahn" - not meant ironically)) but, through addressing them directly, include them in their train of thought: ("you see ..." ("sehen sie ...") or "you can imagine that ..." ("sie können sich denken, dass ...")). Politicians speak of their feelings and impressions ("so that I am in fact amazed ..."; "I look upon this with mixed feelings"; "whereas I fear here..."). Journalists also put personal questions and formulate them similarly: "This is a more personal question" ("das ist eine mehr persönliche frage"). They ask politicians after a mission to foreign parts what has been their "strongest impression". In one instance a politician calls the interview a "conversation" ("Unterhaltung").
- **Interviewers thank** politicians at the beginning of an interview for their readiness to participate: "It is very nice of you to join us today for a few minutes ..." ("es ist nett, dass sie heute ... einige minuten zu uns gekommen sind"). This particular statement nowadays represents no more than an empty gesture at the end of an interview.
- **Interviewers praise** politicians and express admiration for them; they wish them success: "Let me wish you well. I am sure I can say this in the name of our German colleagues who for many years have come to you here in Washington in order to be briefed by you. We have all appreciated this collaboration and wish you every success for the future". All these examples betoken a personal, indeed at times a warm relationship between journalists and politicians.
- Politicians very often take up statements in a **positive** manner. In this small collection I detected 10 sets of expressions of consensus amongst some 70 turns by politicians (in the 1984 collection the relationship was only two out of 80 contributions).

Politicians in those days were, in fact, prepared to offer information of their own accord:

Politician: "I should be very happy to enlarge upon this particular subject, if that is your wish ..."
Interviewer: "Yes, please! ..." ("über dieses kapitel würde ich ihnen ganz gerne auskünfte geben, wenn sie solche

wünschen - ja, sehr gerne").

- Interviewers formulate their questions with caution, reserve and politeness. Their questions are often formulated as interrogative sentences with "you" as the subject and a verbum dicendi as the predicate. Just as in the case of polite requests vis-a-vis strangers they play down the urgency of the question by means of a subjunctive, through modal verbs and adverbs ("perhaps", "please"):
  "Would you be able to tell us something about that?" ("können sie uns darüber etwas sagen?"); Would you perhaps wish to make a brief closing statement about the Federal Republic's fundamental position ...?" ("wollen sie vielleicht abschliessend kurz den grundsätzlichen standpunkt der bundesregierung umreissen?"); "Please would you be so kind as to enlarge on this, Herr Blank?" ("bitte, würden sie darüber noch etwas sagen, Herr Blank?"); "Finally, if you please: How do you assess the EEC timetable?" ("zuletzt bitte: wie übersehen sie den evg-zeitplan?").
- Where a direct question is put, it is accompanied by an apology. They court understanding metacommunicatively and give reasons for such direct questioning:
  "Just one last question, if you please, simply because the answer does not appear to have been altogether complete. Otherwise I shall be accused of being a bad reporter("ich werde sonst als schlechter reporter gescholten"). How then do you conceive this timetable in the light of your Paris experience ...?"
- Interviewers portray facts as seen through the politician's eyes. One interview with the then Federal Republic Minister for Agriculture, Heinrich Lübke, virtually reverses the present-day negative/positive distribution (i.e. Interviewers put their finger on the negative side of events; politicians point to the positive side of the situation): Lübke states that on average farm workers earn less than their counterparts in industry. The journalist then evaluates the overall situation for the Minister as positive: "and I feel sure, Minister, that there is a certain measure of satisfaction for you inasmuch as agriculture has received new impulses through this measure ...".
- The feature which the reader perhaps finds most striking in the light of a 30-year time gap is the almost total absence of critical questions on the part of the inter-

viewer, questions requiring justification and the formulation of political alternatives. Policies are taken as given. For instance, Theodor Blank, who was instrumental in organizing the rearmament in the Federal Republic, is not confronted with the opinions and arguments of the opposition of the day but is asked instead to comment on the uniforms to be worn by soldiers in the future. Heinrich Lübke is not placed squarely before the question whether his project of a Green Plan might not be unfair for small farmers. In almost all cases the modern reader is put in mind of alternative policies which found no place in the interviews of the period under review.

It becomes apparent that interviews were clearly based in the '50s on quite different expectations and conventions than is the case in the '70s and '80s. In brief: Where there is questioning, similar standards continue to apply for an open exchange of views. Politics as such were then further removed from the curiosity and incursion of the media than is now the case. It is for this reason that politicians resorted to their own committee rooms in order to debate controversial issues. They were not in the habit of using public interviews as a means to this end.

It would currently be of great value to be able to substantiate,by means of comprehensive documentation, an analysis tracing the revolution which has taken place in interviewing techniques whereby a journalist stands by his entitlement to persist in a question and so to bring politicians to account. Such research should also extend to vocal patterns and intonation and their significance in terms of communication. Moreover, we require a survey on the subject of other text types available within the media, in which protest vis-a-vis present-day politics finds expression. Only in this way are we able to assess the real relevance and significance of political interviews in the overall spectrum of the various tyes of political communication.

4. Conclusion

Finally, I would like to point out three aims and methods of analyzing political interviews which may illuminate their social and political functions in a society:

1. comparative studies on political interviews in different countries,

2. ethnographical research on how a political interview is prepared and how it is carried out,
3. research on institutional conditions for political interviews, and the effects they have on the linguistic realization of the latter.

As the comparison with interviews of the 1950s may show, interviews are a kind of public demonstration of how to deal with politicians. That is why interviews state a lot about how a society works, what rights its members have in public affairs and how politicians stage their public presence.

Appendix

Interview: Werner Matthöfer (SPD, ehemaliger Bundesfinanzminister) - Peter Gatter (Journalist, Panorama, 20.11.1984, ARD).

1 Gatter: ... wenn zum zeitpunkt ihrer entscheidung der hauptgégner der steuerbefreiung im fall grace gerade in urlaub is↘ 00

2 Matth.: also erst einmal → irgendjemand is immer im urlaub ↘ der referent ↗ der referatsléiter der únterabteilungsleiter der abtéilungsleiter der stáatssekretär 0 der (LACHT) parlamentárische staatssekretär der minístet der léiter des ministerbüros↘ 0 die arbeit muss ja wéitergehen ↘ und sie íst auch weitergegangen ↗ ich kann mich aber nur wundern ↗ mit wélcher 00 genáuigkeit hier sie brauchitsch vermerke vorlegen ↗ die längst widerlegt sind und zwar von den betréffenden beamten → natürlich sind diese 0 vermerke alle masslos übertrieben und wichtigtuerisch ↗ äh 0 von brauchitsch gegenüber seinem chef ↗ 0 brauchitsch war víel zu gut bezahlt ↗ er verdiente gut fünf mal soviel wie ein bundesfinánzminister ↗ hat nicht ein dríttel wahrscheinlich gearbeitet sonst hätte der diese ganzen 0 vermérke nicht diktieren können ↗ aber die stímmen hinten und vorne nicht ... ...

3 Gatter: aber wár denn herr 0 wár denn herr von brauchitsch am fünfzehnten august achtundsiebzig bei ihnen ↘

4 Matth.: was weiss ích wo waren síe am fünfzehnten august neunzehnhundertachtundsiebzig ↘

5 Gatter: in pólen (LACHT)

6 Matth.: (LEISE) ich bitte um entschuldigung aber das is 0 das ist séchs jahre her → und das ist auch ganz und gar 0 únwichtich ↘ au- natürlich hab ich mit herrn von brauchitsch gesprochen ich hab 0 tächlich 0 und mit húnderten äh 0 ich meine mit 0 viélen personen gesprochen ↗ sie müssen bedenken der bundesfinanzminister ↘ 0 entscheidet 0 an jédem arbeitstach ↘ 0 durch tu:n oder níchtstu:n durch di:rekt oder índirekt 0 über víele tau:sende von millionen mark ↘ 0 tächlich ↘ 0 tau:sende von millionen mark ↘ 0 u:nd da war díese entscheidung damals die heute so ungeheuer wichtich erscheint → 0 éine von dutzenden routíneentscheidungen →

7 Gatter: aber da ging's doch um fünfhundert millionen márk das kann doch keine routíneentsch-

8 Matth.: aber das ist doch nicht ríchtich↘0 aber ist doch nicht ríchtich was sie da sagen ↘ das waren víer entscheidungen 0 da war da war die féldmühle da war die ...

9 Gatter: nee es ging damals núr um grace ↘ (SCHNELL)

10 Matth.: bitteschön ↗

11 Gatter: es ging damals núr um grace↘

12 Matth.: ja nich nur um grace ↗ sondern es war éine von zwei graceentscheidungen ↘ nich wahr ↗ da ging es ein drittel waren feldmühle dynamit nobel und budérus↘ dann war die érste graceentscheidung die mein vórgänger getroffen hat↘0 dann kam die gérlingentscheidung ↘ dann kam ús-filter ↘ dann kamen äh 00 pcv oder wie die dinger alle geheissen haben

13 Gatter: dynamít nobel

14 Matth.: es waren eine ga:nze reihe 0 von von entscheidungen ↘ und díese entscheidung über die wir jetzt sprechen ↗ und über die böhme berichtet hat →

Gatter: mhm

Matth.: in seiner grundsätzlichen einstimmung↘äh äh stellungnahme stimm ich ja mit ihnen überéin ↗ wir haben ja auch die rechtsgrundlage geändert ↘ nachdem wír fertich waren wäre eine flickentscheidung ü:berhaupt nich mehr möglich gewesen weil böhme und ich 0 zum beispiel im paragraphen vier auslandsinvestitionsgesetz 0 zur ábschaffung vorgeschlagen haben ↗ und diese abschaffung auch dúrchgesetzt haben neben vielem anderem auch ↗

15 Gatter: aber herr matthöfer ↗ hat ihnen 0 stimmt denn der vermerk von brauchitsch insofern als síe herrn von brauchitsch versprochen haben 00 oder 0 gesagt haben wir werden sie informíeren wenn es noch widerstände im hause gibt ↘ äh:

16 Matth.: is ábsoluter únsinn ↘ wie kómm ich denn dazu ↗ dem herrn brauchitsch zu sagen ich werd ihn über widerstände informieren ↘ ích war der bundesfinanzminister ↘ ích habe dies ministerium geführt ↗ und ích musste mít meinen beamten eine entschéidung treffen↘ nun kommt das manchmal vor ↗ dass sie unterschiedliche 0 éinstellungen bekommen ↘ sie haben gehört der unterabteilungsleiter soll dagégen gewesen sein ↘ die ab-

17 Gatter: das ist ziemlich sícher dass herr ölner dagegen

war war↘ 0

18 Matth.: aber das 0 interessánte is ↗ ob ích zu diesem zeitpunkt darüber unterríchtet war dass er dagegen war ↘ und die akten weisen aus dass (...) keine bedenken hätten und da hat der 0 abteilungs- leiter

Gatter: aber herr

Matth.: war der meinung ja: er möge díese seine mei-

Gatter: ...

Matth.: nung dem wirtschaftsminister ja auch (...) präjudiziert hatte alle anderen waren dafür und böhme hatte im widerspruch gegen díese entscheidung mír gegenüber nicht zur kenntnis gebracht (...)

Transkriptionszeichen:		Transcript symbols
0	kurze Pause	Short pause
00	mittlere Pause	Long pause
↗	steigende Intonation	Rising tone
↘	fallende Intonation	Falling tone
→	gleichbleibende Intonation	Sustained tone
:	Dehnung	Stretching of sound
ʹ	Akzent	Accent

1 Journalist: ... if at the time of your decision the most important opponent is just on vacation.

2 Matthöfer: first of all: there is always somebody on vacation. the consultant, the chief consultant, the subhead of department, the head of the department, the secretary of state, the parliamentary secretary of state, the minister, the head of the ministerial office. the work must go on. and it has gone on. but I am very astonished, how exactly you present notes from brauchitsch which were refuted a long time ago, actually by the officials in question. of course these notes are all extremely exaggerated and pompous, brauchitsch's notes to his chief. brauchitsch was paid too well. he earned five times as much as a federal minister of finance. (but) probably, (he) didn't work a third. otherwise he could not have dictated all these notes. but they are not right at all.

3 J: but was herr but was herr von brauchitsch with you on the 15th of august 1978?

4 M: how do I know? where have you been on the 15th of august 1978?

5 J: in poland.

6 M: I beg your pardon. but that was that was six years ago. and that is totally unimportant. of course, I spoke with von brauchitsch. I spoke with hundreds - I mean, with many people. you should consider the fact that every working day the federal minister of finance decides - by acting or not-acting, directly or indirectly - on many thousands of millions marks. every day. thousands of millions marks. and the decision at that time, which seems to be so enormously important today, was one of dozens of routine-decisions.

7 J: but it was about 500 millions marks that cannot be a routine-deci-

8 M: but that is not correct. but that is not correct, what you say. there were many decisions. there was the feldmühle. there was the

9 J: no, at that time it was only about grace

10 M: pardon?

11 J: at that time it was only about grace.

12 M: not only about grace, but it was one of two decisions concerning grace, wasn't it? it was about - one third (was) feldmühle, dynamit nobel and buderus. then there was the first decision concerning grace, that my predecessor came to. then there was the second decision concerning grace then there was the decisionconcerning gerling. then there was us-filters. then there were, uh, pcv, or what all these things were called.

13 J: dynamit nobel.

14 M: there was a whole lot of decisions. and that decision, we talk about now, and böhme has reported on

J: mhm

M: as to his fundamental ... uh statement, I agree with you. we changed the legal basis too. a decision about flick would not have been possible, because böhme and I suggested the abolition in the paragraph 4 of the law for investments in other countries. and we succeeded with the abolition besides many other things.

15 J: but herr minister, has - is the note of v. brauchitsch right insofar, as you have promised v. brauchitsch, or you have said: we shall inform you, if there is any opposition in our department.

16 M: (this) is absolute nonsense. what should have induced me to tell v. brauchitsch, that I would inform him about oppositions? I was the federal minister of finance. I have lead this ministry, and I had to make

decisions with many officials. now it happens sometimes that there are different opinions. you heard the sub-head of the department was supposed to be against it.

17 J: that is quite sure that herr ölner was against it.

18 M: but the interesting fact is, if, at that time, I was informed that he was against it. and the files say (...) that there were no objections. and then the head of the department has.

J: but herr

M: was of the opinion that, yes! he should his own opinion (...) also to the minister of trade and commerce (...) had prejudged all the others were in favour. and böhme did not inform me about his opposing decision (...)

Interview: Schwarz-Schilling (CDU, Bundespostminister) (25.22.1985, ZDF)

1 Journalist: landáuf 0 landab herr minístér↗0 hört man die fráge ↗ wárum hat der postminister nicht gewártet 0 auf die glásfaser 0 warum investiert er 0 ein milliárdenprogramm in kúpferverkabelung↘00

2 Schw.-Sch.: weil die ánwendungsgebiete der glasfaser für die nächsten zehn jáh:re 0 fast áusschliesslich auf die geschäftliche kommunikation bezogen sind↘0 äh es is heute noch úngeheuer teuer die wandler für 0 licht oder elektrizität zu bauen ↗ sodass ein anschluss etwa auf sechzich, siebzich tausen mark kommt→0 und wenn sie das einmal für prívate haushalte úmrechnen↗0 dann würden wir mit der einen milliarde→0 die wir héute für die privàten haushalte zur verteilung für funk und férnsehen ausgeben→0 ganze zwanzichtausend wohnungen→0 das sind nullkommaein prozent wenn man von zwanzichmillionen pótentiellen haushalten ausgeht ↘0 bei der kúpferkoaxialverkabelung werden wir mit dieser einen milliarde↗0 einskommaviermillionen 00 äh pro jahr 0 versorgbar machen↘0 und das bedeutet↗0 dass in der zéitlichen im zéitlichen áusbau 0 wir bis neunzehnhundertneunzich etwa die hälfte aller privaten haushalte verkabeln können→0 währenddessen wir mit der glásfaser erst im jahre neunzehnhundertfünfundneunzich etwa auf éine million ánschlüsse kommen↘ und dánn erst 0 wahrschéinlich in eine kostendegres-

sion↗0 zu gerîngeren kosten kommen ↗ dass vielleicht
der privâte anschluss etwa dréi- bis viermal so teuer
is wie heute der kúpferanschluss↘

3 J: das wird der zéitpunkt sein, wo man kupfer auswechseln
muss gegen glasfaser ↗ oder auswechseln

Schw.-Sch: man wird

J: wird mit glasfaser↗

4 Schw.-Sch: man wird nichts áuswechseln 0 denn-
diese vertéilkommunikation wird für sich eine noch
lange phase der amortisation haben 0 denn wir setzen
ja dann für die privaten haushalte erst in neunzehn-
hundertfünfundneunzig ein↗0 und bis dáhin sind schon
elf millionen etwa verkabelt ↗ äh in kupferkoaxial-
technik ↗ und zwar bílliger 0 als die néuen die im
jahre fünfundneunzich für die privaten haushalte
kommt↘ ích muss sagen 0 ich fréue mich dass diese
diskussion eigentlich mehr und mehr versáchlicht wird
0 äh: ich habe heute gánz klare indizien dafür↗ 0 dass
der dass diese dogmátische polémik in dieser fráge in
déutschland entstanden ist → weil man mit dem argument
gla:sfaser 0 die verkábelung der privâten haushalte
nicht nur in den siebziger jahren → sondern bis wéit
in die néunziger jahre unterbinden wollte ↗ um die
möglichkeiten von méhr 0 rundfunk und fernsehen in
deutschland nícht 0 entstehen zú lassen↘

5 J: mich intressiert noch was wird héute schon 0 alles mit
glasfaser gemacht↘

6 Schw.-Sch: wir haben als die bundesregierung neunzehnhun-
dertzweiundachtzig von helmut kóhl 0 gestéllt wurde
und wir gleich gesagt haben dass wir die modernen
techniken benützen werden ↗ nich nur von glásfaser
geredet↗0 sondern ich habe bereits im novémber neun-
zehnhundertzweiundachtzig 0 die ersten aufträge an die
industrie gegeben sofórt mit der erstellung des
fernnetzes zu beginnen↘ 0 das war die eröffnung jetzt
von hamburg hannóver am anfang dieser woche am móntag
↗ äh dies fernnetz was wir bis neunzehnhundertsieben-
undachtzich durch die gesámte bundesrepublik 0 als in-
frastruktur gebaut haben werden↘ 00 äh wir haben
weiterhin↗0 äh mit grósser schnellichkeit im órtsnetz
0 pilotprojekte begonnen ↗ in sie:ben städten zehn
verschiedene 0 äh äh 0 pilotprojekte ↗ äh die etwa
sechsundachtzig, siebenundachtzig ausgewertet
werden → (BLICK SCHRÄG NACH UNTEN) da ist also bild-

telefon 0 schnelle datenkommunikation→0 äh 0 rundfunk und fernsehn→ das wird dort alles ausprobiert↘ und dann↗0 und das (BLICK NACH UNTEN) habe ich bereits im vorigen jahr begónnen und dieses jahr verstärkt fortgesetzt↗ werden wir (BLICK NACH UNTEN) im jahr fünfundachtzich sechsundachtzich bereits (BLICK NACH UNTEN) die dírekten 0 teilnehmerleitungen an potentielle 0 kommerzielle anwender für schnellen datenverkehr 0 videokonferenzen 0 äh bild- äh dokumentationsaustausch, bildaustausch 0 beginnen↗ (BLICK NACH UNTEN) und zwar in fünfzehn städten↗0 die pótentiell die stärksten ánwender sein werden→ wo bánken, versicherungen, komputerunternehmen 0 die für so etwas äh äh in entsprechnender weise gebrauch haben↗ und im jahre neunzehnhundertsiebenundachtzig werden wir etwa auf über dréissich städte kommen↘ 0

7 J: noch eine kurze frage zum ábschluss↗ äh sie hatten die glasfaserexperten um sich versammelt zur anhörung↗ gibt es schon ergebnisse gibt es schon schlussfolgerungen↘

8 Schw.-Sch: ja ich glaube es war ein áusserordentlich intressantes hearing↗ ähm 0 ich 0 habe zu meiner befríedigung festgestellt↗ dass unsere entscheidung richtich war↗ dass die industrie dies voll mitträgt↗ dass wir mit an der spítze marschieren werden am in der infrastruktur und im schnellen austausch zu verschiedenen städten↗ wir werden allerdings zwei dinge zu tun haben→ einmal die sogenannte óptoelektronik licht in elektrizität↗ díese wándler 0 müssen noch gánz anders erforscht werden um zu kóstengünstigen preisen zu kommen↗ und die póst muss vor allen dingen die standardisierungen wéltweit voranbringen→ 0 um hier eine entsprechende 0 internationale 0 technik hervorzubringen↘

9 J: vielen dank herr minister↘

1 Journalist: all over the country, herr minister, one hears that question: why did'nt the postsecretary wait for the glass fibre cable? why does he invest millions of marks into the copper cable?

2 Schwarz-Schilling: because for the next ten years the fibre cable is applied exclusively to business communication. today it is still enormously expensive to construct the converters for light or electricity, so

that one connection costs 60, 70 thousand marks. and if you calculate this for private households, then, with the one billion that today we spend for private households in radio and tv, we could only provide for 20 thousand apartments. That is 0.1 percent, proceeding on the assumption of potentially 20 millions of private households. using the copper-coaxial-cable, we can supply 1.4 million per annum with this one billion and this means that until 1990, we are able to supply with cable one half of the private households. whereas, using the glass fibre, we could not achieve more than 1 million connections until 1995. And only then (we) might come to a degression of costs, to lower costs (so) that perhaps a private connection is about three to four times as expensive as today a connection with copper.

3 J: this will be the moment when one must replace copper by fibre cable, or (when one) is going to replace (it) by fibre cable?

4 Schw: one is going to replace nothing. for this distributive communication will have a long time for amortisation. Because we begin for the private households only in 1995. and till then, already 11 millions will be connected, with the technology of copper-coaxial(-cable), (which is) actually cheaper than the new (fibre cable), that we will have in 1995 for the private households. I must say, I am glad, that this discussion is going to become more and more objective. today, I have quite clear evidence that this dogmatic polemic in germany has arisen because with the argument: fibre cable one wanted to stop the connections of private households, not only in the seventies but (also) far into the nineties, in order to prevent more radio and tv in germany.

5 J: I am interested in something else. what can be done with fibre cable already today?

6 Schw: we have - when the federal government was constituted by helmut kohl in 1982, and (when) we said that we wanted to use the modern technologies - not only talked about the fibre cable, but already in november 1982 I gave the first orders to industry to begin immediately with the construction of far-spread networks. this was the inauguration from hamburg to hannover at the beginning of this week, on monday. this

network, which we shall have distributed throughout the federal republic until 1987. furthermore, very quickly we began with pilot projects in local networks, in seven cities ten different pilot projects, which will be evaluated in 86/87. **(looks down as if he reads in a paper)** there is visual telephone, rapid transmission of data, radio and tv. all this is tested there and then **(glance down)**, and I began this already last year, and I continued it forcedly this year. **(glance down)** we shall begin in 1985/1986 already **(glance down)** with the direct lines to potential commercial users for rapid data communication, video-conferences, exchange of pictures and documents. and this **(glance down)** in 15 cities, where will be the most users, where (there are) banks, insurances, computer firms, which need these (communications) for their objectives. and in 1987 we shall have more than 30 cities (with such local networks).

7 J: to conclude with, just one short question. you had a hearing of the experts of fibre cable. are there any results already? are there any inferences already?

8 Schw: yes, I think it was an extraordinarily interesting hearing. to my satisfaction I found out, that our decision was right, that the industry supports it completely, that we shall be at the top (with regard to) infrastructure and rapid exchange to various cities. nevertheless, we have to do two things: first the so called optic technology: (converting) light into electricity. these converters have to be developed quite differently in order to get cheaper prices. and the post has to promote standardization all over the world, in order to produce a corresponding international technology.

9 J: thank you very much, herr minister.

COMMENTS ON JOHANNES SCHWITALLA

Rob Grootendorst

One of the aims of Schwitalla's paper is to shed some light upon the techniques and strategies used by politicians and journalists in so-called political interviews. In his paper Schwitalla presents, among other things, the main outcomes of an analysis of twenty-three political interviews which appeared on German television in 1984.

On the part of the interviewers he observes for example that they asked more informative questions than evaluative or critical ones, that they did not often interrupt the politician interviewed, and that they were not very persistent when the politician did not answer their questions satisfactorily. Also, they hardly contradicted him, even if they had every reason to do so.

Of course there were exceptions, but this was the general picture. On their part the politicians disagreed with the interviewer more often than they used to do ten years ago; they sometimes refused to provide an answer, and they frequently contradicted the interviewer. More than once they also took the opportunity to make propaganda for their own policy, to build a positive self-image, and to attack political adversaries.

In order to get a clear picture of what is going on in political interviews nowadays as compared with ten or (as Schwitalla proposes to do) thirty years ago, it will be necessary to find out whether the observed techniques and strategies used by the participants are really characteristic of political interviews. Do they occur exclusively in political interviews, or can they also be found in non-political interviews or even in verbal activities or speech events of a totally different kind? Without a conclusive answer to this question it will not be possible, to determine for example, whether the historical differences, if any, are specific to political interviews or arise from developments which are more general in nature.

In his paper Schwitalla does not give any definition of political interviews as a specific type of speech event. Neither does he pay attention in detail to the similarities or differences between political interviews and other speech events. He just hints once or twice at possible differences. For example, he observes that in ordinary life it would be embarrassing to praise oneself in a manner which is customary in political interviews. Furthermore he notes that in political interviews, as opposed to everyday conversations, the interviewee addresses himself not always to the interviewer or the audience, but to some representative of another political party, for example.

Regarding the possible differences between political interviews and other types of related speech events like everyday conversations, discussions and debates, Schwitalla leaves it at these rather casual remarks. I deem this insufficient and unsatisfactory. No doubt, one of the prerequisites for a thorough historical comparison is a clear understanding of the phenomenon in question. In my opinion Schwitalla does not satisfy this **conditio sine qua non**.

My second point is connected with the first. Schwitalla discusses two examples at some length. The first interview held was with the former Finance Minister, Matthöfer, the second with the present Minister of Telecommunication, Schwarz-Schilling. In the first interview the interviewer chose to take a tough approach, in the second the approach was softish. Schwitalla characterizes the first interview as an argumentative dispute or even a fight in which the interviewer confronts the interviewee with critical questions and objections which serve as arguments against the latter's point of view.

One can legitimately raise the question as to whether such an approach can still be called an **interview**. For what is the difference in that case with an everyday argumentative discussion? It seems more appropriate, to limit as some authors do, the use of the term **interview** to 'a conversation between a reporter and one from whom he seeks information' (cf. Ensink's contribution to this volume). In the case of the tough interview it is clear that the interviewer is not so much concerned with the acquisition of information as with the critical assessment of the information he gets from the interviewee.

As I mentioned earlier, Schwitalla does not give any definition of political interviews. So we are left in the dark as to where he would draw the line, if any, between an interview and a discussion. For the sake of clarity it would be wise to treat argumentative discussions separately from interviews, whether they be political or not. Naturally, this is partly a matter of terminology. And everybody is entitled to do as he thinks is best.

But if one chooses to incorporate argumentative discussions in political interviews, as Schwitalla tends to do, it would be logical to pay more attention to the argumentative features than he in fact does. For example, it would be fruitful to discuss some strategies used by the participants as specimens of a fallacious way of arguing. Thus Schwitalla mentions the strategy of some politicians to attack political adversaries instead of defending their own policy. This strategy can easily be analysed as a combination of the fallacies of **ignoratio elenchi** (misconception of refutation), **argumentum ad ignorantiam** (from the fact that something has not been proved to be not the case, it is concluded that it is the case or vice versa) and **argumentum ad hominem** (personal attack). This last label can also be applied to an attack against a person who has given incriminating information about the interviewee, as according to Schwitalla is the case in the interview with Matthöfer.

I think it will be illuminating to identify fallacies as they occur in political discussions. However, as I demonstrated above, I think it is equally useful to clearly differentiate between interviews and discussions. In his paper Schwitalla fails to do either.

My third point pertains to the practical relevance of carrying out an analysis of the mechanisms operating in political interviews. In my opinion such an analysis is important in its own right. But Schwitalla points out that he hopes that the audience and the interviewer would benefit from it. The knowledgeof the techniques and strategies used in a political interview can lead to a better understanding of what is happening on the part of the audience, while the interviewers can benefit from this knowledge by improving their skills in asking the right questions and in adequately responding to the answers.

One wonders whether politicians cannot also benefit from the acquired insights according to Schwitalla. He does not say anything about this. More important, however, is the question as to how the practical applications of the insights are supposed to be gained. Schwitalla argues in favour of a thorough historical comparison of political interviews from the 'fifties' to the present day. I fail to see how such a comparison can contribute directly to the improvement of, for example, the skills of the interviewer.

To mention only one of the problems I find myself up against in this respect: it must be acknowledged that a historical comparison is primarily a descriptive activity, while giving instructions presupposes a normative attitude. Besides, I think it will be necessary to specify the features which are to be compared. Otherwise one does not know what to look for. In that case there is the real danger that the observations remain accidental and arbitrary.

What deeper insight can be gained, for example, from the remark that interviewers in the fifties were much more polite or even humble with respect to the politicians whom they interviewed? Without any clear criteria that can serve as guidelines for the comparison, this observation runs the risk of being totally trivial. For example, what purpose can possibly be served by stating that it is the interviewer who as a rule asks the questions and introduces new topics?

This scepticism of mine does not imply, however, that I consider any historical comparison to be useless. On the contrary. But without the required criteria it will be impossible to trace any interesting developments or trends. As a consequence it will also be impossible to establish any important differences between the present and the past, let alone to trace any 'essential' differences, which is nevertheless what Schwitalla wants to do. As he again fails to provide us with the necessary information, we cannot help fearing that the ambitious project is doomed to failure.

11

Fantasy theme analysis of presidential debates

E.G. Bormann

Fantasy theme analysis is a humanistic method of rhetorical criticism that can be combined with the general theory of communication (symbolic convergence) in such a way that together they can unify the humanistic and scientific studies of rhetoric and communication. This combination of social scientific and humanistic perspectives facilitates applications of the theory to practice in such areas as political and medical communication.[1]

In this paper I will explain the uses of fantasy theme analysis based on the theory of symbolic convergence for the study of political communication. I shall illustrate practical applications of the theory with a brief analysis of the Presidential Debates of 1984 between Ronald Reagan and Walter Mondale.

Alternative Meanings for Communication Theory

Scholars studying rhetoric and communication have used the term **theory** rather loosely. Sometimes scholars have used **theory** to mean any systematic analysis of communication whether based on empirical data, philosophical analysis, or conventional wisdom; sometimes to mean the systematized collection of rules-of-thumb, criteria for evaluation, and ideal models of recurrent forms of communication developed for and used by practitioners; and, sometimes to mean social scientific formulations of a general nature designed to account for broad classes of communication events.

The first use of the term **theory** is essentially trivial and simply makes a distinction between practical information and all other thought structures. It is illustrated by the comment "That is all very good in theory but it will not work in practice." I shall ignore that usage in this paper. The first and second usages are the important ones and one way to sort out the differences and avoid the confusions surrounding the notion of theory is to distinguish between them. I use the concepts of **special** and **general** theories to keep them separate.[2]

Special theories are those artistic formulations that specify the nature of conventional forms and usages and provide practical advice on how to use and criticize such forms. Special theories are, thus, the second sort of coherent and organized sets of ideas explained above.

General theories of communication are more analogous to theories of the natural sciences that account for broad classes of events. In the case of communications, general theories are those that relate to communicative practices that cut across the conventional usages and recurring forms that result from the applications of special theories. A general communication theory might, for example, be one that would explain how special theories came into being, evolved, and functioned.

The rhetorical study of fantasy theme analysis has resulted in the development of a general theory of communications called **symbolic convergence**.

The Symbolic Convergence General Communication Theory

The process of symbolic convergence is one in which the dynamic chaining of group fantasies brings about symbolic convergence for the participants. As Newtonian gravity cuts across time, geography, and culture so, too, symbolic convergence holds for the communicative processes that create and maintain social consciousnesses in different cultures and across time. Indeed, the process of symbolic convergence plays a large role in the creation of cultures.

Investigators in small group communication laboratories discovered the process of sharing fantasies when they investigated dramatizing messages and their effect on the group.[3]

A dramatizing message is one that contains one or more of the following: a pun or other word play, a double entendre, a figure of speech such as a metaphor, simile, or personification, an analogy, an anecdote, allegory, fable, or narrative.

If in the middle of a group discussion several members come into conflict the situation would be dramatic but because the action is unfolding in the immediate experience of the group it would not qualify as a basis for the sharing of a group fantasy. If, however, the group members begin talking about a conflict some of them had in the past or if they envision a future conflict, these comments would be dramatizing messages.

Group fantasy sharing. As they studied these messages, small group investigators found that some of them seemed to fall on deaf ears: the group members did not pay much attention to the comments. Some of the dramatizing, however, caused a greater or lesser symbolic explosion in the form of a chain reaction. As the members shared the fantasy the tempo of the conversation would pick up. People grew excited, interrupted one another, laughed, showed emotion, and forgot their self-consciousness. The people who shared the fantasy did so with the appropriate responses.

When a fantasy is shared by a larger audience the members of the audience will indicate nonverbal participation by facial expression, bodily posture, nonverbal evidence of rapt attention, and by laughter, moans, groanings, sobbings, and, if the communication style encourages and sanctions it, by verbal exclamations such as "Hallelujah!" and "Hear! Hear!"

Fantasy themes. A scholar working to reconstruct the consciousness embodied in the sharing of rhetorical fantasies of the past must depend heavily upon the traces left in the messages that created those fantasies. What is the nature of the content of rhetorical fantasies? Fantasies may include fanciful and fictitious scripts of imaginary characters but they often deal with things that have actually happened to members of the community or that are reported in authenticated works of history, in the news media, or in the oral history and folklore of the group. The content of the dramatizing message that sparks the fantasy chain is called a **fantasy theme.**

The power of the symbolic convergence theory stems from the human tendency to try to understand events in terms of people with certain personality traits and motivations, making decisions, taking actions, and causing things to happen.[4] We understand a person making plans in order to achieve goals and succeeding or failing to do so because our personal fantasies and daydreams often interpret our own behavior in that way.

Fantasy themes, in contrast with the way we experience the here-and-now, are organized and artistic. Because fantasy themes are always slanted, ordered, and interpretative, they provide a rhetorical means for people to account for and explain an experience or an event in different ways. The way several or more people come to some meeting of the minds and emotions is by participating in dramatizations in which an explanation of the events is acted out by the personae in the drama.

When we share a fantasy we make sense out of what prior to that time may well have been a confusing state of affairs and we do so in common with the others who share the fantasy with us. We have created a group consciousness and have come to share some symbolic common ground. We can then talk with one another about that shared interpretation with code words or brief allusions along the lines of the inside joke phenomenon in a small group.

The scholar's main task in making a fantasy theme analysis is to find evidence that symbolic convergence has taken place, that groups of people have shared a fantasy. Such evidence is provided by the repetition of fantasy themes in a variety of messages in different contexts; by cryptic allusions to symbolic common ground; and, by the appearance of fantasy types.

Inside cues. When a group of people have shared a fantasy theme they have come to share a consciousness with similar meanings and emotions that can be set off by a commonly agreed upon cryptic symbolic cue.

The inside-joke phenomenon is an example of such a trigger. Only those who have shared the fantasy theme that the inside-joke refers to will respond in an appropriate fashion. But the symbolic cue need not be only an inside-joke. The allusion to a previously shared fantasy may arouse tears or evoke anger, hatred, love, and affection as well as laughter and humor. Among the best evidence available to a scholar that fantasies have been shared is the presence of such inside cues.[5]

Fantasy types. The symbolic cue phenomenon makes possible the development of **fantasy types**. When a number of similar scenarios or outlines of the plot of the fantasies, including particulars of the scenes, characters and situations have been shared by members of a group or larger community they form a **fantasy type**.

A **fantasy type** is a stock scenario repeated again and again by the same characters or by similar characters. Rhetoricians often use the fantasy type as a rhetorical device in their discourse. Rather than dramatizing a fantasy theme with specific characters in a specific setting they presented the general plot line.

Rhetoricians also used an archetypal fantasy as a way to fit the breaking news and the unfolding of experience comfortably into the community's social reality. Thus, if the members of a community share an archetypal fantasy portraying the Republican Party candidates as being in the pocket of the wealthy and the corporations they can interpret new events such as a Republican Administration's pushing for tax changes as an attempt to help the wealthy at the expense of the poor and needy. By portraying the new experience as an instance of an archetypal drama the rhetoricians explain and evaluate the new events and bring them into line with the overall values and emotions of their rhetorical vision.

Rhetorical vision. When a number of people come to share a group of fantasy themes and types they may integrate them into a coherent rhetorical vision of some aspect of their social reality. A **rhetorical vision** is a unified putting-together of the various scripts that gives the participants a broader view of things.

Rhetorical visions are often integrated by the sharing of a dramatizing message that contains a master analogy. The master analogy pulls the various elements together into a more or less elegant and meaningful whole.

Usually a rhetorical vision is indexed by a key word, a slogan, or a label. Such indexing is a special case of the symbolic cuing phenomenon but in this instance the cryptic allusion is not just to details of fantasy themes and types but to a total coherent view of an aspect of their social reality.

Rhetorical Criticism

Fantasy theme analysis is a humanistic approach to the rhetorical criticism of human communication. Fantasy theme analysts use the symbolic convergence theory as part of their basic scholarly perspective when studying communication events. They, thus, bring to their criticisms all of the explanatory power of the general theory. However, rhetorical criticism involves more than descriptions of discourse and accounts of how it came into being and functioned. A critic needs also to evaluate and judge the discourse and provide added insight into how it works.

Criticism as coaching. Fantasy theme analysis is a form of metacriticism and should be distinguished from another form of criticism that consists of the expert evaluation of the specialists in a style who continually relate theory to practice. All teachers of communication, whether in an academic setting or not, practice criticism vital to a rhetorical community. This is the level of criticism of the instructor and the class in public speaking. Criticism at the basic level is ephemeral and of enduring scholarly interest only as history. To say that such criticism is ephemeral is not to deny its importance in practice but simply to note its scope, nature, and function.[6]

Criticism as social corrective. Another form of ephemeral criticism is for the critic to take part in contemporary political, social position by evaluating the communication in support of the preferred position favorably and attacking the shoddy quality of the communication of the opposition. Advocates have also used rhetorical criticism to examine how communication contributes to undesirable conditions in society in general. In the first instance the critic as advocate, for example, attacks the president or foreign minister for his or her foreign policy by attacking the leader's speeches relating to that policy, in the second instance the critic as advocate may examine a culture's communication in more general terms in relation to how racism is embedded in the language in metaphors of light and darkness or black and white or how sexism is embedded in terms using the inclusive masculine pronoun, or how the power structures of capitalism or socialism are embedded in language and control behavior in behalf of the elites.

Social criticism as a corrective for society's ills is important and certainly communication is such a vital part of any culture that criticism of society's communication by scholars especially trained for the task is necessary. Important as it is, however, rhetorical criticism that deals with transitory problems is as ephemeral as the criticism which trains neophytes to appreciate and practice a given style of communication.

Metacriticism. The more enduring critical scholarship results from a metacritical perspective that views the entire process of communication including practice, criticism, and special theory as the object of analysis. The fantasy theme analyst begins by making a study of the communication practices of a group of people by means of qualitative and content analysis of messages to discover the fantasy themes, fantasy types, and rhetorical vision in the material.[7] The critic then makes a critical qualitative analysis of the consciousness of the members of the rhetorical community that shares the vision.

Metacriticism aims at discovering knowledge about human communication that transcends the communication styles and the transitory issues facing the community using the rhetoric. Rhetorical criticism thus takes its place as a liberal and humanizing art, a scholarly endeavor that aims to illuminate the human condition by providing understanding of human communication.

Fantasy Theme Analysis of the Presidential Debates Media Fantasies Prior to the Debates. While President Reagan enjoyed a brief period of relatively positive coverage at the beginning of his first term in office the media honeymoon did not last long. Soon the media journalists were again searching for weaknesses, reporting presidential misstatements, and other evidence of ignorance, stupidity, and errors of judgment. They portrayed the Reagan persona as so stupid it thought that missiles once launched could be recalled. The Reagan persona without a script was at such a loss to answer a question that the Nancy Reagan persona had to prompt it with a suitable answer.

The media rhetorical vision has a relatively simple and pragmatic standard for the success of the Presidential persona as a politician. It looks to polls as the ultimate legitimization of political skill.

The Reagan persona continued popular with the electorate despite the negative fantasy themes and types reported in the media much to the surprise of the journalists. Searching for an explanation that would account for these confusing results media professionals began to share interpretive fantasy that portrayed Reagan as a "great communicator" and his persona as a teflon one to which no media arrows would stick.

In a sense Reagan's persona in the media was a great communicator because the team that created it used the persona to project a coherent saga and big-picture vision of the nation. The high point of this campaign was represented by the anniversary ceremonies of the invasion of France in 1944. Here the Reagan persona conducted a celebration ceremony of one of the great moments of one of the good wars of the nation's history. The media reports of that ceremony to the American people were lengthy, reverential, and showed the Reagan persona to good advantage. The culmination of the Reagan presidential campaign in 1984 consisted of a series of skillfully produced short political documentaries narrated by Ronald Reagan and shown on television that portrayed the saga that the Reagan persona symbolized.

Still the media characterization of the Reagan persona as

a "great communicator" when it became widely accepted by the American electorate proved a handicap in the joint press conferences usually called "debates" of the campaign of 1984. Polls indicated that before the first joint appearance about twothirds of the general public expected that Reagan would win handily because he was the great communicator. Neither the public nor the media observers had any criteria to use in judging who won the joint appearance and yet the most newsworthy question seemed to be "Who won the debate?" Given the confusion surrounding winning and with the public expecting an easy Reagan victory a good performance by Walter Mondale was bound to make his persona more attractive. Indeed, this was the result of the first program.

After the first joint appearance, the Reagan team announced that the Mondale persona had done better than expected in the "debate" but had not delivered a "knockout blow". At the time I evaluated this tactic as a mistake but whether by accident or design it turned out to work to the advantage of the Reagan persona when the media, also apparently thinking it was an error, gleefully focused on the comment and picked up the phrase. When polls were equivocal as to whether or not the Mondale persona had picked up enough ground on the front runner the media began to suggest that Mondale not only needed to "win" the second "debate" but to deliver a "knockout blow". This reversed the expectations for a substantial portion of the audience and the focus was now on Mondale doing so well in the second program that he would clearly beat Reagan. The Mondale team apparently shared the fantasy that to win the election Mondale would have to deliver a knockout blow.

Mondale's communication team drove their candidate hard in preparation to try to achieve the knockout. The end result was an overtrained candidate who appeared tired and Mondale performed in a way very similar to what he had done in the first program. Since no one knew for sure what would constitute a knockout in these circumstances and since Reagan also performed in a way quite similar to what he had done in the first program and in addition looked better and seemed more relaxed, affable, and lively the media professionals tended to discount the influence of both "debates". The media groups began to share fantasies that interpreted the joint appearances as not substantially changing the course of events which before the debates they had cast into the fantasy type of a landslide, one of their favorite explanatory scenarios.

Postelection analysis. In much postmortem analysis of the campaign of 1984 in the United States the discussion has revolved around the question of how it could be that poll results indicated that voters approved of Walter Mondale's stand on the issues but preferred to vote for Ronald Reagan. The conventional wisdom was that Ronald Reagan projected a leadership image and that his communication technologists knew how to manipulate the electronic media. More careful analysis by people intimately involved in both campaigns resulted in the conclusion that there was something deeper and more symbolic at stake. Ronald Reagan had been systematically communicating a coherent rhetorical vision since 1964 and the Barry Goldwater campaign. Walter Mondale by contrast did not dramatize a coherent vision for the American people.

A fantasy theme analysis of Mondale's answers to the questioning of reporters during the two debates reveals why it was that his messages failed the rhetorically crucial task of projecting an attractive and coherent rhetorical vision, one that a majority of voters could share.

Mondale and the New Deal rhetorical vision. Walter Mondale grew up in my state of Minnesota and came to power as a protege of Hubert Humphrey. Humphrey was powerfully drawn to the rhetorical vision of the New Deal as promulgated by such rhetoricians as Franklin Roosevelt. For much of his political life Mondale shared the same vision as his mentor.

The publicists who developed the rhetorical vision that brought Franklin Roosevelt to power used many of the old progressive fantasies of the turn of the century including the fantasy type of the masses against the classes. The New Deal rhetoric portrayed the depression as largely resulting from the selfishness of the economic royalists. The few very wealthy controlled the fate of the rest. When the Administration of Franklin Roosevelt took office the Roosevelt team created and added to the old progressive fantasies a series of new fantasy themes and types that portrayed the Federal Government as having the right and the moral duty to move into areas of human rights and economic security. The Federal Government should control farm production, provide direct relief through monetary assistance to people out of work, provide government work programs for young people and for older unemployed workers, provide a pension for older Americans, a bonus for veterans, aid for young people to get education. In the rhetoric of Franklin Roosevelt such inside-cues as the "Four Freedoms" including the freedom from want alluded to the new vision of government's role in society. The New Deal rhetorical vision served to unify a disparate group of participants including minorities, union members, and Southern Democrats for fifty years.

In the beginning of the primary campaign the messages of Mondale team reflected their candidate's participation in the New Deal rhetorical vision. Indeed that team shared the basic fantasy themes and types of the New Deal so strongly that they took the values and assumptions embedded in them as givens. When they prepared speeches and television commercials for their candidate they did so in the traditional manner of New Deal rhetoricians. They examined specific problem areas such as poverty, women's rights, and rights of minorities, and reasoned about them without ever examining the underlying symbolic common ground - that is the rhetorical vision of the New Deal. They never brought to the surface the basic fantasy type of the New Deal vision that the Reagan publicists had for twenty years been attacking with repeated and graphic fantasy themes and types portraying the Federal Government as too large, too expensive, too repressive, and too inefficient. Did the Mondale rhetoricians still share the fantasies of the Lyndon Johnson Administration which had portrayed the fantasy that the American people no longer had to fear the ogre of big government? The American people never found out.

Mondale's rhetorical problems. The Mondale publicists discovered early in the primary campaign that there was something rhetorically amiss. For many years the standard practice for candidates enacting the New Deal vision was to approach each audience with a list of its member's grievances and needs and assure them that the candidate had a plan to take care of their problems. Many critics, including other candidates in the Democratic Party primary, characterized this rhetoric as the "old politics" and charged the Mondale persona with appealing to the selfish concerns of special interest groups. In addition, after the primary election in New Hampshire many voters apparently were attracted to the persona of Gary Hart who was dramatizing fantasies about a new politics for the future.

The Mondale rhetoricians were apparently thrown into disarray. They began to seek material for their messages that would be more effective at enticing voters into sharing their fantasies. They picked up dramas on an ad hoc basis. These rhetorical decisions were often made because polling results suggested that they would be advantageous rather than because they were an integral part of a new rhetorical vision. In this hit or miss fashion the Mondale team began to have their candidate dramatize new fantasies that were often at odds with the rhetorical vision of the New Deal. However, the New Deal rhetorical vision remained the solid symbolic ground that held the partisan Mondale supporters together and they continued using many inside-cues to that symbolic common ground. The net result was that they projected a confused and contradictory vision to the American electorate.

The Mondale team's general confusion as to what rhetorical vision they believed in is revealed in graphic detail in the two joint press conferences that Walter Mondale had with Ronald Reagan on October 7 and 21 of 1984.

The first "debate". The first program was devoted to domestic policy. Each political party in the United States had a firmly established fantasy type that portrayed their emotions, values, and motives in regard to financial deficits of the Federal Government. The fantasy type of the Republican Party portrayed the Democrats as the party of fiscal irresponsibility that fueled inflation by running up huge deficits with giveaway programs for foreign countries and welfare chiselers at home and thus mortgaging the future of the country's children and grandchildren. The Democratic Party, on the other hand, had shared a fantasy type that portrayed the deficits as, at worst, a necessary evil, and at best a tool for the fine-tuning of the economy. Certainly the Federal Government's role in taking care of those in want and need far outweighed monetary considerations such as a growing national debt.

Mondale leaped to the attack in answer to the first question by saying, "And perhaps the dominant domestic issue of our times is what do we do about these enormous deficits." He then proceeded to dramatize the old Republican fantasy type of the danger of an unbalanced budget. "There is no question that we face this massive deficit, and almost everybody agrees unless we get it down, the chances for long-term healthy growth are nil. And it's also unfair to dump these tremendous bills on our children."[8]

But in the same answers in which he sounded more Republican than his conservative opponent on the deficit question

Mondale made a series of stirring inside-cue allusions to basic fantasy types of the New Deal rhetorical vision when he said, "And I have proposed over $ 100 billion in cuts in federal spending over four years. But I am not going to cut it out of Social Security and Medicare and Student assistance and things that people need."[9] While his old-line Democratic listeners were probably confused by the Republican sounding attack on deficit spending and the promise to cut the budget they could cheer the allusions to the old shared fantasies of the Federal Government providing things that people need.

Over the years the major difference between the rhetorical vision of the two parties was reflected in the way the Republicans dramatized the increasing size of the Federal Government as a bloated bureaucracy that threatened individual freedom and ineffectively threw money at problems while the Democrats were dramatizing a scenario in which, by assuring civil rights, waging war on poverty, and dealing with other humanitarian needs a large Federal Government was a positive good.

In the October 7th television appearance Mondale, sounding more Republican than Reagan, said, "The president just said that his government is shrinking. It's not. It's now the largest peacetime government ever in terms of the take from the total economy. Instead of retreating, instead of being strong where we should be strong, he wants to make it strong and intervene in the most private and personal questions in American life. That's where government should not be."[10]

Shortly after redramatizing the traditional Republican Party fantasy type about the evils of big government Mondale listed a string of powerful inside cues to traditional Democratic Party fantasy types when he said, "The American people want this environment protected ... The American people want their children educated ... They want those civil rights laws enforced, they want the Equal Rights Amendment ratified, they want equal pay for comparable effort for women ..."[11]

The confusion was compounded because running through many of Mondale's comments were allusions to the core fantasy type of the New Deal vision in regard to the Republican Party, namely that it is the heartless selfish party of the wealthy exploiting the poor, women, the minorities, the elderly, and the handicapped. In his conclusion Mondale said:

> The president's favorite question is, 'Are you better

off?' Well, if you're wealthy, you're better off. If you're middle income, you are about where you were. And if you are of modest income, you are worse of ... I don't think this nation is composed of people who care only for themselves ... When we terminated 400,000 desperate hopeless, defenseless Americans who were on disability, confused and unable to defend themselves, and just laid them out on the street, as we did for four years. I don't think that's what America is all about. America is a fair society. And it is not right that Vice President Bush pays less in taxes than the janitor who helps him.[12]

The second "debate". The second program which took place on the evening of November 21, 1984 was devoted to foreign policy. The foreign policy fantasy types of the traditional Republican and Democratic Party rhetorical visions had their roots in the Cold War rhetoric that caught up many Americans in the years immediately following the second world war. In one fantasy type the Republicans portrayed the Democrats as soft on communism and dangerous because of their willingness to appease aggressive totalitarian communism. Reagan's campaign in 1980 had dramatized the Carter Administration's response to Russia's invasion of Afghanistan in these term. In the other fantasy type the Democrats portrayed the Republicans as trigger-happy doctrinaire anti-communists liable to plunge the country into war. Carter's campaign in 1980 had shown a political announcement of the president's chair in the oval office in the White House and suggested that Reagan would be a risky president to have sitting in that chair close to the nuclear button.

The Mondale team had redramatized the war and peace issue in terms of the old Democratic fantasy type during the campaign but in the second meeting with Reagan, Mondale's message further confused his listeners when he repeatedly enacted the basic Republican party fantasy type about the evil nature of communism and the need to be tough on communist aggression.

On Central America, Mondale said, "Our objectives ought to be to strengthen the democracies, to stop communist and other extremist influences and stabilize the community in that area". On presidential leadership in foreign policy he said, "A president must not only assure that we're tough but we must also be wise and smart in the exercise of that power. We saw the same thing in Lebanon ... because the leadership of this government did not use wise policies. We have been humiliated, and our opponents are stronger."[13]

Reagan responded to a question about his description of the Soviet Union as a powerful, evil empire intent on world domination by saying "I retract nothing that I have said" he went on a bit later to suggest that "I know that Mr. Mondale in the past has made statements as if they were just people like ourselves and, if we were kind and good and did something nice, they would respond accordingly. And the result was unilateral disarmament."[14]

At the next opportunity, Mondale portrayed the Soviet Union using the same fantasy type as Reagan had used. He said, "I have no illusions about the Soviet Union leadership or the nature of that state. They are a tough and ruthless adversary, and we must be prepared to meet that challenge. And I would ... There will be no unilateral disarmament under my administration. I will keep this nation strong. I understand exactly what the Soviets are up to."[15]

Conclusions

The Mondale messages in the two "debates" of 1984 illustrate in miniature the confusions as to a coherent and consistent rhetorical vision that characterized his entire campaign. It was as though being challenged by an opponent who attacked basic fantasies of the New Deal rhetorical vision the Mondale rhetoricians were at a loss as to how to proceed. They seemingly had internalized the fantasy themes and types of that vision to such an extent that they were barely conscious of them and their response was not to bring their symbolic common ground back to the level of consciousness for systematic examination and evaluation but to draft messages in knee-jerk fashion either alluding to old shared fantasies from the New Deal vision or drafting new ones on the basis of polling data. They continued to go to audiences theyanalyzed in terms of such characteristics as being women, minorities, needy, and Union rank-and-file and in line with the New Deal rhetorical vision present them with a list of grievances and governmental programs to meet those grievances. They also seemed to adopt new fantasies from the opposition vision which were implausible in the same dramatic scene as the New Deal fantasies. The net result was an unwillingness on the part of many in the audience to suspend disbelief and become caught up in the drama. Instead Mondale's rhetoric often did not play and it seemed that his team rhetoricians had no vision; that the campaign was in disarray, and that the Democratic Party did not know what it was about.

NOTES

[1]. For more detailed analysis of practical applications see Cragan and Shields (1981). For a full development of the method of fantasy theme analysis in rhetorical critisicm see Bormann (1972); Bormann (1982) and Bormann (1983).

[2]. For a full discussion of general and special communication theories see Bormann (1980).

[3]. See particularly Bales (1970); Bormann (1975); Gibbard, Hartman and Mann (1974); Bormann, Pratt and Putnam (1978).

[4]. For further evidence of how human beings attribute motives to human actors see psychological studies conducted under the label of **attribution processes**. For a survey of these matters in terms of persuasion see Smith (1982) pp. 117-141.

[5]. For an examination and explanation of the inside cue phenomenon in political communication see Bormann, Koester and Bennett (1978).

[7]. The critic may also gather data about the consciousness of the community of people who share the rhetorical vision by means of observational techniques such as Q-sort interviews, focused group interviews, individual interviews, questionnaires, and applying other instruments in both small sample and large sample surveys. For a study employing a number of these other observational techniques see Bormann et al. (1984).

[8]. The quotations from the debates are taken from the reports of the texts in **The Washington Post** of October 8 and 22, 1984. This quotation is from October 8, P.A. 22.See Appendix.

[9].Ibid.

[10]. Ibid., p. A23.

[11]. Ibid., p. A24.

[12]. Ibid., p. A25.

[13]. October, 22, p. A10.

[14]. Ibid.

[15]. Ibid., p. A11.

EXCERPTS FROM THE TEXT OF THE FIRST REAGAN-MONDALE DEBATE
The Washington Post, Monday, October 8, 1984.

QUESTION : Mr. Mondale, the Carter-Mondale administration didn't come close to balancing the budget in its four years in office, either, despite the fact that president Carter did promise a balanced budget during his term. You have proposed a plan combining tax increases and budgetary cuts and other changes in the administration of the government that would reduce the projected budget deficit by two-thirds, to approximately $87 billion in 1989. That still is an enormous budget that we'll be running for those four years. What other steps do you think should be taken to reduce this deficit and position the country for economic growth?

MONDALE: One of the key tests of leadership is whether one sees clearly the nature of the problems confronted by our nation. And perhaps the dominant domestic issue of our time is what do we do about these enormous deficits ...
There is no question that we face this massive deficit, and almost everybody agrees unless we get it down, the changes for long-term healthy growth are nil. And it's also unfair to dump these tremendous bills on our children. The president says it will disappear overnight because of some reason. No one else believes that's the case. I do and I'm standing up to the issue with an answer that's fair. I think that's what leadership is all about. There's a difference between being a quarterback and a cheerleader. And when there's real problem, a president must confront it. (p. A22).

MONDALE: ... The president just said that his government is shrinking. It's not. It's now the largest peacetime government ever in terms of the take from the total economy. Instead of retreating, instead of being strong when we should be strong, he wants to make it strong and intervene in the most private and personal questions in American life. That's where government should not be. (p. A23).

MONDALE: ... The American people want this environment protected. They know that these toxic waste dumps should have been cleaned up a long time ago. and they know that people's lives and health are being risked because we've had an administration that has been totally insensitive to the law and the demand for the protection of the environment. The American people want their children educated,

they want to get our edge back in science and they want a policy headed by the president that helps close this gap that's widening between the United States and Europe and Japan. The American people want to keep opening doors. They want those civil rights laws enforced, they want the Equal Rights Amendments ratified, they want equal pay for comparable effort for women, and they want it because they understood from the beginning that when we open doors we're all stronger ... (p. A23).
MONDALE: ... The president's favorite question is, "are you better of?" Well, if you're wealthy, you're better off. If you're middle income, you are about where you were. And if you are of modest income, you are worse off. That's what the economists tell us ... I don't think this nation is composed of people who care only for themselves. And when we assault Social Security and Medicare, as the record shows we did, I think that was mean-spirited. When we terminated 400,000 desperate, hopeless, defenseless Americans who were on disability, confused and unable to defend themselves, and just laid them out on the street, as we did for four years, I don't think that's what America is all about. America is a fair society. And it is not right that Vice President Bush pays less in taxes than the janitor who helps him. (p. A24)

EXCERPT FROM THE TEXT OF THE SECOND REAGAN-MONDALE DEBATE

The Washington Post, Monday, October 22, 1984.
MONDALE: ... (On Central America) Our objectives ought to be to strengthen the democracies, to stop communist and other extremist influences and stabilize the community in that area ... A president must not only assure that we're tough but we must also be wise and smart in the exercise of that power. We saw the same thing in Lebanon, where we spent a good deal of America's assets, because the leadership of this government did not pursue wise policies. We have been humiliated and our opponents are stronger. (p. A10).
REAGAN: ... I have said on a number of occasions exactly what I believe about the Soviet Union. I retract nothing that I have said. I believe that many of things they have done are evil in my concept of morality that we have, but I also recognize that as the two great superpowers in the world, we have to live with each other ... I think that,

in dealing with the Soviet Union, one has to be realistic. I know that Mr. Mondale in the past has made statements as if they were just people like ourselves and, if we were kind and good and did something nice, they would respond accordingly. And the result was unilateral disarmament. We canceled the B1 under the previous administration. What did we get for it? Nothing. The Soviet Union has been engaged in the biggest military buildup in the history of man at the same time that we tried unilateral disarmament ... (p. A10).
MONDALE: ... I have no illusions about the Soviet Union leadership or the nature of that state. They are a tough and ruthless adversary, and we must be prepared to meet that challenge. And I would ... There will be no unilateral disarmament under my administration. I will keep this nation strong. I understand exactly what the Soviets are up to.

COMMENTS ON BORMANN

Dick Springorum

One of the essential elements, and perhaps the most essential in the convergence theory of communication is the dynamic of **sharing group fantasies.** Sharing group fantasies is realised in participating in dramatizations. In small groups this process of sharing fantasies is observable in the ongoing process of real interaction: in small groups people may search for common ground (value, opinions) directly by discussing their values and interests. The way people react in sharing opinions, telling second stories, commenting on political statements and so on is defined by the author as the empirical basis for the process of chaining opinions or fantasies. His theory of fantasy theme or fantasy type as based on the detailed analysis of the process of interaction seems to be a firm part of the vast area of the theory of the social construction of reality. The social world people suppose to be living in, or are supposed to live in, is also based on processes of interaction in daily life. The author's fantasy-theme approach is a valuable contribution in this area.

However, in analysing the results of the November elections in the USA, the speaker presupposes the existence of fantasy themes or fantasy types in rather large groups. My first question, then, is: how small or large is the difference between small and large groups in this respect? Is there the same empirical basis, the same recognizable interactional basis for the supposition that in large groups or communities like 'the people in the state of Minnesota', or 'the people in western Europe' people really share fantasies? Furthermore, how can the empirical basis in both groups - the small and the large one - be brought together, or in what respects are both groups comparable? What or where is the evidence that the audiences before the mass media also 'share fantasies'? My second question has to do with the analysis given of the press conferences as a theory. So this question concerns a methodological point.

In my opinion the author's post-factum analysis is rather plausible; and observing my own feelings after reading his paper, I feel rather convinced, and maybe other people with me. In some way or other I was impressed by the way he analyzed how Reagan and Mondale dramatized or just failed to dramatize the distinct and different political fantasy types. It is an intuitively attractive description of both the press conferences, and the results of the elections. But in what sense is the author's description an explanation? How does it 'explain' the outcome of the debates and/or the election? Is it possible for his theory to be tested, and to be falsified? And if not, in what sense is his theory a theory? In my opinion at least it is not impossible that the description and interpretation "Mondale has dramatized his opponents fantasy type", or "Mondale has failed to dramatize a or his own or the democratic fantasy type" is, at least partially, based on the results of the election. In other words: what exactly does the author mean by the description or interpretation "to dramatize the opponents fantasy type" or "to fail to dramatize your own fantasy type"? If the outcome of the elections had been the reverse, what would have been the basis for an interpretation of the press conferences in terms of 'dramatizing fantasy types'?

12

The normative reconstruction of argumentative discourse

An illustration of its efficacy in the analysis of the confrontation stage in a political discussion

F. van Eemeren

1. A normative extension of the description of discourse

In recent years a lot of attention has been paid to language use,be it oral or written, formal or informal, institutional or spontaneous.[1] Whether the research is done in vivo or in vitro, and whatever research methods are employed, in all cases this research is guided by an empirical disposition leading to a description of things going on or noticeable in the actual processes and products of language use.[2] I share this empirical attitude.[3] As long as descriptive research is based on solid ground, with the observations made being not merely ad hoc, nothing would seem to be wrong with this.[4] Nevertheless, I would like to make a plea for a more normative-oriented point of view. Hazardous as it may be, when dealing with certain problems, a normative policy is, in my opinion, a useful supplement to a purely descriptive procedure.

According to Russell, a theory may be tested by its capacity for dealing with puzzles.[5] Of course, it depends on the kind of puzzle to be solved, as to what sort of theory will work. If the problem that faces us is that reality at some point does not come up to standard, it will not suffice merely to describe the state of affairs from a theoretical point of view alien to the standard at stake - no matter how revealing this description per se may be, viewed linguistically or otherwise. To solve this sort of problem it is necessary to judge reality from a well-defined normative point of view, appropriate to the standard concerned. This means that a theory of language use which concerns itself, for instance, with the adequacy of verbal communication and interaction, by the very nature of its **raison d'être**, must include a component related to the standards to be upheld.

In my opinion, for all practical purposes it is necessary that a theory of verbal communication and interaction which purports to be of importance for discussants be normative as well as descriptive. In order to comment constructively on a particular specimen of language use one has to know what purpose has to be served by the verbal utterances and to what extent the verbal behaviour is adequate in view of this purpose. Language use is a form of goal-directed behaviour and has to be judged and described as such. This normative element has to be incorporated in the theorizing.

The normative supplement to the description of discourse I propose does not simply consist of an enumeration of norms, like the Gricean maxims, which are operative in language use. Any and all norms which further the pursuit of the language goal concerned have to be taken into account. This means that a system of norms is developed which may comprise norms that are disregarded by the discussants in question or that are even unknown to them. As a matter of course the norms proposed need not be accepted at face value. They might, for example, display inconsistencies. Therefore, the system of norms must be scrutinized with respect to both its 'problem validity' and its 'intersubjective validity'.[6] A normative construct evaluated in this way can be employed in describing (and appreciating!) a particular specimen of language use, demonstrating, as we already know from other disciplines, that systems of norms, once established, can be made to play a part in the fulfilment of (analytical) descriptive purposes.Later on, I will use an example of political discourse to show what I mean by this.

2. A dialectical approach to argumentation

At this point I will make some remarks on argumentation, as I have been invited to do. This means that I shall focus my attention on just one, be it rather important, phenomenon in the field of discourse.[7] First of all, I would like to define my position.

By argumentation I mean, roughly speaking, any attempt to justify or refute an opinion by verbal means. Put more precisely: argumentation is a complex speech act consisting of a constellation of statements designed to justify or refute an opinion. Argumentation is directed towards obtaining the approbation of an audience. In the dialectical perspective offered by my colleague Rob Grootendorst and myself one could also say: argumentation is calculated in a critical discussion to convince a rational judge of a particular standpoint with regard to the acceptability or unacceptability of an opinion.[8]

What is dialectical about this? It is, to put it briefly, mainly the premise that argumentation must always be considered part of a critical discussion between language users to resolve a conflict of opinion. A discussion which is critical in a dialectical sense takes place between a protagonist of a standpoint and one or more language users who, rightly or wrongly, are considered to fulfil the interactional role of antagonist. In the most simple form of a fully-fledged dispute, one language user has explicitly cast doubt upon another language user's explicitly avowed positive or negative standpoint.[9] Unfortunately, life is seldom that simple and real discourse as a rule does not simply reflect the dialectical ideal. Nevertheless, this definition supplies us with a practical starting point for further considerations.

Characteristic of the normative conception of the dialectical approach to argumentation is that, as a matter of principle, every argumentation is considered part of a critical discussion aimed at resolving a dispute, regardless of whether this dispute and this discussion are actually externalized or not. It may be the case that the protagonist happens to anticipate a discussion which will never be verbalized; he is just trying to parry an imaginary attack. Putting it even more strongly: he may be trying to solve a dispute which does not exist. But in all these cases, the moment he argues, the very fact of his argumentation testifies to the legitimacy of a dialectical approach to argumentation. In my opinion, this dialectical approach needs to be allied (among other allies) to the functionalist speech act approach, in a so-called normative pragmatics.[10]

3. Dialectical characterization of disputes about opinions

Language users who have externalized a difference of opinion and have embarked on a dispute about an opinion could, of course, leave it at that, but very often they will undertake an attempt to resolve the dispute, as postulated in dialectical theory. Disputes are resolved when the language users who have expressed doubt about points of view have withdrawn these expressions of doubt or when language users who have advanced points of view retract those points of view. To resolve a dispute by way of a critical discussion several **stages of discussion** have to be gone through, which correspond to the stages in the resolving of the dispute, although they need not always be explicit.[11]

According to our dialectical theory a critical discussion passes through four discussion stages: the **confrontation stage** during which the dispute is externalized, the **opening stage** during which agreements are reached concerning the manner in which the dispute and the discussion are to be conducted, the **argumentation stage** during which argumentation is advanced and reacted to, and the **concluding stage** during which it is established how the discussion is concluded. Although all four stages are indispensable, on this occasion I will occupy myself only with the confrontation stage.

In the confrontation stage of a discourse analysed dialectically as a critical discussion a difference of opinion becomes apparent between a language user advancing a point of view and a language user (in many cases a different one) casting doubt on that point of view or, in more complex cases, even arguing against it. The language users than have a dispute about an expressed opinion, and an analysis of the confrontation stage consist of **identifying the type of dispute**.

Disputes may be categorized according to their complexity.[12] I shall here identify four **standard types of dispute**. In the first place, I believe, it is necessary to differentiate between **single** and **multiple** disputes. Single disputes have to do with **one and no more than one opinion**. Multiple disputes have to do with **more than one opinion**. Multiple disputes can always be broken down into a number of single disputes. The situation is then, for example, as follows:

Peter: "You should never take an aspirin with milk, and you shouldn't drink so much either."

Agnes: "Are you sure about the aspirin? And why shouldn't I drink when I feel like it?"

In the second place, I believe it necessary, when analysing disputes, to distinguish between **simple** and **compound** disputes. In simple disputes only one **(positive or negative) point of view** is advanced with respect to an opinion, and in compound disputes **two contradictory points of view** (one positive and one negative) are propounded with respect to one and the same opinion, as in the following example:

Peter: "You should never take an aspirin with milk."
Agnes: "On the contrary: you should!"

Simple single disputes, in which a single positive or negative point of view with regard to a single opinion is advanced and subjected to doubt, represent the **basic form** of dispute. All the other standard types of dispute can be analysed as a **composite** of simple single disputes. If we indicate the expression of doubt with a question mark, we can then characterize the two variants of the basic form of a dispute as follows:

(*a*) Peter: "You should take an aspirin with milk!"
Agnes: "Should I?"

Analysis of (*a*) as a simple single dispute:

party I: +/*p* (party I = Peter)
party II: ?/(+/*p*) (party II = Agnes)

(*b*) Peter: "You should never take an aspirin with milk!"
Agnes: "Shouldn't I?"

Analysis of (*b*) as a simple single dispute:

party I: -/*p* (party I = Peter)
party II: ?/(-/*p*) (party II = Agnes)

It is important to observe that expressing doubt, while it may **accompany** the adoption of the opposite point of view, **is not identical** to propounding the adoption of the opposite point of view. In variant (*a*) of the basic form of dispute, for example, Agnes does not necessarily have to take the position that you should **not** take an aspirin with milk, and in variant (*b*) she does not necessarily have to take the position that you should. Not every dispute must always be compound. Besides **compound multiple disputes** and **compound single disputes**, **simple multiple disputes** and even **simple single disputes** can also occur.

As a dialectical analysis of the confrontation stage of a critical discussion consists of an identification of the type of dispute at the heart of the discussion, the analysis amounts to establishing the exact composition of the conflict of opinion underlying the discussion. Crucial for this is the detection of standpoints, positive or negative, and expressions of doubt, explicit or implicit. When these are known, further analysis is as easy as shelling peas. Unfortunately, in real discourse standpoints and doubts are often only implicated or tacitly assumed, so that serious problems of interpretation may arise.

4. Analysis of a sample of political discourse

Let us now analyse the confrontation stage in a sample of political discourse. For the sake of clarity, in this institutional context I will concentrate on a deliberation of party representatives trying to reach agreement on the question of whether or not to vote for a proposal concerning the abolition of a certain provision of the Act of Settlement. Before revealing their standpoint to the public, they have to reach a unanimous position on the matter, and this means there is no need for them yet to play up to the audience, as politicians so often do, but they must try to even out their differences of opinion. This example is particularly suitable for the things I want to illustrate, the reason being that I made it up for the occasion. I based myself on real life cases, but for demonstrative purposes I have concentrated a number of exemplary peculiarities in one piece of discourse.

Refraining from the peculiarities of oral presentation, this is how the discussion on the Act of Settlement amendment develops:

Mr. Starfield

"How about the Act of Settlement amendment?"

Miss Jones

"I'm all for it."

Mrs. Harrison

"I am not."

Mrs. Williams

I don't know yet. It's not that easy."

Miss Frankel

"Oh, but I'm sure we ought to sustain it."

Mrs. Williams

"Should we, really? I think not. As liberal-minded people, in my opinion, we have to reconsider."

Mr. Parsons

"I would be ashamed if we voted for it."

Mrs. Goulding

"Would you? And why exactly, I wonder?"

Miss Jones

"Our young voters would be very disappointed if we didn't join in."

Mr. Vanderberg

"Speaking of young voters, I'm due to address the Union of Railwaymen next Friday, and they are mostly a rather young lot, so, as this question is in everybody's mind at the moment, it is important to me, or I should rather say to the party as a whole, that I make a clear statement, and it had better not be some kind of pretext for not giving support to the amendment. I can't see why we shouldn't sustain it wholeheartedly. Everybody who thinks otherwise is a blockhead. To put it more carefully: why should we not vote for the amendment?"

Mrs. Harrison

"I would like to vote against the amendment, but that doesn't mean that I'm totally free from doubt. I'm afraid I'm not as sure about my own point of view as some of my political associates seem to be. Maybe I am overlooking something important that tells for the amendment. I could have drawn an overhasty conclusion. Now that I come to think of it I am beginning to wonder. Perhaps I am wrong - as I have been in the past. Could anybody tell what it is that argues for the abolition of the provision?"

Mr. Starfield

"If everybody changes his mind continually we can't possibly come to an agreement."

Mr. Parsons

"Hear, hear!"

Mrs. Harrison

"Isn't that the whole point of a party deliberation?"

Miss Jones

"Don't we want to eliminate abuses? Don't we strive after a fair constitution, without any discriminatory stipulations? Then, why aren't we all, whithout any hesitation, in favour of the proposed amendment?"

Mrs. Goulding (frowning)

"I don't know. I really wonder why we shouldn't vote against it. I really don't know.

Mr. Starfield

"I think we'd better start a formal discussion on this subject. I myself am prepared to be chairman."

At this point the opening stage of the discussion seems about to begin, so I will leave it here.[13] For a dialectical analysis of the confrontation stage of a critical discussion it is necessary to trace the protagonists and the antagonists of the opinions under discussion. There is just one opinion (O) under discussion, viz. the Act of Settlement amendment must be sustained. Some take a positive view with regard to this opinion, some take a negative point of view, and many participants betray their doubts. The assignment of dialectical roles turns out to be as follows:[14]

(a) **protagonist of a positive point of view about O**
Miss Frankel, Miss Jones, Mr. Vanderberg
antagonist of a positive point of view about O
Mrs. Harrison, Mrs. Williams, Mr. Parsons

(b) **protagonist of a negative point of view about O**
Mrs. Harrison, Mrs. Williams, Mr. Parsons
antagonist of a negative point of view about O
Miss Frankel, Miss Jones, Mrs. Goulding, Mrs. Harrison, Mr. Vanderberg

As the dispute as a whole is not resolved until all doubts have disappeared and all participants hold the same view on the disputed opinion, all positions being taken into account, with Miss Frankel, Miss Jones, Mrs. Goulding, Mrs. Harrison and Mr. Vanderberg participating in party I and Mrs. Harrison, Mrs. Williams and Mr. Parsons in party II, whatever the outcome of the discussion, for all concerned a dialectical analysis of the complex dispute to be resolved is as follows:

party I: +/O , ?/(-/O)
party II: ?/(+/O), -/O

This dispute can be characterized as a **compound single dispute**.

Some amplification may be wished for. Let me make a few explanatory remarks.

For one thing, it is important to realize that a dispute by definition entails that a standpoint is being cast into doubt. The parties involved need not necessarily hold contradictory positions (so that the dispute becomes more complex); for a simple dispute it is sufficient that doubt is cast upon the other party's point of view. Not every dispute is a compound one. Mrs. Goulding, for example, in the discussion just reported, does not hold any standpoint of her own, but is, by virtue of the articulation of her doubt, involved in the dispute all the same. Mr. Starfield, on the other hand, does not even venture any doubt and he is therefore not involved in the dispute.

Doubting a point of view is a sufficient but also a necessary condition for a dispute. This means, among other things, that in a technical sense the articulation of a contradictory point of view automatically implies casting doubt upon the point of view contested. Otherwise, by definition there would be no dispute but merely a coincidental externalization of different viewpoints which happen to be contradictory. That would be, so to speak, as if you were to say in Chicago that it is a sunny day today and I say in Amsterdam that it is not, while we are not talking to each other.

Reciprocal doubt must be assumed in the analysis of any compound dispute to do justice to the complex nature of this kind of dispute. Without this assumption the analysis would be as if there were no real dispute at all. Suppose, for instance, that the negative Mrs. Harrison has completely changed her position in favour of a positive point of view, owing to the mere fact that the charming Mr. Vanderberg holds a positive point of view. In that case there is no doubt left and the compound dispute between them has indeed disappeared. This could even be rational if Mr. Vanderberg is a famous expert on the matter concerned. In both cases the dispute comes to a stop in the confrontation stage.[15] With Mr. Vanderberg as party I and Mrs. Harrison as party II, viewed in a dialectical perspective, the situation develops like this:

Mrs. Harrison (party II): -/0
Mr. Vanderberg (party I): ?/(-/0), +/0
Mrs. Harrison (party II): +/0

Therefore, if the compound dispute is to be fully maintained, the dispute must be analysed in this way:

party I: +/0, ?/(-/0) (Frankel, Goulding, Harrison, Jones, Vanderberg)
party II: ?/(+/0), -/0 (Harrison, Parsons, Williams)

Unfortunately, the presentation of standpoints and the expression of doubt are seldom unambiguous. Very often the intended communicative force of utterances and series of utterances is only implicitly indicated and must be made explicit with the help of the verbal and non-verbal context, whether or not institutionally determined, and with the help of other kinds of background knowledge. This may pose some problems for the analysis of discourse, political and otherwise.[16]

One such problem arises when a point of view advanced earlier is repeated, summarized or formulated anew and at the same time rephrased or reworded, so that it is not clear whether a "new" standpoint is being advanced. If this were the case, a previously single dispute may become multiple. This would, for example, be the case if Miss Jones, after having stated her approval of the Act of Settlement amendment, had ventured to say that every sensible person should support the amendment.

Differences of opinion are sometimes difficult to detect. Here insight of an empirical descriptive kind into the verbal and non-verbal cues for interpretation can come in handy.[17] Knowledge of the institutional context can create a well-defined framework for anticipation which facilitated interpretation.[18] A normative model, like our dialectical model of a critical discussion, may play a similar anticipatory role.[19] But that is not what I have chosen to talk about now.

I must confine myself to calling your attention to just one problem of interpretation which is crucial to dialectical analysis. It concerns the difference between an expression of doubt and a negative point of view. These can be difficult to discern, as is shown by the reaction of Mrs. Williams to the positive standpoint of Miss Frankel ("Should we, really?"), but in this case the expression of doubt, as frequently occurs, is followed immediately by a negative statement, so that the expression of doubt acts as a preliminary to the advancing of a negative point of view contradicting a positive statement put forward earlier by the interlocutor.[20] Sometimes the institutional context makes clear that an expression of doubt may be taken as a negative point of view as well, as when a politician in a public debate doubts whether his opponent's standpoints are acceptable.

5. A comparison between dialectical analysis and pure description

As you can see, dialectical analysis clearly differs from so-called pure description. Bearing in mind that even a "pure" description, if it is to be of any significance, has to be theoretically motivated, one must realize that the difference is not just between theory-loaded and not theory-loaded. It is rather a difference between a descriptive record and a normative reconstruction, both equally based on theoretical considerations. The normative perspective, however, as it manifests itself in the dialectical approach to argumentation, by its very nature, has its own characteristic impact. A comparison between dialectical analysis and pure description may show what this distinctive impact results in.

The first difference between a normative reconstruction and a descriptive recording is one of selection. Depending on the criterion of relevance supplied by the theoretical framework serving as a starting point, some data are deemed worth noting while other data are left aside as immaterial. This means that all redundance is removed, so that the discourse can be reported in the dialectical garb of a dialogical tableau.[21] This removal of redundance is why the transformation which has taken place can also be called **deletion**.

The specimen of political discourse quoted earlier provides us with numerous examples of deletion in this sense. Apart from such more superficial phenomena as stammering and hesitation, which were already left out, the analysis leaves out repetitions and paraphrases, and - in my view, more importantly - selects from the utterances made in the discourse only those which have a dialectical role to fulfil in the confrontation stage of a critical discussion. This means that certain speech acts can be excluded beforehand.[22] Abstracting from the persons who play the parts, only the parties involved in the dispute are registered, together with their contributions to the creation of the dispute, without any need to record all speech acts of different persons amounting to the same dialectical contribution.

The second noticeable difference is one of completion. This is partly a question of making explicit, externalizing implicit elements which are required to fill the dialectical gaps, as when by contradicting a standpoint somebody implicitly expresses his doubt with regard to that standpoint. Completion is also partly a question of adding elements whose presence has to be assumed in the case of a fully-fledged dispute of the type implicated by the way the discussion develops, as when somebody defends his position without any attacks being made. Because of this supplementary character, this transformation may also be called **addition**. In compliance with the dialectical theory adhered to, in certain cases the addition may even involve assigning an argumentative communicative force to a constellation of speech acts which seems to lack such force in its literal utterance.[23]

In the discussion quoted earlier, completion is accomplished by addition of statements of doubt where, **expressis verbis**, no doubt is articulated. This applies to the casting of doubt on a positive point of view by persons who put forth a negative point of view against a positive point of view about the same opinion, as Mr. Parsons does indirectly and Mrs. Harrison in a more direct way, when she opposes Miss Jones at the beginning of the discussion, by setting a negative standpoint against the positive point of view of Miss Jones. It also applies, of course, the other way around. But it is even more strongly the case when, in the absence of evidence to the contrary, it is assumed that persons who are contradicted, not only maintain their originally expressed point of view, but also feel doubt about the opposite viewpoints which are posed against theirs.[24]

The third difference between dialectical analysis and pure description to be mentioned here is one of **arrangement**. In contrast to the procedure in a descriptive recording, the normative reconstruction of a dispute need not directly reflect the linear course of events in the sequential order of their actual occurrence. In the dialectical analysis the arrangement is organized in order to bring out as clearly as possible the composition of the dispute, the facts reported corresponding to dialectically relevant factors. Because of the alterations it may bring about, this transformation may also be called **permutation**.

The effects of permutation in the analysis of the political discussion quoted earlier are clear. Abstracting from the individuals who are participating in the dispute and from the order in which their contributions are put forward, an arrangement is made in accordance with dialectical party membership. Thus Miss Frankel, Miss Jones and Mr. Vanderberg, for instance, are put together as protagonists of a positive point of view about the Act of Settlement amendment and Mrs. Harrison, Mrs. Williams and Mr. Parsons as protagonists of a negative point of view. The order in which they expressed their positions is immaterial to the analysis. The same holds for the order in which different aspects of the position of the same person (doubts and standpoints) are expressed, as long as it does not affect this position.[25]

The fourth and last difference I will mention is one of **notation**. It is completely in line with the points just made to provide for an adequate notation of the analysis. It is advisable to report the findings in such a way that the things which are theoretically noteworthy are expressed clearly. Similar cases need to be recognizable as similar, dialectically relevant distinctions need to be easily identifiable, and so on. In order for a comparison to be possible, it is necessary to create a notation system and reformulate the various contributions to the dispute in terms of this system.[26] In consequence of this procedure diffuse and ambiguous wordings have to be replaced by standard formulations. For this reason this transformation can also be called **substitution**. Different ways of expressing which, dialectically speaking, amount to the same thing, have one and the same substitute, so that identical cases are treated alike. In a purely descriptive notation differences of expression are maintained and dialectical similarities may easily escape attention.

In the analysis under consideration the notational differences are immediately clear from the use of question marks, parentheses, plus and minus signs, and slants. They reflect the effort being made to standardize the formulation. In addition to this, however, it must be recognized that non-relevant differences of expression in the analysis are also abolished. Mr. Parson's indirect speech act "I would be ashamed if we voted for it", which means something like "The Act of Settlement amendment must not be supported", for example, is treated in exactly the same way as Mrs. Harrison's "I am not", which is - for our purposes - equivalent to it.

6. Some advantages of normative reconstruction

I opened my exposition with a plea for a normative extension of the description of discourse, exemplified in the dialectical approach to argumentation. Subsequently I discussed some of the characteristics of dialectical analysis, confining myself to the identification of the type of dispute characterizing the confrontation stage of a critical discussion. The analytical instrument was applied to a specimen of political discourse, the purpose of this exemplary analysis being to compare dialectical analysis with pure description. The remaining question is: what might be the advantages of this normative reconstruction of the dispute?

These advantages are mainly of two kinds: **surveyability**

and **discernment**. The increase in both stems from the selection, completion, arrangement and notation which are the result of analysis. Especially in more complex discourse the transformations of deletion, addition, permutation and substitution can alter an inextricable tangle into a clear picture of the very thing we are looking for. Something of this is already evident in the analysis of the Act of Settlement discussion.[27]

For example, it is noteworthy that the analysis of the complex discussion reported clarifies the dispute under discussion. It explains what exactly the points of difference are, as far as these differences are maintained during the confrontation stage and eventually constitute the dispute to be resolved. Doubt which no longer exists need not give cause for argumentation and the same holds, **mutatis mutandis**, for points of view which are already abandoned.

The analysis of the confrontation stage also gives us insight into the particular positions of the discussants with regard to the various components of the dispute and the likeliest distribution of roles in the dialectical role play resulting from it. It supplies us with an overview of the commitments which each of the discussants has accepted in advancing his own statements. Someone who has advanced a positive point of view about an opinion has thereby accepted a positive commitment with regard to that opinion and someone who has advanced a negative point of view, a negative commitment, while someone who has expressed doubt has accepted no commitment at all. A positive commitment may lead to an obligation to defend a positive point of view (if challenged) and a negative commitment to an obligation to defend a negative point of view (if challenged). An expression of doubt creates no obligation at all, whether conditional or unconditional.

The analysis of the confrontation stage makes it possible to check afterwards (preferably in the concluding stage) to what extent the dispute has been resolved and in so far as this is not the case, what components are not resolved. In this way it can be established what the remaining obligations are, and whose duty it is to oblige. This helps to solve the burden of proof problem and may prevent the fallacy of **shifting the burden of proof**. A protagonist who does not acknowledge that, because he has voluntarily advanced a point of view which has been called into question by the antagonist, the burden of proof with regard to that point of view rests on him, retreats from a discussion in which his point of view can be tested critically. And a protagonist who tries to evade his burden of proof by passing it on to the antagonist is guilty of the fallacy of shifting the burden of proof. This fallacy of forcing the other party to suggest a better proof if an alleged proof is not admitted, is also called (by Locke) the **argumentum ad ignorantiam.** It occurs in its strongest form when from the fact that it is not possible, or seems not to be possible, to justify a positive point of view about an opinion, the conclusion is drawn that the contradictory negative point of view must hold, or vice versa. Especially in the case of a compound dispute, it is necessary to take care that this unjustified simplification does not take place. Just as an adequate analysis of the confrontation stage prevents a multiple dispute from not being recognized as such (or a single dispute from being regarded as multiple), the analysis prevents a compound dispute from being regarded as simple, or the other way round, so that the analysis can act as a fallacy-detecting safeguard in the evaluation of the discussion.

The approach to argumentation in political discourse and other kinds of discourse that is proposed here is profitable to discussants and potential discussants, and also to people who act as chairpersons or who, as supervisors or otherwise, have an interest in the quality of discussions. Practitioners of speech communication, in particular, will want to take this interest to heart. That is why I was so bold as to draw your attention to dialectical analysis of argumentation.

Notes

1. Many recent publications bear witness of this attention. To name just a few interesting ones: Clark and Clark (1977), Cole (1981), Edmondson (1981), Leech (1983), Levinson (1983), Searle, Kiefer and Bierwisch (1980). Cf. also Verschueren's bibliography (1978) and its annual supplements in **Journal of Pragmatics.**

2. Cf. for instance **Mental Models** by Johnson-Laird (1983) and **Discourse Analysis** by Stubbs (1983).

3. See Van Eemeren, Grootendorst and Meuffels (1984).

4. Especially not if the research is part of a more-embracing research program.

5. See Russell (1968).

[6]. Cf. Barth and Krabbe (1982: 19-22) and Van Eemeren and Grootendorst (1984: 134).
[7]. In fact I can only give a glimpse of a preliminary round of the real thing, for as I will explain argumentation is put forward in the 'argumentation stage' of a critical discussion, while I must confine myself here to a preceding stage, the 'confrontation stage'.
[8]. Cf. Van Eemeren and Grootendorst (1984: 18), Van Eemeren, Grootendorst and Kruiger (1984: 7) and Krabbe in Barth and Martens (1982: 123-132).
[9]. Note that words like **standpoint** and **doubt** are used here as technical terms in a dialectical theory, not necessarily referring to any well-delineated 'psychological state' of the language users playing their parts in the dialectical role-play, although they may also be regarded as 'psycho-pragmatical primitives'.
[10]. For a more extensive account of this view, see Van Eemeren and Grootendorst (1984).
[11]. This is explained in Van Eemeren and Grootendorst (1984) and Van Eemeren, Grootendorst and Kruiger (1983).
[12]. Cf. Barth and Krabbe (1982) and Van Eemeren and Grootendorst (1984).
[13]. Systematic demarcation of the stages is facilitated by reliance on a well-defined framework of a dialectical theory about the development of a critical discussion.
[14]. For the sake of brevity I have refrained from a textual justification of the assignment of dialectical roles.
[15]. In my opinion it is an interesting task for discourse analysts to examine the ways in which in real discourse confrontation is sought or, for that matter, averted.
[16]. Cf. Van Eemeren, Grootendorst and Kruiger (1983). Of course, in this paper I can not deal with the many problems of interpretation which may arise.
[17]. That is why I think it important for those who want to improve speech communication systematically to participate in empirical research like that reported in Van Eemeren, Grootendorst and research like that reported in Van Eemeren, Grootendorst and Meuffels (1984).
[18]. Cf., among others, Schank and Abelson (1977).
[19]. Cf. Van Eemeren and Grootendorst (1984).
[20]. Other problems arise, for example, from the fact that standpoints are often put forward in an indirect way ("Wouldn't it be better to stop?") and from the fact that the non-explicit stating of a positive standpoint is often

indistinguishable from mere informing ("Learning French is more difficult than learning Dutch").

[21]. Cf. Beth (1962) and Barth and Krabbe (1982) for formal dialogical tableaux. This notion is here interpreted in a rather informal way, as in Van Eemeren and Grootendorst (1984). As I confine myself in this paper to characterizing the type of dispute, in this case the question of dialogical tableau notation does not really come up.

[22]. For a detailed discussion of this cf. Van Eemeren and Grootendorst (1984).

[23]. Cf. Van Eemeren and Grootendorst (1984: 117) and Van Eemeren, Grootendorst and Kruiger (1983: 139-144) for the 'strategy of maximum argumentative interpretation'.

[24]. To say nothing of the rather more complicated possibility of completing some arguments by making explicit unexpressed arguments with a complex structure, as is sometimes necessary when analysing the argumentation stage of a critical discussion.

[25]. As the same person, like Mrs. Harrison, may belong to different dialectical parties at the same time, no permutation is called for in that case. It is quite another matter that such a position will be difficult to maintain.

[26]. Cf. Van Eemeren and Grootendorst (1984) and also Van Eemeren, Grootendorst and Kruiger (1983).

[27]. It must be stressed that each dialectical transformation has its own specific advantages to offer, but for the sake of brevity I cannot explain those here in full detail.

COMMENTS ON FRANS VAN EEMEREN

Arrie van Berkel

In Wim Wender's film **Room 666** in which film-directors explained their ideas about the future of cinematography, Jean Luc Godard declared that a movie is nothing but the representation of a reality that does not exist. From an epistemological point of view this contradictory statement is rather puzzling and therefore needs further explanation. This need is also felt when Frans van Eemeren (henceforth: FvE) emphazises his empirical attitude towards the normative description of language use whereas his demonstration of such a description is based on a constructed discussion. Epistemologically the relation between the dialogue and its description according to the theoretical and normative rules must be clarified.

In several of his publications Popper has developed his Three-World Theory, assuming the existence of three subworlds of knowledge: the first world of physical objects, the second world of mental states and the third world of "objective contents of thought" being "theories in themselves, and their logical relations" (Popper 1974: 106). As this third world is also the world of poetic thought and works of art, we may include movies following Godard's definition, which we might re-interpret so that a movie is a third-world object that is not the representation of the first world but of the second. This agrees with Popper's remark that the relation between the first and the third world can only be made through the second world (Popper 1974: 155).

In applying this global framework to FvE's paper we need an explicit statement about the relation between the theoretically-contructed norms and the language used in the real world of physical objects. I assume that the link between those worlds is something that Labov called the Consensus Principle (Labov 1975). As long as we agree that mental representations of physical events are able to replace the real events, nothing can be brought against it, even when we know that the reality thus represented does not exist. Most linguistic material presented in order to be analyzed can be classified as pseudo-empirical, that is: we act as if it is empirical in a strict sense.

FvE's paper begins with a question that is strongly connected with the point mentioned above: what to do when reality does not come up to a standard? If such a standard or norm is part of a theoretical system that is consistent in itself (cf. the third world), then we need our mental world as a mediator to reality in the physical-empirical sense. In my opinion argumentation theory, being a set of more or less formalized systematic intuitions, leads downward to common intuitions about how language behaviour in discussions ought to be. A serious problem arises when pseudo-empirical data are used as empirical evidence for the correctness of both kinds of intuitions. This also leads to the widely known problem that language behaviour can not be described according to the rules so that an intuitive-interpretative transformation must be carried out. Let us assume that pseudo-empirical data are constructed according to the rules from a reality that does not exist at all. In this connection Mr. Starfield's proposal "I think we'd better start a formal discussion on this subject" is quite remarkable in FvE's political discussion.

When we look at FvE's normative description of the dispute, then the results are rather poor, even when we realize that the dispute under consideration is only the confrontation stage of a full dispute. At the very point where disputes become more and more complicated, and that is just the point where normative descriptions fail, Mr. Starfield is speaking his immortal words. FvE's remark that "if the compound dispute is to be fully maintained, the dispute must be analyzed in this way (...)" is not convincing, on the one hand because the presentations "are seldom unambiguous" (FvE), on the other hand because it is not clear what else the participants could add. I must admit, however, that FvE proved elsewhere that a normative dialectical approach can be extremely useful as a tool to decompose complex discussions for evaluative reasons and as the provisional basis for a set of maxims that enable participants to control their argumentative conduct (Van Eemeren & Grootendorst 1984).

Another limitation in FvE's approach, and in argumentation

theory in general, is the absence of a theory about cognition and actions. Argumentative behaviour is treated in isolation from situation and context merely as a set of independent normative rules. When FvE's concept about language use is also one of "goal-directed behaviour", then it is to be expected that argumentative moves will be treated as goal-directed actions, e.g. what language devices participants use to what ends, or what do participants do with words even beyond the level of speech acts (cf. Van Eemeren & Grootendorst 1984). In this way I will elaborate FvE's example as a sort of counter-demonstration.

According to FvE it is situationally given that the participants have to achieve a unanimous standpoint towards the voting dichotomy whether to vote for the amendment or (exclusively) against it. This goal, that need not be shared by all participants, generally requires an action focus of cooperation and persuasion. The participants have to focus on agreement and not on adversability. Theoretically, the participants may adopt three goal-directed attitudes: (1) voting for, (2) not voting for (= voting against), and (3) other goals or not clear. Other goals may be not voting at all or divided individual voting. The third attitude is realized when participants express doubts about a goal-directed opinion without expressing their own goal-directed opinion. I agree with FvE that expressions of doubt need much attention in a dialectical description, and I also agree that doubters keep themselves free from obligations. Doubts express planned or unplanned absence of goal-directed behaviour, and under the action focus of cooperation it may be considered dereliction that serves other (noncooperative) goals (cf. Rehbein 1977: 299ff.). In this dispute however the doubters may be object of the persuasive actions carried on by the goalsetters. A global action scheme of the dispute in which FvE's categories have been adopted, may look as Fig. 1 (see pag.323).

Note that the positions need not necessarily be equal to positions of individual participants. A participant may act goal-less as a tactic for achieving a tacit goal. The action scheme involves two possible action patterns: A persuades both B and C, and B persuades both A and C, or A and B persuade C but not each other. In the last case A and B have to act adversatively towards each other which leaves out their cooperative focus of action. The complexity of the constellation will increase if position C is taken by par-

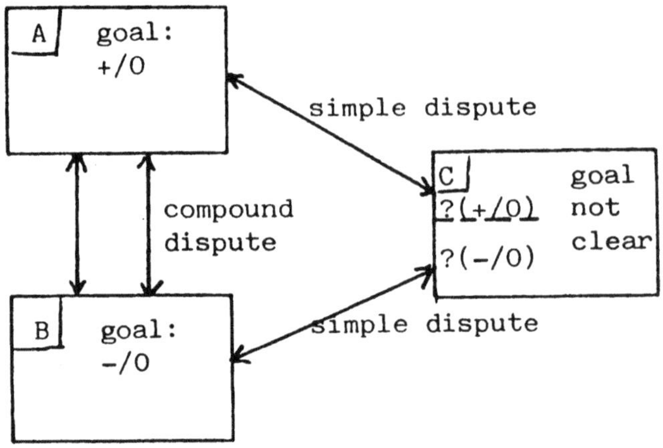

ticipants as a strategy to achieve goal (+/0) or (-/0). Such a fifth column of discussants in political discourse looks rather common to me.

If we take a closer look at the goals and doubts as they are expressed, then the following observations can be made:

(1) from position A some global results of goal (+/0) are summed up as arguments;

(2) from position B a subgoal ("reconsidering") is proposed twice (by Williams and Harrison) and a personal global result ("I should be ashamed if we voted for (+/0)")

The outcome of the confrontation stage is that the subgoal as proposed from position B has been implicitly accepted. This outcome may be normatively correct, but it is in fact very improbable in real-life discussions.

This global and loose description of a decision-making process that never took place, roughly shows that dialectical normative descriptions become richer when they are connected with goal-determined positions that participants could possibly take. It stresses the assumption that dialectics as expressed by participants in real discussions not only represent argumentative patterns but also goal-directed action patterns.

13
Political interviews

T. Ensink

Political interviews play an important role in society, both in establishing the 'image' of politics and politicians, and in informing (and disinforming, for that matter) the public. In view of this fact, it is surprising to see that little research has been done on political interviews in their quality of speech events. To be sure, political language has been the object of inquiry many times, but it is mainly studied from a rhetorical or critical point of view. In a rhetorical perspective, political language is seen in its persuasive function; here it is often noted that political language is similar in function to the language of advertising (Hudson, 1978). In a critical perspective, political language is evaluated against some standard; standards are found in ideology (as in Marxism, e.g. Pateman, 1975), in general concepts such as 'truth' or 'credibility' (e.g. Orwell, 1946; Hudson, 1978), or in a general question pertaining to some field of analysis, as in the sociological question of why the status quo of inequal distribution of wealth and income is so readily accepted (Edelman, 1977).

Linguistically the most interesting analyses of political language are conducted by British critical linguists (Fowler et al., 1979; Kress and Trew, 1978; Kress and Hodge, 1981). In general, their analyses presuppose a Whorfian idea about the ideological function of language. In detail, they analyze language materials on the basis of a functional approach (borrowed mainly from Halliday); they try to show how options made at the level of the ideational function affect ideological pre-suppositions concerning the 'facts' talked about.

As far as language is concerned, these studies either address political language on a general cultural level, or on the detailed level of lexical and syntactic structures. I think, however, that important aspects of the functioning of political language can be found on a different level: interaction and negotiation processes in which political matters are discussed; contextual and cognitive presuppositions that are fundamental to political discourse. In this paper, I want to discuss a few phenomena on this level, the level of discourse analysis. I will concentrate on political interviews.

The term 'political interview' denotes a type of speech event (Hymes, 1972) or an activity type (Levinson, 1979). The term 'interview' as such refers to a conversation between a reporter and one from whom he seeks information; in the speech event two active participants are involved (as roles; there can be more than one person per role): the Interviewer (Ir) and the Interviewee (Ie). The general goal of the speech event is that Ir obtain some information from Ie, either for himself, but mostly in behalf of a public. This creates interactional rights and duties for Ir and Ie, and it presupposes a specific distribution of knowledge between Ir and Ie, or between Ie and the public. A political interview is one in which Ie has (or eventually had) some political function. Typically, political interviews are held in order to inform the public about the performing of this function by the politician. The public is, generally speaking, the people represented by the politician.

At this point, some clarifications are called for.

First of all,it makes a great difference in which 'political culture' an interview takes place. In a totalitarian political culture, there is hardly any freedom for Ir to ask what he wants to ask; here, the interview is just one other medium in the hands of the leaders in order to get their points of view across. The medium cannot be critical or revealing. This can be different in a democratic political culture, but not necessarily so; in Western democracies deals are very often made between Ir and Ie as to which questions can be asked (or, if they are asked, which can be shown to the public). Furthermore, interviews can be refused if, for whatever reason, Ie does not like to be interviewed. Nevertheless: where there is, both legally and practically, freedom of press, political interviews are such that Ie, by entering into the interaction of the interview, is obliged to go along to the end of the interaction, without being able to take other punitive measures than refusing to answer questions or in the last resort refusing to finish the interview. In democracies there can furthermore be an important difference in the organization of the democracy, and hence in the type of political function about which politicians can be interviewed; there can be differences as for direct presidential elections or indirect ones: one-party majorities or coalitions between several parties.

Secondly, the channel through which the interview is presented to the public, can be either direct or indirect. If the channel is direct (as in radio or television broadcasting) the public is able to witness directly the interaction between Ir and Ie. If the channel is indirect (the written press) the public should depend on the way the interview is mediated by the reporter, typically Ir. The importance of the directness of the channel is demonstrated in the different judgement of the Kennedy - Nixon-debates by people who watched the debate on television, in comparison with those who listened to it on the radio (Chaffee, 1978: 331). I will restrict my discussion to the direct channel, because I want to concentrate on directly observable discourse structures.

Thirdly, the relationship between Ir and Ie can vary. Ir can be a political adherent of Ie (even to the extent of licking his boots), or Ir can be a political adversary. As a consequence, the interaction in the interview can vary from harmless questioning to an occasional debate or verbal combat.

Finally, interviews can vary as to the political functions of Ie, and as to the political issues to be addressed. Each variation has implications for the extent to which the politician might want to show himself, and for the kind of questions that can be asked. The political function of Ie can vary from regional to national, or even international; from legislative to executive functions; from being in power to being in opposition; and from being in office to being out of office (as in the case of the Nixon-interviews after his resignation). - The issues to be talked about in the interview can range from current, pertaining to the day (as in press conferences or in short interviews made for the daily newsreel), to general conversations in which the politician is to be portrayed and in which principles of his policy are to be discussed.

I will now discuss a few aspects of the discourse analysis of political interviews. I will illustrate my discussion with a few examples from the political scene of the Netherlands.[1]

As I have indicated, political interviews have inherently three participants: Ir, Ie, and the public. Ir and Ie are the jointly acting participants, and their interaction is constrained by the public: Ir represents the public in expressing what it wishes to know, and Ie is providing this desired information. At least, this is the ideal picture.

The relationship between Ie and the public, however, makes this picture more complicated: 1. As a representative of the public, the politician is obliged to account for his policies; many policies, however, have sensitive spots that ask for secrecy. 2. The public itself is not a monolithic, undifferentiated whole. Part of the public consists of adversaries, part of allies, part of rank and file. Different parts of the public have different interests in certain policies. 3. The interview itself can play a role in the execution of policies (as exemplified by the interview (October 1984) of the Soviet leader Chernienko given to an American reporter; an official reaction to this interview was given two days later by Secretary of State Shultz).

These considerations explain why the political interview is not a straightforward interaction (if ever any is). The interview is most straightforward in its 'technical' functioning qua interview, i.e. that Ir and Ie both know and expect from each other to participate in an interaction in which Ir has the right to ask questions and Ie the interactional obligation to answer these questions. On this level, a cooperation principle is in operation between Ir and Ie (Grice, 1975). In other respects, however, political interviews do not necessarily have a cooperative character. (An argument in favor of the view that political interviews are essentially cooperative is provided, on the basis of data from Israeli television, by Blum-Kulka 1983). The participants, especially Ie, are not in the same way interested in a smooth flow of information; Grice's maxims are not fully operative (cf. Bolinger, 1980; Lakoff, 1982). The public (or parts of it) have many strong preferences, or strong aversions, to specific sorts of information. The politician on the other hand has a great interest in presenting information which is favorable to his policy (or to keep silent about sensitive aspects of it).

I will now consider **Example 1.** In lines 1 and 2 Ie points out that a specific formulation ("it can be talked about now"; the original Dutch expression bears a strong connotation that what can be talked about was previously a taboo topic) used by the rival political party of the Christian Democrats amounts to a furtive, maybe even mendacious, way of putting things. A few minutes later in the interview, however, Ir is asking what the Labor party -of which Ie is the leader- is going to do after the next elections (in 1986), in view of the fact that Ie has stated in line 13 that the Labor party is going to "contribute to prevent" the construction of new nuclear power plants. It may be the case that the planning is implemented already, and what is the Labor party going to do about it? Now it is important to know that in the Dutch political situation no party has a chance of getting an absolute majority in elections. A coalition has to be formed if a party wants to get into power. Now, when pressed by Ir to say what the Labor party is going to do when it will be in power, the statement made in lines 12-13, 'the Labor party will contribute to prevent it' is changed into: 'the Labor party will insist on reconsideration of such a decision' (lines 30-31). Because Ir2 takes over and changes the topic of the interview, the point isn't pressed further. But Ir could have made a similar point as the one Ie made about the Christian Democrats in lines 1-2: 'insist on reconsideration' means: 'you will ultimately accept the decision but you won't tell it'.

Now Ie is not utterly self-contradictory by stating both 13 and 30-31: 'to contribute to prevent it' and 'insist on reconsideration' are not necessarily incompatible formulations. The motives behind the two formulations, and inferences that can be made from these formulations, however, are incompetible. The reaction of the audience after line 13 (a rather massive applause) shows that the audience consists of adherents of the Labor party, or in any case of opponents of the use of nuclear energy. To them, to this considerable part of the electorate (according to reliable counts, more than 50% of the Dutch public) the statement in line 13 is addressed: the ultimate rationale of this statement, is to be in accord with this part of the electorate.

The rationale of line 31 is quite different. If the Labor party wants to get into power after the elections, the Christian Democrats are the most likely partner (at least, traditionally they are) to form a coalition with. For this reason, they cannot be put off too bluntly: the antagonistic attitude of the Labor party in the nuclear energy debate cannot be put in absolute terms. So, looking back from line 31 to line 13, it can be seen that line 31 really means: 'will contribute to prevent it, not, however, do everything to prevent it'. But this is not the way line 13 was intended. Materially, lines 13 and 31 are compatible, in their intended consequences they are not.

How can an interpretation like this be warranted? Discourse in political interviews is to be treated as discourse by partial informants (cf. May 1981). Generally, speech in discourse is treated as cooperative discourse. Speech of partial informants is not cooperative in the sense in which Grice (1975) used this word: participants are willing to participate in a verbal encounter, and they intend all their contributions to be "such as is required, at the stage at which it occurs, by the accepted purpose or direction of the talk exchange in which/they/are engaged" (Grice 1975: 45). In normal conditions, this cooperative principle leads to the obedience to a set of maxims. Violations of these maxims by the speaker lead to inferential processes, under the assumption that the cooperative principle is still being followed. The speaker intends these violations as an invitation to these inferential processes.

May (1981) has analyzed discourse in which (one of) the participants is/are partial (meaning both incomplete and biased, May 1981: 56). He proposes a set of maxims for the interpretation of this type of discourse.[2] These maxims are not on a par with the maxims proposed by Grice:

1. Grice's maxims are essentially speaker's maxims: the speaker is following or possibly violating, the maxims; the speaker's behavior yields grounds for interpretation. May's maxims are interpreter's maxims: they tell the interpreter what can be inferred from observed verbal behavior (but this behavior is not intended to lead to these inferences).
2. Underlying both sets of maxims are different assumptions. Grice's maxims are based on cooperativeness, May's on partiality. As a consequence, to choose one or the other set of maxims as a basis for interpretation, means that one makes different assumptions about the psychological attitude of the speaker: if the speaker can be supposed to have rather strong motives and/or interests which force him to speak in a certain direction, he can be supposed to speak partially and not cooperatively.
3. Grice's maxims presuppose the credibility of the speaker: he is cooperative. May's maxims do not presuppose credibi-

lity; the maxims are intended to make possible an assessment of what can be believed or not. The speaker can be believed in what he actually states. Inferences from what the speaker says that could be believed in a cooperative context, should not be believed.

In politics, information that is generally accessible from the press and media about the actual political situation, provides a basis on which motives and interests of politicians can be 'calculated': the kind of interest they have in statements of one type or another, has to be inferred from this general knowledge.

The fact that partners in a political interview are cooperative only to a certain extent, has further consequences. In most speech situations, a mutual attitude of face preservation exists (cf. Goffman 1967; Brown and Levinson 1978). In the case of the political interview, however, there is more to this than just trying to be nice and polite to each other. To be sure, as argued before, in the technical sense of the interview qua interview, normal discourse conditions hold. Questions are asked, or interruptions are made, with due payment to (negative) face (e.g., Example 1, line 17).

But in other respects political interviews show peculiarities of their own. Politicians have a strong tendency to putting up the best face they can, and to trying to put the face of adversaries as far down as possible. This can be done directly, by straightforwardly railing at the adversaries or indirectly, by showing defects in the line of action that is taken by the adversaries (remember that face is inherently tied up with the line of action one takes, cf. Goffman 1967). The most effective, of course, is the indirect way: one does not insult directly but leaves it to the public to find the proper qualifications for the now exposed bad actions of the adversary. Of course, Ie can only do this to the extent to which it is deemed justified by Ir and the public.

More important, however, is the way in which face is connected with the action scheme of the political interview: the way in which individual speech acts in the interview are considered to be a face threatening action (cf. Brown and Levinson 1978: 70-73. The basic structure of the interview is a series of questions of Ir, answered by Ie (or topics determined by Ir, commented upon by Ie). The nature of the interview itself legitimizes the questions of Ir, provided that they do not touch upon issues that are out of order. In other words: the nature of the interview compensates for the face threatening aspects of the questions. Ie, on the other hand, is interactionally obliged to answer the questions. But in many cases Ie is not willing to answer. Ie is not in a position to claim consideration with his face: as a public functionary, he does not have too much of a 'negative face', a safe and granted territory of his own. So, evasive strategies have to be used, or answers have to be refused with a specific legitimization; e.g. the interests of the state, promises of secrecy or confidentiality made to others involved, the fact that an answer might endanger some current affair, or lack of competency.[3] The strongest strategy however is to give an answer which is after all no answer at all. Because of the complexity of politics, this strategy is not difficult to follow. It is easy to comment upon an issue associated with the question, in such a way that the answer shows connectedness with the question without however answering it; a sensitive answer has been avoided.

Ir has to choose, in this case, between either swallowing the answer, or insisting upon a true answer to the question. If Ir takes his job seriously, he should insist. But this it not easy. Ir runs the risk of being tricked out a second time, or being rebuffed. To insist for the third time may very well give the impression of being pedantic, disputatious or insolent. The public does not always like the truth-hunter, the public often likes decent good manners. And Ir runs the risk of not being backed up by the superiors of the broadcasting organization for which he is working.

I will consider now Examples 2 and 3, in which a lenient and a stubborn Ir are involved, respectively. (I have pointed out already that in Ex. 1 after line 31 Ir drops the issue which is not yet fully clear.)

In Ex. 2, the Dutch Prime Minister is questioned about his alleged mixing up of private and state affairs. During his official visit to Kuwait, it is told, he has brought up problems concerning the payment of almost 25 million dollars (60 million Hfl.) to the concern of which he is a major stockholder. Ir brings up this issue, but not by asking whether the allegations are true or not, but by indicating that such a line of action would be, in his opinion, just efficient. The only utterly marked question that Ir asks is: 'Isn't this possible in politics?' (line 7) The way this question is framed can be interpreted in 2 ways:

1. Ir knows that it is inadmissible to act as the Prime

Minister allegedly has done, according to regulations which prohibit politicians to have incompatible political and private functions. He frames his question however in such a way that this action seems a harmless, natural thing to do. The Prime Minister is invited to agree (or: to explain why this point of view is not correct) but if he would do so, he would expose himself as not acting according to the rules of political decency.

2. The question can be interpreted at face value: Ir does not know that these regulations exist (or: he assumes that the public does not know), and his opinion is that it would be a normal and efficient way of acting.

For 3 reasons, this second interpretation can be assumed to be correct:

1. Ir's attitude in the rest of the interview is very lenient toward the views presented by Ie (look at lines 23 and 29-30: in 23 Ir is eager to accept an excuse; in 30 he assumes the incorrectness of suspicions);

2. Ir does not ask a question that is sensible to ask in view of Ie's answer; did Ie have prior knowledge of or responsibility for the visit of Junior Minister Bolkestein when he drew the attention of the Kuwaitis to the problems of the business concern of Ie's family?;

3. According to a newspaper article published a few days after this interview,[4] there had been an earlier version in which the Prime Minister answered this same question in a way that could easily be understood as being affirmative. Under pressure of the State Information Service Ir agreed to do the interview a second time.

Notwithstanding this pliable (to the point of bootlicking) attitude of Ir, Ie takes the issue of allegedly mixing up state and private affairs to be the real question to which he should react. Instead of giving a straightforward affirmation or denial, the answer is framed in a wordy way in which many related topics are brought up: it belongs to state visits to take care of business interests, although not this business; it was already put to the attention of the Kuwaitis in an earlier visit by a secretary of state; the Kuwaitis brought it up themselves; it has to be left to experts; it is better not to discuss the contents of the problem. The answer is not completely clear; what can be inferred is: because I did not bring it up myself I am not responsible. On the other hand: we have made procedural appointments and this belongs to my job. Ir never presses for a completely clear answer, but accepts the inferences of innocence.

In Ex. 3 is shown what happens interactionally if Ir takes on an aggressive rather than pliable attitude. This particular Ir has a reputation of having no consideration whatever with his Interviewees. His approach is, to ask for principles that are valid in politics, and then how they are put into practice. Questions that are asked by him do not just ask for information, but they presuppose information. The questions themselves are directed to attitudes toward and consequences of this information.

In Ex. 3, Ie is the minister of social affairs, member of the Christian Democratic party, and known to have a Calvinistic conviction. This fragment is from an interview in which already during 1/2 hour Ir and Ie have discussed the political consequences of a Christian conviction, and principles of justice. Because Ie is minister of social affairs, he is responsible in the first place for the cutting down on welfare. In this rather extensive fragment, Ir is questioning Ie why people on welfare have to pay, while the circuit of black money is almost left free. This question is related to the minister's Christian convictions (1-5). Ie does not address the question concerning his principles, but he answers pragmatically: fraud is difficult to discover, and fraud is stimulated by high tax pressure (5-15). Ir however does not accept the first part of this answer: he alleges that in the official policy the battle against fraud never had a high priority and Ir quotes official functionaries on this issue (15-23). Ie answers by pointing out once more that there is not enough personnel for fighting against fraud while fraud is difficult to discover, and once more pointing to the fact of the heavy burden of taxes (23-35). Now, in 35, Ir insists on his initial question (asked in 1-5), and he reformulates the same question (36-44). Ie starts his answer with a remark on what is said in the Bible about thieves, associatively connected to the last words of Ir. Once more Ie points out that there are limited possibilities for fighting against fraud (47). Ir immediately takes this remark as a starting point for repeating that official policy was never interested in the battle against fraud (48-49). Ie argues that the attention has grown ever since the extent of fraud has grown, and that measures are needed: more personnel, but especially more control (51-56). More control, however, is socially unwanted. Justice however forces to choose for more control (56-60). Ir makes his point by comparing this approach to the control already exerted on the people who have to live on a minimum welfare income. In contrast, he gives an inventory of possibilities of practising fraud (61-65). Ie admits that fraud exists on too large a scale (66-68). Now, once again Ir insists on his initial question. Since Ie has admitted the extent of fraud, Ir asks the almost rhetorical question: 'How do you corrupt' if you admit this and at the same time are cutting down on the money for the poorest (68-71). Ie does not accept this way of putting things: the financing of the welfare state is one thing, the battle against fraud another, and you fight against fraud because it is evil, not in order to get the welfare state financed (71-77).

In this fragment, Ir is pressing his point very strongly. This is shown not only in his insistence on the same question three times over, but also in his interruptions during Ie's turns at each moment at which Ir disagrees (lines 35, 48, 58, 60 and 68); and it is shown in the strong way of formulating his points of view: Ir has no consideration whatsoever with the face of Ie: his rhetorical use of the term 'christian politician' (5), the reproving way of indicating not to have received an answer (35-36), the almost explicit accusation of being corrupt (68).

Nevertheless, nowhere is a direct answer given by Ie to the three times repeated question. Ie makes clear, however, on which point he does not want to accept the presuppositions on which the question is based: the two issues of fighting against fraud and financing the welfare state should be kept separate. This means, ultimately, that the huge amounts of money involved in both issues, do not directly bear upon each other, as Ir would have it, and should be kept separate in decisions about policy.

The strategy that is followed by Ir is about the strongest that can be imagined. No respect other than formal is shown to threaten Ie's face to a far greater extent than is possiformation to the contrary can be brought in, it is done by Ir. Ir insists on getting an answer to the questions he asks. The strategy shows that the Interviewer can afford to threaten Ir's face to a far greater extent than is possible in many other discourse types. The strategy seems to be overpowered, however, if one considers where it leads the Ir. These interviews are not very popular. Not every politician is willing to enter into these interviews. And these interviews are received by many as being offensive, pedantic and selfrighteous, while Ir is seen as a man who is not looking for information but knows already what he should think, and who pretends to have the position of a public prosecutor.

Interviews like Ex. 3 are not comparable to the first two fragments, which are taken from interviews where Ir just tries to get information from Ie. The borderline between 'interview' and 'argumentative debate' is almost obliterated in Ex. 3. Nevertheless, Ex. 3 shows an interview in the sense that the conversation has its prime value not because of the intrinsic value of the arguments, but because Ie is an important public person. Ir and Ie are not on a par as in the case of a debate. And the goal of the conversation is not to reach a solution, but to put Ie in the position in which he is forced - because he is confronted not just with questions, but with an opposite world view from which politics is investigated - to show in which way the political world is put together and which political actions should be, and can be, undertaken, and why.

Political interviews are one of the most frequently used ways of providing information about the political world, which destines to a large extent the lives of everybody. The important question is what the quality is of the information that is provided in this way. The information should be verifiable. The information is provided not just in propositions or in statements, but in the interactional and textual structures of discourse as well. Political discourse is sponging to a large extent on the everyday cooperative type of conversational discourse: there is a pretense that we are sitting happily together, that you like me and I like you, that I believe you because you are a nice hard-working person. From this pretense, politicians try to get part of their credibility.

The central problem is one of power and of knowledge, and their relation. Politicians are the people who usually possess the best part of both. Ideally, from the point of view of democracy, both should be shared as far as possible with the people that are represented - the public.

Now, what relevance does discourse analysis have?

In general, the problem is how insights gained from interactional analysis, can be implemented into interaction. There is the mind with its subconscious and conscious, and its automatically functioning, parts. The mind lets people act in interaction in a certain way. It would be too simple to suppose that knowledge gained from analysis of this interaction, can be provided to the mind in a straightforward way, so as to play a desired and controlled role in subsequent interaction.

More specifically, power structures in politics, or policies, are not directly influenced by interviews. Discourse analysis can just show the way in which politicians present themselves and their policies in discourse. Such an analysis could yield a few guide-lines for interviewers:

- Do not accept the presented line-and-face too readily; insist on getting an answer to your questions;
- Always analyze which presuppositions are being made, and which knowledge is presupposed. If a presupposition does not seem to be warranted, mention it, and give reasons for it. If the public in general has no access to this knowledge, mention it.

Subsequently, it should be analyzed what the interactional results of these guide-lines are.

Discourse analysis can be the most important, I think, by being of service to the public. By analyzing implications of what is said, by analyzing strategies, and motives behind strategies, by analyzing the ways of presenting and withholding information, grounds can be found on which information can be believed or has to be discredited. Working in this direction, discourse analysis should be a part of political education, as a part of the education in the mother tongue.

NOTES

[1]. In order to understand the examples to be discussed in the text, the following information is necessary:
In the Netherlands, the major political parties are:

pvda (Labor Party, social democrats) leader:	Den Uyl	% of voters: 32
cda (Christian Democrats) leader:	Lubbers	30
vvd (Conservative Liberals) leader:	Nijpels	25

In 1982,after the last elections, the formation of the government was based on a coalition between cda and vvd. Prime Minister is Lubbers.

The next elections will be in 1986.

The three examples of interviews discussed in the text, are part of a larger sample of interviews recorded from Dutch radio and television. I assume that, in general, the examples I discuss are representative of political interviews as such. Details, of course, can be typical of a 'national political culture'. For reasons of space, I cannot go into methodological questions concerning the question of how representativeness is to be established.

The three examples discussed in the text appear in the Appendix to this paper. Examples 1 and 2 are presented in the original Dutch version; an approximating English translation is also given. The 3rd example is too extensive; for reasons of space, I left out the original Dutch version, while the first part of the example is presented in a summarized form.

[2]. The maxims proposed by May (1981: 55-58) are:

veracity: Take plain statements of fact by vulnerable authors at face value.

best face: Treat the case that is put as the strongest case that can be made.

The 'best face' maxim is elaborated in three submaxims.

[3]. Schwitalla (1979b) gives an inventory of (types of and grounds for) evasive answers to questions.

[4]. De Volkskrant, november 20, 1984.

Appendix

Ex. 1: interview Den Uyl, radio, 3 november 1984 (topic: nuclear power plants)

1 Ie: en een paar weken later komt de fractie en zegt JA we zijn er niet VOOR
and a few weeks later the party comes and says WELL we don't FAVOR it

2 maar 't is wel bespreekbaar geworden / lacht / weet u wel 't is bespreek-
but it can be talked about now / laughs / you know it can be talked about

3 baar geworden dat beteke je je bent er voor maar je houdt 't nog effe
it mean you you do favor it but you still hide it behind your back for

4 achter je rug en en
a while and and

Ir: maar ja ALS ze ALS ze voor zijn en de vvd is ook voor dat
but o.k. IF they IF they do favor it and the vvd too that

5 is wel duidelijk (...) dan komen ze er dus eigenlijk he
is rather clear (...) then there will be new power plants isn't it
nee dat hoeft niet
no not necessarily

6 kijk eh die zaak is nou net iets te belangrijk om op die cda vvd manier
look uh this issue is just a bit too important to be wangled in that cda

7 geritseld te worden (...) ((haalt resultaten brede maatschappelijke dis-
vvd fashion (...) ((quotes results of national discussion on energy

8 cussie aan)) en ik DENK dat cda (en) vvd . dat 't kabinet LUBbers zich
policies)) and I THINK that cda (and) vvd . that the LUBbers government

9 royaal vergist als men denkt dat men in DIT DICHTST bevolkte land van
makes a great mistake if one thinks that in THIS most DENSELY populated

10 europa er nou maar weer een paar kerncentrales bij kan gaan plaatsen
country of europe just a few new nuclear power plants can be built

11 dan zal blijken dat dat een ZO GROOT verzet gaat stuiten dat ik niet
then it will appear that it will hit on SUCH a GREAT resistance that

12 zie dat dat gebeurt in elk geval zal de partij van de arbeid 'rtoe
I do not see that happen in any case the labor party will

13 bijdragen om daar een stokje voor te steken kijk in de eerste
contribute to prevent it look in de first
Ir: HOE
HOW
Pu: /applause---------/

14 Ie: plaats en misschien ook in de laatste plaats op de manier waar ik aan
place and maybe also in the last place in the way that I believe

15 HECHT dat is door de goede arguMENten te geBRUIKen (...) ((argumenten:
in that is by Using the right ARGUments ((arguments:

16 om verschillende redenen hebben we ze niet nodig en het afvalprobleem
for several reasons we don't need them; the problem of nuclear

17 is onopgelost)) e en
waste is as yet unresolved)) a and
Ir: maar als ik u mag onderbreken kijk de
but if I may interrupt you look the

18 bezwaren tegen kernenergie die zijn binnen de partij van de arbeid eh
objections against nuclear energy are within the labor party uh well

19 bekend de vraag is alleen of als c d a en v v d die samen een meer-
known the question is just whether if cda and vvd which have together

20 Ir: derheid hebben in de kamer en beSLUIten dat die kerncentrales d'r
a majority in the chamber and deCIDE that those nuclear power plants

21 komen de partij van de arbeid nog de mogelijkheden heeft om dat TEgen
will be built the labor party still has the possibilities to STOP it

22 te houden dat KAN natuurlijk . als de partij van de arbeid na zes-
it CAN be of course . if the labor party after eighty-six

23 entachtig in een kabinet komt . luidt dan de conclusie een kabinet met
will join in the government . is the conclusion valid a government with

24 de partij van de arbeid is ondenkbaar als er kerncentrales komen
the labor party if there are going to be nuclear power plants

25 Ie: /haalt adem / ja eh daar u kun wel een heleboel van die eh veronderstel-
/draws a breath/ yes uh there you can a lot of those uh presuppositions

26 lingen uiten iedere keer lijkt het wel alsof u erop uit bent te horen
you can utter every time it looks as if you want to hear when the

27 wanneer de partij van de arbeid NIET zal regeren ik hecht er meer aan om
labor party will NOT take part in the government I prefer to say what

28 te zeggen wat de partij van de arbeid WEL doet als we gaan regeren
the labor party WILL do if we take part in the government

29 Ir: n geen kerncentrales bouwen
n no building of nuclear power plants
Ie: en dat is dat is als er zo'n besluit komt
and that is that is if there will be such a

30 dan staat 't vast dat de partij van de arbeid op heroverweging van zo'n
decision then it is for sure that the labor party will insist on recon-

31 besluit zal staan
sideration of such a decision
Ir: ((initieert nieuw onderwerp))
((initiates new topic))

Ex. 2: interview Lubbers, tv, 9 november 1984 (topic: mixing up of state and private affairs)

1 Ir: eh u kwam zelf deze week in het nieuws eh meneer Lubbers
uh you yourself became this week a news topic uh mr. Lubbers

2 Ie: dat komt regelmatig voor / lacht /
that occurs regurlarly / laughs /
Ir: ja maar u als persoon eeh was in koeweit
yes but you as a person uh you were in

3 en u zou daar eheigen belangen 't belang ook van 't bedrijf van uw broer
kuwait and you allegedly stood up there uh for your own interests the inte-
rest also of the business of your brother

4 hebben verdedigd nou daar worden dan vragen over gesteld in de kamer u
well questions are asked about that in the chamber you

5 hebt de kamer geantwoord ik ZELF denk gewoon nou als ik dan toch in koe-
have answered the chamber I mySELF think just well if I am in kuwait

6 weit ben laat ik dan ook dat stukje even meenemen want ik ben er toch
anyway just let me handle this piece also I am there anyway.

7 dat is toch eeh is dat . maar kan dat niet in de politiek
isn't that uh is that . but isn't that possible in politics

8 Ie: eh dat zie ik een slag anders ik ben daar als als minister president vanuit
uh I see it a bit differently I am there as as prime minister because of

9 mijn ffunctie met de minister van buitenlandse zaken ter goed begrip
my ffunction with the minister of foreign affairs for a clear understan-

10 in zo'n delegatie zitten dan ook mensen eh van het bedrijfsleven niet
ding in such a delegation there are also people from business life not

11 van dit bedrijf maar van andere bedrijven en de belangen van het bedrijfs-
from this business but from other business concerns and the interests of

12 leven worden tijdens zo'n reis ook behartigd maar als tijdens de reis
business life are taken care of during such a visit but if during the

13 van de kant van mijn gastheren die hier in een vorig bezoek van staats-
journey on the part of my hosts the attention of who was drawn to this

14 secretaris bolkestein op geattendeerd waren de vraag komt
during an earlier visit of junior minister bolkestein the question is

15 eh stelt u 't misschien op prijs daarover te praten dan heb ik toch de
asked uh would you perhaps appreciate to discuss this then I am inclined

16 neiging om te zeggen eeh . daar is dan geen aanleiding voor want dan ga
to say uh . there is no occasion for it because then you

17 je er als het ware TE concreet in een bepaald geval waarvan je ook alle
are going into it as it were TOO concretely in a certain case of which

18 details niet kent en wat beter overgelaten kan worden aan deskundigen
you do not know every detail and which better can be left to experts

19 eh daar . die afspraak is dan ook gemaakt en dat heb ik ook aan de kamer
uh there . that agreement has been made and that I have informed to the

20 bericht ik vond 't dus inderdaad niet juist om er echt inHOUDelijk op
chamber I thought it indeed not justified to go into it subSTANTially

21 in te gaan en ter goed begrip de de de man aan de andere kant de ministers
and for a good understanding the the the man on the other side the minis-

22 van koeweit vonden 't zeer voor de hand liggend dus we waren er in twee
sters of kuwait thought indeed that it went without saying so in two

23 minuten over uitgepraat zij brachten 't ter sprake
minutes we had finished about it they brought it up
Ir: en zij brachten 't ter sprake
and they brought it up

24 Ie: en dat vind ik ook heel hoffelijk en verstandig van hun omdat 't eerder
and I do find it very courteous and sensible of them because it was

25 van nederlandse zijde een keer aandacht voor was gevraagd dus ze komen
earlier from the dutch side one time attention for it was asked so they

26 dat bij de voorbereiding natuurlijk tegen en wij hebben gezegd op hun
come accross this point of course during preparations and we have said

27 voorstel laten daar deskundigen over praten JA laat dat inderdaad op
on their proposal let experts talk about it YES let that happen at

28 korte termijn gebeuren want zo'n geschil kan beter de wereld uit
short notice for such a conflict be better solved

29 Ir: ja maar de als men in nederland zou reageren zoals nederlanders vaak
yes but th if one in holland would react as dutchmen often do like uh

30 Ir: reageren van eh waar rook is is vuur d dan heb ik 't helemaal mis
were there is smoke there is fire then I am completely wrong

31 Ie: /2 sec./ ik k ik weet niet eh ik weet niet waar waar u op doelt maa 't
I I I don't know uh I don't know what you are aiming at bu it

32 is natuurlijk wel zo dat er altijd zoiets is van eh is er iets
is of course the case that there is always a question of uh is some-

33 scheefs nou in dit geval ben ik daar erg simpel in eeh eh je moet
thing wrong well in this case I take a quite simple stand uh uh you
Ir: ja
yes

34 Ie: natuurlijk eh ALS zoiets aan de orde komt wel zorgvuldig zijn maar ik
should of course uh IF such a thing comes up be careful but I

35 zou me niet voor kunnen stellen dat ik daar gezegd had . HOOW . eeh
could not imagine that I there would have said . STOP . uuh

36 ik mag zelfs geen procedure (afspraken) da's natuurlijk gewoon ONzin
I may not even agree on a procedure that's of course just NONsense

37 ik moet mijn werk doen als minister president dat heb ik gewoon weer
I must do my job as prime minister that is just what I

38 gedaan
have done
Ir: ehhuh nogn andere zaak die ik nog (...)
uhhuh still' 'nother case that I (...)

Ex. 3: interview De Koning, tv, 26 september 1984 (topic: ethics of cutting on welfare)

1 Ir: but may I ask you then ((you take measures against a group that is on
2 record. That makes it easy. Why don't you take action against the not-
3 registered group of the black money circuit; this group pinches 10 to
4 12 % of the national income, 30 to 60 billion guilders. Why doesn't a
5 christian politician put his first priority there?
Ie: Two remarks: fraud is
6 seized upon, not enough discovered. If it is discovered, then it is
7 seized upon forcibly. It could be more forcible but it IS seized upon.
Just it is not enough discovered.
Ir: Because there is not enough personnel.
8 Ie: Because there are too many opportunities for practising fraud. That is
9 the second point: WHY does fraud exist? Because in many circles people
10 say: solidarity is fine, but not too much of it. I withdraw as soon as

solidarity demands too much. Earlier there was a ratio of 1 person on welfare to 7 with paid jobs, now this ratio is 1 : 2.8. That makes the burden of solidarity heavy; it should be, because it is necessary. Now we hit again upon the bad traits of man. People say: the last guilders

Ie: I do not return anymore.

Ir: The last guilders! It is nonsense if you say: we seize upon it forcibly. District attorneys take action on their own initiative, not because of the official policy.

Ie: They do, of course.

Ir: Van Bijstervelt writes in a report: two out of three people who CAN practise fraud do it. An estimation made by Hofstra is: 15 billion fraud in building trade and metal industry. According to him the authorities are ladling with a sieve out of a barrel without a bottom. Nóthing happens against fraud, in no sector, to be sure neither as for abuse of social security)) (there evil is hiding)

Ie: I think that (our whole ivestigation department) at this moment uh is heavily overburdened especially as fighting fraud is concerned huh but it uh to fight fraud to disCOVer fraud is terribly complicated in a complicated society swindlers are extremely skilful people uh when fraud should be covered up but again people have always been inclined to all evil so fraud too they have practised it always too but they practise (it) now to a VERY great extent and then you should as authorities rather start thinking about it why is it expanding so much well I can mention an obvious reason the average em-

ployee with thirty-two thirty-three thousand guilders bruto income pays
over his LAST guilder which is then taxed in the highest terriff that
applies to him NOW fifty-seven cents for taxes and premium that was ten
years ago thirty-three cents that makes a considerable difference
Ir: you do
not answer my question in my opinion uh my question was if you
Ie: I think I do
Ir: you talk about justice which you need not do as for me but you DO it.
why do you seize upon the group that is on record and which has already
almost nothing anymore and why is also from this policy of the govern-
ment for it is really just a drop in the ocean what you now have stated in
the declaration of policy to do about fraud why is this group where
Ie: yes
Ir: billions and billions and billions are embezzled every year why was
Ie: yes
Ir: there no policy to collect the money THERE that you collect now from
(the naked old and needy) just to speak in biblical terms
Ie: yes . the bible
has something to say about thieves too that's uh no joke so you can find
there CERtainly starting points for a very intensive battle against fraud
that battle is on this moment with the LIMIted possibilities that we
Ie: have in personnel and apparatus ( )
why is that why are those possibilities
Ir: LIMIted because there was no interest for it
Ie: we:ell that interest has

50 grown of course because fraud (phenomena) expanded so much
Ir: from NOTHing

51 to something
Ie: huh from nothing to something . compared with fraud it is

52 something right . it is also ( ) rather much but compared with the

53 extent of fraud it is indeed just a trifle so it must be reinforced and

54 improved that means more personnel but that is a problem for the author-

55 ities but especially better administrative techniques such that you are

56 more able to follow a bigger group of people and as I said resistance is

57 rising immediately against that for people do not want to be followed . I

58 think that it is from the point of view of justice necessary
Ir: that holds for the lowest income too

59 Ie: to apply that technique anyhow in our society in order to push back

60 that horrible extent of fraud and the chance of being caught ( )
Ir: but the lowest

61 income people are purSUED . you could say . they are (controlled by)
Ie: yes ( )

62 Ir: social security offices even spied upon in their neighbourhood EVERYbody

63 is sitting in their neck the SWINDlers . be it ((a list of possibilities
Ie: yes that that

64 Ir: of practising fraud is enumerated)) a giGANTic reservoir of people who

65 just mess around . NOTHing ( ) yes read the
Ie: you have read the catechism well

66 Ir: catechism well but I have ( ) it
Ie: (you must understand) that there is no difference of

67 opinion it is indeed a giGANTic circuit and we have to take care of it

68 BEIter and for that we must provide the means
Ir: but how do you corrupt if you

69 know THAT and define it that way and then at the same time seize upon

70 those people who really have nothing anymore to lose . because of that

71 you can seize upon them easily for they are on record
Ie: uhhuh uhhuh no that

72 is of course no right line of reasoning right reasoning is that there

73 where evil is it should be seized upon because it is EVil
Ir: well but that

74 doesn't happen
Ie: the second point is the question of financing the system of

75 social security the financing of the welfare state but you shouldn't

76 say if we uh uh we we seize upon fraud in ORDER to finance the welfare

77 state we seize upon fraud because it is wrong (...)
Ir: no but I just say

Legenda:
text UPPER CASE: spoken with stress
(text): not clearly intelligible text
( ): unintelligible
(...) : part of text skipped
. : pause
/ / paralingual or contextual information
((text)): summarized text

COMMENTS ON TITUS ENSINK

Rob Grootendorst

Most parts of Ensink's paper are, in my opinion, very interesting. In particular I like his ideas on the role of 'face preservation' and 'face threatening' in respect of political interviews. I have serious doubts, however, about some of his other ideas and proposals.

First a minor point. Ensink wants to limit the use of the term **interview** to 'a conversation between a reporter and one from whom he seeks information'. Referring to his third example, in which the persistent interviewer Wim Kayser appears, Ensink observes that here the borderline between an interview pur sang and an argumentative debate is almost obliterated. Following Ensink's own characterization it would be a more appropriate conclusion to say, however, that the line is clearly crossed. But Ensink nevertheless prefers to use the term **interview** in this case, because the interviewee 'is forced (...) to show in which way the political world is put together and which political actions should be, and can be, undertaken, and why'. I find this explanation extremely unclear and, as a consequence, I fail to see why this apparent counter-example should be considered an interview at all, in the sense that Ensink himself uses this word.

My second point has to do with the applicability of the Gricean Cooperative Principle and the maxims connected with it to political interviews. Ensink is not quite clear on this matter. On the one hand he says that in a 'technical' sense the Cooperative Principle is operating in political interviews, on the other hand he claims that the maxims are 'somewhat out of operation', because the participants are not in the same way interested in a 'smooth flow of information'.

Elsewhere Ensink seems to be more positive when he says that the participants are 'not cooperative in the sense in which Grice used this word'. The main reason for this is that the participants engaged in a political interview are supposed to be 'partial informants'. I would like to make three comments on this.

(1) I disagree with Ensink's view that the participants in a political interview are not cooperative in the Gricean sense. Grice admits that his maxims are stated as if the purpose of a talk exchange 'were a maximally effective exchange of information' (1975: 47), but that does not mean automatically that in all other cases, in which the purpose is different, the participants are non-cooperative. Cooperation is not a matter of black and white, but a matter of degree, as Grice explains: 'Our talk exchanges (...) are, to **some degree at least**, cooperative efforts; and each participant recognizes in them, **to some extent**, a common purpose or set of purposes, **or at least a mutually accepted direction**' (1975: 45; my italics). Given this explanation, I see no good reason whatsoever why political interviews could not be taken, **to some extent**, as cooperative speech events, just like e.g. argumentative discussions (cf. Van Eemeren & Grootendorst 1984: 121). This view coincides with that expressed by Holdcroft in his paper 'Speech Acts and Conversation', in which he argues that even in quarrels, cross examinations, and interrogations the Cooperative Principle and the maxims are operating. Holdcroft claims that cooperation 'for a limited purpose against a background of conflict and general suspicion is surely intelligible' (1979: 133).

(2) Ensink refers to the **technical** sense with respect to the scope of the Cooperative Principle. He does not explain, however, what other senses there are. Besides, it is doubtful if any other senses but technical ones can be of any significance for the problem in question.

(3) If it would be true that partiality as such is always incompatible with the concept of cooperation (which is a matter Ensink leaves unexplained), one can cast serious doubts on the possibility whether to apply the cooperative Principle to everyday discourse at all. For conversations in daily life are hardly ever totally free of partiality. In my opinion it would be absurd to conclude from this that the language users engaged in such conversations are guilty of a non-cooperative attitude. Perhaps they are, but if so, it must be due to something else than their alleged partiality.

My third point pertains to the alternative which Ensink proposes for the Gricean Cooperative Principle and the maxims. Instead of the Gricean maxims, Ensink prefers May's maxims of veracity and best face, which (1) are connected with the listener, (2) are based on partiality, and (3) do not presuppose any credibility on the part of the speaker. The preoccupation with partiality leads the interpreter, according to Ensink, to an analysis of the motives behind the speaker's utterances. Ensink thinks that this is a great advantage, I do not. On the contrary, I feel very uneasy about it, to say the least.

The first problem is how the listener is supposed to detect the motives behind the speaker's words, especially when the latter does not bring them into the open, which normally will be the case in political interviews as well as in many other types of conversation. I think Ensink is unjustified in neglecting this problem. In his first example, the interview with Den Uyl, Ensink jumps too easily to the conclusion that Den Uyl's words, literally taken, may not be necessarily contradictory, but the motives behind them are incompatible. The reader is left in the dark as to how Ensink has managed to discover these hidden motives. Has he any secret access to them that we have not?

Secondly, Ensink tells us that May's maxims make it possible to make an assessment of the credibility of the speaker's words. If that would be the case, which I doubt, then May's maxims are not to be taken as an alternative for the Gricean maxims, but must be placed on a totally different level. The Gricean maxims are an essential part in the process of working out a conversational implicature, i.e. they serve as important aids for the interpretation of the speaker's utterances, and not for the assessment of them.

Thirdly, from the perspective of the theory of argumentation, it is imperative to warn against the dangers connected with the so-called detecting of motives behind the speaker's words. In particular, the hunting for motives can be very dangerous, when it replaces a fair interpretation of what the speaker has actually said. Among other things, it makes it possible and easier to divide the world into two kinds of people: the good guys (whose motives are respectable) and the bad guys (whose motives are despicable). This technique is frequently used in argumentative disputes in which emotions rise high. According to a longstanding tradition, this practice is condemned as (the circumstantial variety of) the fallacy of argumentum ad hominem (cf. Van

Eemeren, Grootendorst & Kruiger 1984: 83 ff.). It is rather disappointing to see that Ensink wants to upgrade this fallacy to a guiding principle in the interpretation of political interviews.

14

The expressive stragegy in the political interview: A system error

P. van Lint

Introduction

Studies on politics mushroom in the Netherlands, but studies on political rhetorics are hard to find, are mostly journalistic in character[1], and concentrate on style, lexicon and semantics, as do the rare studies with more pretentions (Meddens/Sturm 1977). This applies to foreign studies as well. In The Tyranny of Words Stuart Chase already asked the question: "What is a nation, a people, national honor, democracy", if said by "Statesmen" (Stuart Chase 1938). These elocutionary aspects are easily connected with suppositions about intentions, persuasion, manipulation or even cheating or repression as do Trevor Pateman in his **Language, Truth and Politics** (Pateman 1980), Murray Edelman in his **Political Language** (Edelman 1977), or long before them, Hans Sperber in his **Expressive Aspects of Political Language** (Sperber in Werner 1955).

Essays like these usually do not deal with rhetorical, but with linguistic or sociological facts, basically. In my view rhetorics is a discipline not only interested in how and why things are as they are, but also in how and why they are made as they are made, and how they should be made. Apart from being a scholarly discipline it is an art, exploring "how it is done and how it is made and what it is made of", wanting to acquire skills, investigating material and structure of texts and the skills needed to construct texts for different occasions. Truly rhetorical therefore are only those studies that treat **texts as a whole**, not only the elements of style, but focusing on all rhetorical aspects, both thematic, structural, interactional and theatrical ones, the classic inventio, dispositio, elocutio and pronuntiatio. Examples of such treatment are Campbell and Jamieson's analysis of Barbara Jordan's convention-speech (Campbell/Jamieson 1977) or Michael Halloran's study about the telecasted debate on Nixon's impeachment (Halloran 1977).

Because this branch of rhetorics has to do with rhetorical processes in society and has social implications, it is a subset of what could be called "socio-rhetorics" in order to distinguish it from more traditional branches moving mainly in the field of stylistics and textstructure. True "socio-rhetorics" has emancipatory aims on top of that: it tries to trace imbalances in powerstructures in communicative scenes and chooses the part of the participant in the communication who can be manipulated or forced by the other party on grounds of imbalance of power, like the accused, the patient, the applicant, the pupil, the unskilled.

In this paper a **method of sociorhetorical analysis** will be proposed based on a **classification** of **text types** and **rhetorical** strategies. The main problem to be faced is: does the **expressive strategy** fit into the **political interview** according to the purpose of that text genre, and if it does not, how can its occurrence be explained? The material will be found mainly in **transcripts of weekly interviews** with former Dutch Prime Minister Van Agt (collected in Van Lint 1981a, part 2).

In order to answer these questions, six termino-theoretical problems will be dealt with in the first part of this paper:

1. What is an interview?
2. What is political?
3. What is a political interview?
4. What is a strategy?
5. What is a rhetorical strategy?
6. What is an expressive strategy?

The second part of this paper will concentrate on the major problem, the **relation between the political interview and the expressive strategy**, and in the third part a possible explanation will be proposed for the fact that this strategy occurs at all in the sophisticated texttype that the political interview is: the expressive strategy is a relict (in an evolutionary or ecological sense) of a **conversational primitive**, the small talk.

1. Interview, politics, texttypes, and strategies

1.1. What is an interview?

In this paper an interview will be regarded as a type of dialogue[2], or if that somewhat hybrid formation is preferred, as a type of duologue (As in Andrew K.Kennedy Dramatic Dialogue. The duologue of personal encounter. Kennedy 1983). Along with other dialogue types such as criminal interrogation, examination, enquiry and others I place it in the group of **investigatory** types, which together with **instructional** types make up the **referential** text genre, distinct from other spoken text genres like the **general** genre (small talk, conversation), the **argumentative** genre (e.g. debate, discussion) the **evaluative** genre (e.g. appraisal interviews, job-interviews) or the **activating** genre (negotiations, therapeutic discourse e.g.) In a graphic model[2]:

(model 1)

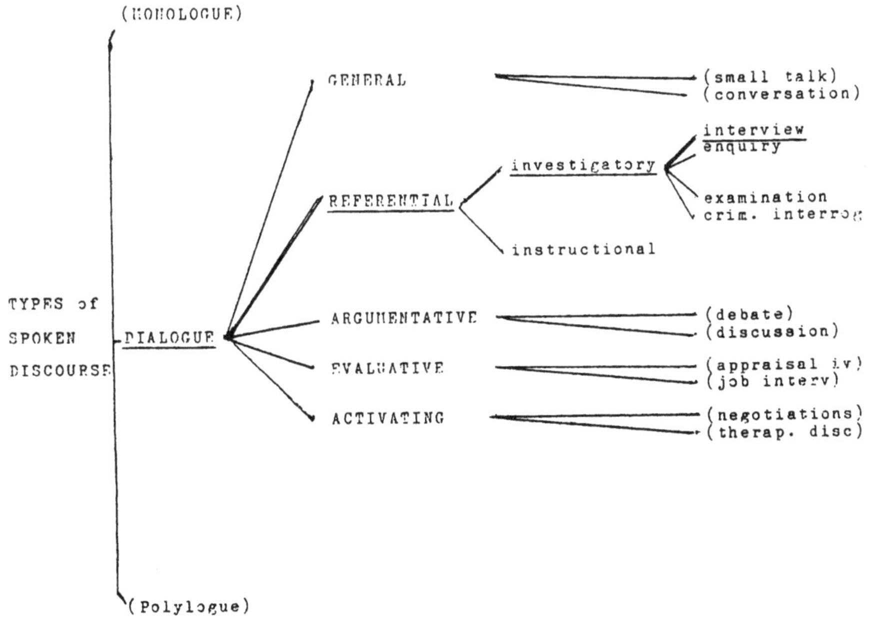

The interview as a texttype is a **dialogue** because as a rule there are two participants ("agonists" in a terminology derived from dramaturgy), it is **referential** because it aims at knowledge of facts and it is **investigatory** because one person tries to get information from the other person by asking questions. In fact I would prefer the Dutch vernacular "vraaggesprek" ("conversation by questions"), as in the title of the book by Hendrik van der Zee: **Het vraaggesprek als instrument bij praktijkonderzoek** (Zee 1979), or Susanne Piët: **Een vraag en een weet. Gereedschap voor het vraaggesprek** (Piët 1980), for which I do not know a good English equivalent. I would prefer "vraaggesprek" because I am aware of the fact that the word "interview" may be used in a much broader sense than I intend to do here. However, I will still use the word interview, which in itself is quite common in Dutch for a "vraaggesprek" in newspapers, or on radio or TV.

It is distinct from other types in the investigatory subgroup, for here both participants are relatively **equivalent in rights and power**, if not in function (Van Lint 1980, p. 69,70)

1.2. What is political?

This is the most crucial question in the research of political rhetoric. We find views such as that expressed by Willy Olmüller (Olmüller 1977, p 24)

> "Unter Politik verstehe ich unter den gegenwärtig in Europa und in der westlichen Welt vorgegebenen Lebens- und Herrschaftsbedingungen all dass, was handelnde und leidende Menschen und soziale Gruppen (z.B. Völker, Klassen, Schichten, Minderheiten) tun müssen und tun können, wenn sie streiten um die öffentliche Anerkennung sowie um die durchsetzung ihrer Vorstellungen vom Überleben und vom guten Leben. Menschen und soziale Gruppen handeln politisch und erleiden Politik unter zeitlich, räumlich und sozial ausserordentlich verschiedenen Lebens- und Herrschaftsbedingungen."

In this view Politics only concerns either Leaders or Groups. A broader view is taken by C. Rogers (according to M. Zappen (Zappen 1980))

> Rogers emphasizes the political character of **On Personal Power**. The work is political in a contemporary sense; that is, it has not so much to do with government as with

"power and control", with "the maneuvers, the strategies and tactics, witting or unwitting, by which such power and control over one's own life and other's is sought and gained - or shared or relinquished", with "the locus of decision-making power", with "the effects of these decisions and these strategies". Such a view is, in fact, traditional in its identification of politics with social relationships and social action. What is distinctive about Rogers' view of politics is that it retains his characteristic attitudes toward individuals and individual relationships even while introducing those attitudes into the multiperson situation.

In the latter view any discourse that is not "herrschaftsfrei" (Habermas 1973, p. 343) is Political, even, or maybe ranking among the first, the therapeutic discourse, as is the opinion of i.a. Murray Edelman in his chapter on the Political Language of the Helping Professions. (Edelman 1977)

I agree with that view. Yet in this paper I will adopt the more restricted sense of politics, no matter how all-important and emancipatory the broader view. I shall use the word politics and political in the sense in which we apply it to the daily work and the profession of statesmen, of politicians. Plainly spoken, I use it in its everyday meaning, which, however, implies quite a specific way of having and using power and struggling for it.

1.3. What is a political interview?

A political interview meets the demands of an interview in the above sense, and aims at investigating political matters, i.e. matters having to do with the daily work of politicians and statesmen in general and the Government and the Administration in particular.

1.4. What is a strategy?

The word "strategy" is used by different authors in quite different ways. The term is derived along with the terms tactics and manoeuvres from military science (Clausewitz in Obermann 1970, p. 139), or, if you prefer, the "art of war", and goes back of course to Greek strat-egia: the leading of the army, the taking of appropriate measures. In everyday life it is used for a whole range of quite different actions

(Wagner 1978, p. 159 ff)
- The Union develops a strategy for a national strike
- Prime Minister Lubbers refuses for strategical reasons to reveal the contents of the letter to German Prime Minister Kohl
- For an important meeting one has to figure out which strategy has to be followed.

Connotations of the meaning are:
1. something well thought out, kept under control, intentional, manageable, aimed at a goal
2. something nog just for the moment, but with at least a medium time-planning.

The military complement to strategy is tactics (Gr. taktike, the art of positioning): the way a strategy is performed: it is an attitudinal concept in order to choose the appropiate means: i.c. the manoeuvres (or, French: man-oeuvre; literally: manual work).

Apart from military strategies it seems that nowadays there are sociological, psychological, and even politeness strategies (Brown/Levinson 1978). Dubber/Weijdema call certain linguistic devices in their research also strategies (Dubber/Weijdema 1980), Harari speaks of "Textual strategies" (Harari 1980), Ferrell/Salerno call their book "Strategies in Prose" (Ferrell/Salerno 1973), and Angenot deals in his chapter "Structures Discursives" with "Stratégies d'ensemble", more specifically "Stratégies et tactiques" and "Deux modeles de stratégie", which are: "Argumentation et narration" (Angenot 1982), Houtkoop writes about "taalgebruik en konversationele strategieën" (Language use and conversational strategies") (Houtkoop 1981), a list which could be expanded infinetely.

All these studies have in common that apart from the very general and broad definition they use the word strategy in an ad-hoc sense, meaning usually not much more than "way", or even "use" itself.

1.5. What is a rhetorical strategy?

Leaving Linguistic and Sociological and even Political Strategies for what they are worth, this paper concentrates on Rhetorical Strategies. Now even rhetorical authors, though acquainted with a stricter use of the word and concept of "strategy", seldom define it and certainly not as a discriminating concept. Yet, as far as "textual strategies" are involved they have to do with

1. "constructed texttypes" or "texttypes to be constructed" and at the same time with
2. the "aims of the text" or the "aims of the communicator" and with
3. certain stylistic features of the text.

This in itself is rhetorically sound, and connects the use of the word strategy with the rhetorical tradition, in which several texttypes are discerned more or less in relation to the aims of communication or to the style.
These aims could be:

1. knowledge
2. emotions, values, or diversion
3. action.

Rhetorical strategies then are the ways and means communicators have at their disposal to achieve goals in communication, (of which, I emphasize, persuasion is by no means the most important, much less the only one). Of course this definition is still too broad and too easy. For reasons of efficiency I will not elaborate on argumentation about how several theories could gradually be combined, but propose to define a rhetorical strategy as a complex of means aimed at the construction of a specific texttype (Van Lint 1980). This only makes sense if these "complexes" and "texttypes" are defined immediately. Otherwise the definition is nearly as broad and prone to ad-hoc uses as the ones attacked above. This is the more important because aim, texttype and strategy do not necessarily have to be compatible: an informative strategy resulting in let us say a news-item about Ethiopia could lead to emotions, an expressive strategy, resulting in a pamphlet, could lead to a change of values, a narrative strategy, resulting in a story at times aims at diversion, at times however at values, at times even at knowledge. This apparent confusion has a long history: docere, movere and delectare are goals an orator can aim at both in narratio or in argumentatio, (Quintillianus, XII, X 58-61). Strange combinations like these we find also in Mediaeval Rhetorics, according to Fumaroli (Fumaroli 1984, p 205).

"La rhétorique, comme art de plaire, encore plus comme art de persuader, est chez elle á la Cour de Rome, ou de toutes façons la langue latine exige de chacun des dignitaires une formation oratoire savante. Les prédications comme les Ora tiones de Christi domini morte, y sont aussi des chefs- d'oeuvre d'art oratoire "démonstratif" (...)."

Usually however strategy, texttype and communicative aim are looked upon as at least closely related and treated as such by several authors. A few examples, not only on rhetoricians: Morris (semanticist) discerns four Use-categories of texts: informative, valuative, incitive, systemic, and four Mode-categories: designative, appraisive, prescriptive, formative (Morris 1971). Klammer sees three ways of writing, depending on the aim: description, narration and expository writing (Klammer 1978); Winkler/McCuen deal with narration, description and argumentation (Winkler/McCuen 1978); Werlich (textlinguist) explains "deskriptive, narrative, expositorische, argumentative, instruktive Texte" (Werlich 1975); Bormann/Bormann discuss several texttypes of the persuasive or informative kind (Bormann/Bormann 1977); Kinneavy speaks of reference, persuasive, scientific and expressive discourse (Kinneavy 1971). Many other examples could be found.

In fact Morris is the only one who makes a real attempt to distinguish between type, use and mode, a distinction possibly comparable though not identical to that in type, strategy and goal.

So there are goals in communication, texttypes to achieve these goals, and strategies to construct these texttypes.

Texttypes then should not cause much trouble, they are given names even in everyday language, and in my above definition of the interview I relied on that fact. For classificatory purposes they could be divided according to the goals they are supposed to achieve[3], as explained above.

The "complexes of means" could be further defined and specified in view of the rhetorical devices the texts-to-be-constructed should possess, using criteria of topic-territory (Latin "res" or "materia") and stylistic representation (Latin "elocutio"). It is then possible to define eight clearly distinct strategies (for a demonstration[4] see Van Lint 1980, 1981), divided in four groups:

1. informative, narrative, descriptive,
2. deliberative, argumentative,
3. imperative, moving,

4. expressive.

Roughly speaking the first group constructs texts that deal with the "res" of the world around the participants in the communication, such as they observe and understand it;

the second group constructs texttypes that question relations in that world;

the third group constructs texttypes that have to do with the relations between the participants themselves;

and the last one, the expressive strategy, constructs texts that deal mainly with the speaker himself.

This last one we want to explore further in this paper.

1.6 The expressive strategy

In spite of the work of Dewey (Dewey 1934), Croce (Croce 1978), Read (Read 1956), and many other philosophers, "self-expression" usually is regarded as something for the classroom, perhaps for psychologists, or, if need be, something for the Arts, but hardly worth the attention of researchers in the field of linguistics or rhetorics. Yet already in 1955 at the Clark University a symposium was held on expressive language (Werner, 1955). The scholars however almost all restricted their definition of the word expressive to word or sentence level. Kinneavy, much later, is among the few who regard expressive discourse as a genre in itself (Kinneavy 1971, p. 393-447).

As a strategy was defined above by the rhetorical devices which the texttype-to-be-constructed (itself classified by aim) should possess in terms of res (theme in a broad sense) and elocutio (of which style is one), I treat each of the components briefly.

In my view the expressive strategy[5] deals with the theme of the speaker's own very personal experiences of life, his feelings or value judgements, which find their realisation at the level of elocution, apart from direct statements about those feelings or judgements, in stylistic-esthetic deviations from plain language like metaphors, figures of style, manners of speaking (Bally 1951), verbal routines, and frequent use of I, me, my, we, our, ours and all constructions that point to the speaker him/herself. "I find" and "I feel" are the central formulas, in many variations.

"Tout ce qui, dans un message écrit ou parlé, trahit la personnalité de l'émetteur, relève de la fonction expressive (la fameuse expression "moi je" par exemple, mais aussi la présence d'interjections a valeur émotive, de jugements subjectifs, d'intonations caractéristiques, etc...). La fonction expressive se manifeste par l'emploi de la premiere personne, mais aussi par l'utilisation de procédés soulignants les affirmations du destinateur: répétitions, emploi de oui". (Vanoye 1973, p. 55,56).

Manoeuvres[6] of this strategy are: sighs, lamentations, effusions, ebullitions, apologies, briefly all verbal manoeuvres by which one may express directly one's feelings or values.

At the level of Texttypes the expressive strategy flourishes of course in small talk and other conversational primitives (meaning nothing depreciative, but referring to types with more general purposes compared to types with more specific purposes, which are derived from the first, just like higher computer languages are derived from lower-level languages), and constructs at a higher level certain texttypes like diaries, pamphlets, poems (Kinneavy 1971, p 424, p 429; Pauw 1984) and even helps in the construction of stories, tales, novels, or drama, starring the speaker, his partner, children, parents, relatives, at times in a direct, autobiographic way, at times in disguise. But it figures in many other texttypes, which in fact it is alien to, but helps at time to enliven, though often it just perverts (corrupts, spoils) the texttype it has invaded.

Now that the six terminological questions are answered, the major problem can be faced: the relation between the political interview and the expressive strategy. Only a small subset of the political interview will be dealt with, viz. weekly TV-interviews with the Prime Minister, mainly with former Prime Minister Van Agt.

2. The expressive strategy and the political interview

2.1. The expressive strategy in the political interview

In the interviews researched, which cover part of the Friday-night interviews of the period in which J. den Uyl was Prime Minister (1976 Jan. to March, Van Lint 1977) and of the first period in which A. van Agt was Prime Minister (December 1977 to June 1978, Van Lint 1981a), the expressive strategy ruling an interview as a whole seldom occurs. The interview of 1977, December 23rd, is a specimen of such an interview: (expressive features are bold-faced).

K3,R3: (Yes I think so. It is obvious every opportunity will be grasped to tackle me, I know that. We are heading for heavy weather. I can take it.)

K5,R5: It was) terribly busy. A bit uneasy of course. One enters a new department, new people. But I did find most able and sympathetic assistants around me. With that crew I'll make it.)

K7,R7: (I got used more or less to being in that position, and after all there was not one moment last week that I realised having power or dwelling in majesty[7] or how such a thing is expressed.Bearing a heavy responsibility, yes, having a good deal of work at hand, having to make work a crew heavily under attack, these are the feelings that arise)

(Part of the protocol of this interview is attached, along with the other quotations)

Often the expressive strategy is part of a larger unit. A kind of complaint can be found in:

20-1, K4,R4: (That was a grave, in fact a very grave accusation. And what of course should have been the natural follow-up of THAT accusation, if he really means that, that he should have asked a verdict of the representatives. And he did not do that. He did table a number of motions about all sorts of matters, not about this main question).

Usually the interpretation of an emotion or a value depends on interpretation of the context[8]. This is easier when it is identified by name in the text itself: Gladness without smugness, but with modesty, in

20-1, K6,R6: (Well, we are of course eh glad, the cabinet came out of the debate without damage (...) we may say apparently, without indulging in smugness, (...) and we do know of course we do not have an exclusive claim to wisdom (...) we got something to learn from the first experience and we have been doing that to our best possibilities).

Indignation we find in other interviews quoted in Van Lint 1981 e.g. in 13-1, K3,R3 or in 27-1, K4R4 and K5R5, quite personal emotions and values in 27-1, K12R12 through R14.

Metaphors, mythical motives, images are abundant in the

interviews with former Vice Prime Minister Wiegel, as in:

3-2, K3,R3: (But the Government of course does not happen to be a body with the tree with golden apples ready to be picked just in the back garden)[9] or in:

K4R4: ("Water has risen to the lips of many companies. And authorities they are not able to just stop all the gaps either. In short, we are facing a situation in this sense that we may have to accept the fact that, generally, things go BADLY in the Netherlands...")

Other manoeuvres found as part of an expressive strategy are:
making restrictions with a positive value-judgment, giving an emotionally coloured evaluation, or a joke mingled with indignation. Other emotions expressed are: frustration, pride, or annoyance. (For examples see Van Lint 1981) Originally narrative manoeuvres like "giving a summary of what happened" or "telling anecdotes" (meaning short stories characterizing a person, happening or situation), by which the speaker tells about his own experiences and adventures, do fit into an expressive strategy. These narrative episodes with an autobiographic touch that makes them expressive, often occur in the interviews. (Examples again in Van Lint 1981).

Of course the expressive strategy does not show only in the subjective formulas, but also in intonation. I regret I cannot elaborate on that aspect here. It is most important, as may be seen a.o. in the research of Atkinson (Atkinson 1984). Though that research is restricted to monologues only, the results hold for dialogues as well.

The examples given here show clearly that the expressive strategy as such, or as a manoeuvre in other strategies, often appears in the interviews. The question to be answered now is whether it is a system error or not.

2.2. The expressive strategy as a system error in an interview: The texttheoretical point of view.

The definition of "interview" given before nearly excludes any other strategy but informative, narrative, descriptive or deliberative strategies. The argumentative could hardly be expected, because that one belongs in a debate or a discussion, not in an interview. Moreover it is not the

Prime Minister's task in these interviews to justify his behavior, at least according to some of the Prime Ministers themselves (and other politicians). The only place to do that is in Parliament, as former Prime Minister Den Uyl often said (Van Lint 1977, 12 maart 1976, R13, p 97) and as the present Prime Minister Lubbers regularly observes. The imperative strategy also has no place in these interviews: there are no commands. But how about the other more subjective strategies? The moving strategy in fact is often used, but I will not treat that one here, but limit myself to the expressive strategy.

Of course the political interview in the strict text-typical definition given above is not intended to entice the politician, in this case the Prime Minister or the Vice Prime Minister, to express their very personal feelings or ideas.

Even if the matters under investigation are these feelings and values, the informative strategy is wanted. The expressive strategy therefore does not fit into an investigatory genre. Within the framework of a socio-rhetorical theory about aim-directed texttypes it follows that the expressive strategy perverts the type. Therefore the expressive strategy is a system error in the system of the interview.

Now who is responsible for the error? Certainly the respondents cannot be held responsible alone. The tactics of the "conagonist" (the answerer, itee in lingua americana) consist of his sequential manoeuvres, but these are provoked by tactics of the "protagonist" ("interviewer"). Questions asking for comments instead of facts provoke comments and views, and these often have a very personal touch. So far we have concentrated on the conagonist and saw his strategies to be at fault with the demands of the genre. But in most cases an expressive strategy or manoeuvre is the reaction to a chain of mainly K-questions, questions demanding Comment, about the personal experiences of the conagonist. These questions of course can be met with other manoeuvres, like evasions or no-comment statements or ignoring. These are the manoeuvres often used by former Prime Minister Den Uyl, but also by present Prime Minister Lubbers. Nevertheless, both use the expressive strategies, too, not so much in order to speak about their experiences or feelings, but to express their value judgements.

2.3 The expressive strategy as a system error in a political interview: The political point of view.

Could the specific nature of "politics" be responsible for the error in the texttype system? Politics is a matter of power. It is also a matter of statesmanship and of policy. But it is in this statesmanship and policy itself that politics shows. And power, and the ways it is dealt with, should be the theme of a political interview. That does not imply that the expressive strategy would not be possible in a political interview. On the contrary, feelings and values direct the politician's behaviour as much as anybody's. However, the petty annoyances of everyday shouldn't be the theme. Mr Van Agt might express his feeling that he "did not realize having power or dwelling in majesty" (1977, December 23rd, K7R7), but in fact he had that power, and was in a high position. And he should have been asked how he dealt with that power instead of how he felt in a new Department or under an attack of his political opponents. And again, his interrogators made it practically impossible for him (or other Prime Ministers) to explain that true political issue. A person asked petty questions gives petty answers.

However, in this case Van Agt may be suspected of not having deplored this state of affairs. In his own words (De Tijd, March 1981):

> "I am, I believe, still not a connoisseur of the political trade, not an artisan in a traditional sense, and still have no intentions of becoming one (...) Things I do not do are designing grand strategies, tactical concepts, holding pre-meetings, preparing plans (...) I am not shrewd enough (...)".

The non-political politician, making believe power is not at stake.

In the examples of the expressive strategy found in these interviews (and in many others) this power-factor is not explained or even discussed. It is obscured as if it did not exist. Therefore these examples do not have any connection with politics at all. This expressive strategy in the political interview is a system error from a political point of view as well, because the res itself is not political.

3 The expressive strategy: a relict of a conversational primitive: small talk

If the expressive strategy is a system error in the political interview, why does it figure in it? Of course there could be many non-rhetorical reasons, but these are not under consideration in the first place. Maybe the thing we call a political interview by any other name would smell better. But that conclusion could only be reached if proof was given that this type of conversation lacked other necessary strategies as well, which in itself would not be difficult, but exceeds the limits of this paper. With these restrictions in mind we shall still regard it as a political interview. To explain the occurrence of the expressive strategy we can only assume the interview shows occasionally qualities of an underlying, more primitive (in the sense of less specified), type of conversation, the **small talk**[10]. From time to time both interrogator and respondent engage in a nice small talk, and that is the type that claims the expressive strategy.

But if that is true, why do the agonists allow that relict of small talk in this highly sophisticated and rule-governed type of communication? Could it be a deliberate choice?

Could it be that in fact the function of the expressive strategy in these interviews is not so much to show the true feelings of the speaker, but to give a show, to help building an image of a human personality, like a neighbour or a good friend, someone you can trust? And what would be the ground for that?

Texttype, aim and strategy, though tightly connected, are not always in line and level. They can be manipulated.

Could it be that these weekly political interviews serve other purposes than just the exchange of information and have also affective aims, which in fact pervert the genre? Could the aim quite simply be to show "the viewers in the country" ("de kijkers in het land" as Vice Prime Minister H. Wiegel was wont to call them) that they have a good government, headed by good people, not so different from the spectator or his family, able to combine reason and emotions and concerned, body and soul, with whatever happens; and what happens is very much like what happens to everybody? Maybe on closer inspection these weekly interviews would turn out to be neither an interview nor political? Maybe again true politics and true political interviews are incompatible.

Only careful study of the way the other strategies are used might give the answer.

NOTES

[1]. E.g. Jan Joost Lindner in De Volkskrant
[2]. See Van Lint 1980 and 1985. In the Netherlands researchers hardly bother about good definitione of texttypes, and innocently even mingle unspecified monologues with unspecified dialogues. I am glad to find some support in a.o. Burger, p 75 to 96 where he works hard to discriminate between "Radio- und Fernsehinterviews" and several varieties therein (Burger 1984). See also Wilhelm Franke: Taxonomie der Dialogtypen (Franke 1984)
[3]. For a discussion of types of discourse on categories of aim, Kinneavy (Kinneavy 1971). I have elaborated that concept in my "Vormen van Taalverkeer" (Van Lint 1980)
[4]. Van Lint: Vormen van Taalverkeer, p 42 ff., idem: Iedereen kijkt mee, hopen we ..., p 137-207, both also based upon Van Lint 1973
[5]. See Van Lint 1981a p 155-177, 1981b, 1984 p 8-28 and p 85-93
[6]. Van Beers (Beers 1982) in his review seems to think I use the word manoeuvre whenever I mean speech-act. If there is a connection at all, of which I am not sure, the speech-act is like the record stored, whereas the manoeuvre is like the record played, on a certain occasion, on a certain equipment, and as part of a certain strategy.
[7]. "In hoogheid te zijn gezeten". Maybe an (ironical?) allusion to Vondel, Lucifer: I, vs 281: "Wie is het die zo hoog gezeten" (Asselbergs 1954, p 48), or to psalm 92, vs 9: "Maar Gij O Here, zetelt in den hoge voor eeuwig" (Bijbelgenootschap 1971), "But thou, Lord, art most high for evermore" (Oxford), or to psalm 93, 1: "Jahwe heeft zich met hoogheid bekleed" (Canisiusvertaling 1955), "He is clothed with majesty" (Oxford), or to psalm 112,5: "Wie is Jahweh gelijk, onze God, die troont in de hoge" (Canisius),"Who is like unto the Lord our God who dwelleth on high" (Oxford)
[8]. A review of possibilities among others in Bally,t II, tableau synoptique, ch. VII, Le sentiment, p 256-260 (Bally 1951)
[9]. This allusion is dealt with in Van Lint 1981, p 262, 262
[10]. For my interpretation of small talk I rely heavily on

the views of Knapp (Knapp 1978) and of Hayakawa (Hayakawa 1972)

I wish to thank Mr. Dolf Hartveldt of Zevenhuizen for his kind help with style and syntax of this paper, and Mr and Mrs Luc and Carol Wagt from The Hague for their final corrections. Of course all responsibility for any errors and other un-English features in language and textstructure remains mine.

APPENDIX

The translated quotations are part of the following original transcripts
(Taken from Van Lint 1977 and Van Lint 1981)
Protocols: Dramaturgic Model / AS-transcription system.
Both Inv. and reaction of the Pair from which a quotation was taken, are given.

23-12-1977 Tros Aktua Extra, Ned 1, 21.50. Geen bandopname.
Protocol RVD.
P/C M. Bruyns/A. van Agt

K3,13,P: (...) is dat een voorproefje geweest van wat u nog te wachten staat aan kritiek?
R3,C: Ja ik denk het wel. Het is duidelijk dat geen gelegenheid onbenut zal worden gelaten om mij te lijf te gaan, dat weet ik. We gaan zwaar weer tegemoet. Ik ben daar wel tegen bestand.
K4,14,P: Hoe was nou die eerste week op Algemene Zaken, is dat meegevallen of tegengevallen, moet je daaraan wennen?
R4,C: Druk
K5,15,P: Druk wel, ja.
R5,C: Ontzettend druk. Ook een beetje onwennig natuurlijk. Je komt binnen op een nieuw departement, nieuwe mensen. Maar ik heb bijzonder bekwame en sympathieke medewerkers om me heen gevonden. Met die ploeg rooi ik het wel.
(...)
K7,17,P: (...)
R7,C: (...) ik ben er min of meer aan gewend geraakt om in die positie te staan en in ieder geval is het in de afgelopen week geen moment zo geweest dat ik me realiseerde van macht te hebben of in hoogheid te zijn gezeten of hoe men dat ook zegt. Wel een zware verantwoordelijkheid te torsen, veel werk te moeten verzetten, een ploeg te moeten waar maken die nogal sterk wordt gecritiseerd, dat zijn de gevoelens die boven drijven.

20-1-1978 Tros Aktua, Ned 1, 21.50. Transcript van video.
P/C: M. Bruyns/A. van Agt

K4,14,P: Nu zit hier een insluiper, een inbreker, een dief

in de nacht (C, b.c.t.: ja) of een premier.

R4,C: Dat was een hele, eigenlijk een heel zware beschuldiging. En wat nu natuurlijk het natuurlijke vervolg van DIE beschuldiging, als hij dat werkelijk meent, had moeten zijn, was, dat hij daarover een uitspraak had gevraagd van de volkvertegenwoordiging. En dat heeft hij niet gedaan. Hij heeft wel, een aantal andere moties ingediend over van ALLERlei zaken, NIET over dit HOOFDpunt.

K5 (...)

K6,I6,P: (...) Wat is het resultaat geweest, zelfkritiek of eh tevredenheid?

R6,C: Nou, wij zijn natuurlijk eh blij dat, het kabinet zonder schade door dit debat is heen gekomen. Het is altijd een avontuur, een risico, om zo'n ontmoeting, die een confrontatie zou KUNnen worden, met de volksvertegenwoordiging, te ondergaan. (...) en wij mogen dus zeggen, zonder in eh in zelfvoldaanheid te vervallen, dat we blijkbaar voldoende argumenten hebben aangevoerd (...), maar we zijn natuurlijk ook bezig geweest in zelfkritiek, want we weten zelf heel goed, dat we de wijsheid NIET in pacht hebben (...), dat we hebben te leren van de eerste ervaring en daarmee zijn we naar best vermogen doende geweest.

3-21978 Televizier Magazine, AVRO, Ned 1, 21.25. Transcript van video
P/C: J. van Meekren/H. Wiegel

K3,13,P: (...) bent u bereid geld te fourneren om de werkgelegenheid bij Hoogovens op peil te houden?

R3,C: Maar de overheid is natuurlijk OOK niet een instantie die de boom met gouden appelen zo maar voor het plukken zo maar in de achter-tuin heeft staan.

K4,14,P: (...) u weet dat als Brussel geld geeft (...) dan verwacht men van de Nederlandse regering in dit geval de andere helft.

R4,C: (...) het water is een heleboel ondernemingen TOT DE LIPpen gestegen. En de overheid, die is ook niet in staat om maar alle gaten te dichten. Kortom, we zitten in DIE zin voor een situatie dat we KUNnen constateren, dat het algemeen in Nederland gewoon SLECHT gaat (...)

12-3-1976 KRO, Brandpunt. Tijdstip niet bekend. Transcript van video
P/C: Ch. Schwietert/J. den Uyl

K13,I13,P: Het is van u bekend dat u niet zo graag met de heer Wiegel in betoog gaat, althans op de televisie, laat ik dat er vooral bij zeggen.
R13,C: Ja heel graag, maar wel in de verkiezingstijd. Maar de ministerpresident debatteert in het parlement
K14,I14,P: In Brandpunt kunnen we dat niet verwachten
R14,C: Nee in het parlement, dat is de plaats.

De Tijd, maart 1981
C: Van Agt
C: Ik ben, geloof ik, nog altijd geen kenner van het politieke métier, geen vakman in de traditionele zin en nog steeds niet voornemens dat te worden (...) Wat ik niet doe is grote strategieën ontwerpen, tactische concepties opstellen, voorvergaderingen houden, plannen voorkoken (...) ik ben er niet handig genoeg voor.

15

General discussion of Political Discourse

J.G. Stappers

I have been asked to comment on the contributions, mainly those treating the political interview, from the perspective of my own discipline, rather than delve into the linguistic aspects as such. This gives me the opportunity to start by stating that what I heard I found both interesting and worthwhile on its own terms; it also gives me the freedom to provide criticism of what went on from an outsider's point of view, remembering of course, that whatever I say will not keep linguists from doing what they are already doing.

Let me begin by doubting the statement that everyone who is studying language is a linguist; if the statement is correct it should not be. Not everyone studying behaviour is a behaviourist and if you think I am being somewhat flippant, then consider sociology, psychology, political science or metaphysics.

Names for disciplines are perhaps not handed out at random, but they are not assigned according to only one logical principle. That disciplines are different from one another is the reason why cooperation is both necessary and fruitful. Members of a discipline who claim to posses the special competences of practitioners from another discipline as well, will show little concern for cooperation. Admitting to being different implies the recognition of the other.

I am a representative of a discipline called publicistics (Publizistikwissenschaft) which in the near future will be known as 'communicatiewetenschap' (Kommunikationswissenschaft, communications). This discipline is not the mere aggregate of those who study communication. In fact, the main theme of this discipline is 'mass communication' - an American term that was totally unsuitable to European traditions.

Incidentally, mass communication is a term which was never satisfactorily defined by the Americans, but which was accepted in Europe in the 1950s.

A literal translation in Dutch or German of the two words separately explains nothing about the nature of mass communication.

Mass communication is not, as many believe, communication to large numbers of recipients, but it is public communication, the dissemination of knowledge (or perhaps information) in society. Not necessarily by the so-called mass media, but to a large extent via these media. The object of **'communicatiewetenschap'** is (in German: **'Veröffentlichung'** or **'Öffentlichkeit'**) in English perhaps best rendered by 'public-making' in the double meaning of that expression (see Stappers 1983). Please note that the word 'public' as used here does not have the broad meaning it has in the title of this conference; it means something like: 'generally available'. Not just linguistics, but several disciplines claim to contribute to the understanding of mass communication.

What distinguishes linguistics from many other disciplines is, that mass communication messages are studied **as they actually are** and not as some experimental simulation. Do not underestimate the positive contribution of this approach: studying reality, not the look-alike. However, some questions about the above procedure should be asked.

In all the papers there seems to me to be a great danger of **'hineininterpretieren'**; not in the explanation of the text, but in the interpretation of the surrounding circumstances or antecedent conditions that are supposed to explain what is happening.

Samples are given but most of the time they are just 'examples' that fit the explanation, but which may easily be explained by other principles. The authors do not justify why these other explanations should be excluded. There we get the situation of the linguist acting as a magician, finding the rabbit in his top hat, and pretending he was not the one who put it there.

This danger is caused, I think, by too little reflection upon research methods and by a lack of theory.

If linguists want their research to be of value for the mass media they should start with a theory or at least with theoretical approaches that are relevant to the mass media, and not take refuge in some post-factum conclusions, even if some of these conclusions are correct. A researcher should state what he is looking for before he starts looking for it. Much of what has been presented here, resembles a kind

of organized serendipity.
As soon as theory, or more modestly, some antecedent principles are introduced, they are of a rather simple nature: "The journalist represents the public ...". That is what journalists like to think - but at best they are self-appointed representatives. 'Cabinet ministers do not have to justify themselves to the media' - of course not, but in practice, they often do, or do so to the general public through the media. After Parliament has been informed there is a lot that politicians can and will tell the public, provided it suits them to do so. Politicians have a lot to account for.
From my point of view, the political interview, whatever it may be is one of many genres of messages. By the way, the study of messages, message analysis, (Aussagenanalyse), very often called content analysis, is a very important area of research, of special interest to the discipline I represent (but not exclusively so) and an area to which linguists could contribute. There exists a wealth of literature on research procedures, and a long standing discussion on several aspects such as quantitative versus qualitative research. It is exactly there that linguistics, as one of the humanities, could be extremely useful. I have, however, not come across any references to the literature on content analysis during this conference, nor have I noticed any explicit connections between this tradition and the research projects discussed here.

To return to the interview as a message. Perhaps the newspaper journalist's interview is a fact-finding mission, undertaken in preparation of a message, but the radio or television interview is a self-contained message as such, and is directed - not just by the interviewer, nor indeed by the politician, but by a collectivity of many persons and not-so-neutral technical equipment - towards the radio listeners or television viewers, sometimes also to a live audience.

The actors play an interview: sometimes well-rehearsed, sometimes badly prepared, but never as spontaneous as it seems to be: the tv interview with the Prime Minister is held on Fridays after all the newspaper journalists have asked their questions.

Whether a particular message is an interview or something else, may be of some value to linguists, but not to me, nor to any audience. The reaction of the audience varies in the case of the same interview from "the politician is unreliable" to "the interviewer is an impolite twit harassing someone who is so earnestly doing what is good for us, the common people". The asymmetry may work both ways. For some politicians it is an advantage, that they can play the role of the underdog. This is certainly true in an environment such as the Dutch broadcasting system, where the media are balanced by making all the programmes unbalanced in all directions (A fact that was not sufficiently explained to the foreign participants in this conference). Anyway, the discourse is only part of the message. If you want to realize how the other components work, you should read Norman Mailer's essay "How to commit murder in the mass media" (in Mailer 1960). Of course it may still be worthwhile to find out how the interview was conducted, but it should be remembered that in broadcasting discourse is a tool; one should, in studying how tools are made, also look at the purposes for which they are made. As I said: the discourse is only one element. Furthermore, if, as has been said here during the workshop, language is a form of goal-directed behaviour, then it should be remembered that mass communication is a form of highly inefficient behaviour. A particular message reaches only a relatively small number of people, many of whom are not interested in, nor receptive to what is in the message.

This does not mean that messages have little importance: once a message is made public, it is part of the public domain, and in the case of political messages, it will be picked up and reacted to by other politicians, who can never be sure how many people - potential voters - may have noticed the original message or will notice the reaction.

Therefore, regardless of the restrictions mentioned, it is worthwhile to study what politicians actually said.

Discourse analysis can serve other purposes. Let me mention two different possibilities. One, hypothesized and mentioned several times during this conference, is that interviewers, politicians, and the public might learn from it. Well, after some time, these three groups of notoriously slow learners will learn from it, and you will discover what the social sciences have already found out, that this knowledge will change their behaviour and that you will have to start all over again.

An altogether different approach - here I come to the second possibility - was implicitly suggested by several speakers. Since linguistics is at its best when it deals with the instruments used in the manufacture of messages, linguistic research procedures could be applied to the old question of impartiality.

It is too often complained that one party gets more attention - i.e. gets more time allotted to it - than the other. Of course there may be obvious political and programmatic reasons for this: "we only pay attention when something worthwhile is being said", that argument will be used whether it is true or not. A linguistic analysis can shed new light on the complaints as such.

To conclude: what linguists do is useful as such, and some of it, perhaps even much of it, may become useful in the long run. But let us remember that possible usefulness starts at the beginning, with theory.

Not all that happens is particularly useful, but in this respect linguistics is not different from other disciplines: we are only just beginning to understand public life.
It will take a long time before full understanding is achieved.

References

Aakster, C.W. & Kuiper, G. (eds.) (1978). Leerboek Medische Sociologie. Sociale wetenschappen toegepast in de gezondheidszorg. Groningen.

Aalderen, H. van & Hollenbeek Brouwer, H. (1982). Methodisch Werken. Amsterdam.

Alban, S.L. & Groman, W.D. (1976). 'Neurotic Anxiety, Pronoun Usage and Stress'. Journal of Clinical Psychology 32, pp. 393-399.

Anderson, R.C. (1977). 'The Notion of Schemata and the Educational Enterprise'. In: R.C. Anderson et al. (eds.) Schooling and the Acquisition of Knowledge. Hillsdale, New Jersey, 1977.

Anderson, R.C. et al. (eds.) (1977). Schooling and The Acquisition of Knowledge. Hillsdale, New Jersey.

Angenot, M. (1982). La parole pamphlétaire. Contribution a la typologie des discours modernes. Paris.

Apeltauer, E. (1978). Elemente und Verlaufsformen von Streitgesprächen. Münster.

Armstrong, D. (1980). An Outline of Sociology as Applied to Medicine. Bristol.

Asselbergs, W.J.M.A. (1954). Joost van den Vondel: Lucifer Treurspel. Zwolle.

Atkinson, J.M. & Drew, P. (1979). Order in Court. The Organisation of Verbal Interaction in Judicial Settings. Atlantic Highlands, New Jersey.

Atkinson, M. (1984). Our Master's Voices. The Language and Body Language of Politics. London.

Atkinson, M. & Heritage, J.C. (eds.) (1984). Structures of Social Action. Cambridge.

Bales, R.F. (1970). Personality and Interpersonal Relations. New York.

Bally, Ch. (1951). Traîté de stylistique française. (3d edition). Geneve/Paris.

Bandura, A. (1976). 'Social Learning Theory'. In: J.T. Spence & R.C. Carson (eds.) Behavioral Approaches to Therapy. Morristown, New Jersey.

Barker-Benfield, G.J. (1976). The Horrors of the Half-Known Life. New York.

Bartlett, F.C. (1932). Remembering. Cambridge.

Bateson, G. (1972). Steps to an Ecology of Mind. New York.

Bax, M. (1981). 'Taalgebruiksverschijnselen bij het aanvaardbaar maken van oordeelsuitspraken in spontane interactie'. In: Steehouder, M.F. & Jansen, C.J.M. (eds.) **Taalbeheersing 1981. Lezingen op het VIOT-taalbeheersingscongres (...)** Enschede, 1981, pp 151-160.

Bax, M.M.H. (1985). **Oordelen in taal. Semantische en pragmatische aspecten van evaluaties in narratieve communicatie.** Groningen.

Beers, W. van & Kusters, T. (1982). 'Boekbespreking van Vormen van taalverkeer.' **Levende Talen 371**, pp 375-380.

Bensing, J. & Sluys, E. (1984) 'Leren luisteren, maar wat dan? Evaluatie van een gesprekstraining voor huisartsen'. **Nederlands Tijdschrift voor de Psychologie 39**, pp. 265-280.

Berens, F.J. (1975). **Analyse des Sprachverhaltens im Redekonstellationstyp "Interview"**. München.

Berenst, J. et al. (to appear). Huisarts-patiënt interactie en de structuur van conversaties. **Nederlands Tijdschrift voor de Psychologie.**

Berger, P.L. & Luckmann, T. (1966). The Social Construction of Reality: A Treatise in the Sociology of Knowledge. Garden City, New York.

Bijsterveld, D.M. van (1985). 'On Accessibility in Conversations with Schizophrenic People'. In: R. Wodak & P. van de Craen (eds.) **Highways and Byways in Communication Disorders.** Clevedon, Avon, 1985. (to appear).

Bishop, Y.M.M., Fienberg, S.E. & Holland, P.W. (1980). **Discrete Multivariate Analysis:** Theory and Practice. Cambridge.

Bliesener, T. (1982). 'Konfliktaustragung in einer schwierigen "therapeutischen Visite"'. In: K. Köhle & H.-H. Raspe (eds.) **Das Gespräch während der ärztlichen Visite.** München, 1982.

Bliesener, T. & Siegrist, J. (1981). 'Greasing the Wheels: Conflicts on the Round and How They are Managed'. **Journal of Pragmatics 5**, pp. 181-204.

Blum-Kulka, S. (1983). 'The Dynamics of Political Interviews'. **Text 3**, pp. 131-153.

Bogue, D.J. (1975). **Twenty-Five Communication Obstacles to the Success of Family Planning Programs.** Community and Family Study Center. Chicago.

Bolinger, D. (1980). 'Fire in a Wooden Stove: On Being Aware in Language'. In: L. Michaels & C. Ricks (eds.) **The State of the Language.** Berkeley/Los Angeles, pp. 379-388.

Bormann, E.G. (1972). 'Fantasy and Rhetorical Vision: The

Rhetorical Criticism of Social Reality'. **Quarterly Journal of Speech** 58, pp. 396-407.
Bormann, E.G. (1975). **Discussion and Group Methods: Theory and Practice.** (2nd edition) New York.
Bormann, E.G. & Bormann, N.C. (1977). **Speech Communication. A Comprehensive Approach.** (2nd edition) New York.
Bormann, E.G., Koester, J. & Bennett, J. (1978). 'Political Cartoons and Salient Rhetorical Fantasies: An Empirical Analysis of the '76 Presidential Campaign'. **Communication Monographs** 45, pp. 317-329.
Bormann, E.G., Pratt, J. & Putnam, L. (1978). 'Power, Author ity, and Sex: Male Response to Female Leadership'. **Communication Monographs** 45, pp. 119-155.
Bormann, E.G. (1980). **Communication Theory.** New York.
Bormann, E.G. (1982). 'Fantasy and Rhetorical Vision: Ten Years Later'. **Quarterly Journal of Speech** 68, pp. 288-305.
Bormann, E.G. (1983). 'Rhetoric as a Way of Knowing: Ernest Bormann and Fantasy Theme Analysis'. In: J.L. Golden, G. Bergquist & W.E. Coleman (eds.) **The Rhetoric of Western Thought.** (3rd edition) Dubuque, Illinois, 1983, pp. 431-449.
Bormann, E.G. et al. (1984). 'Rhetorical Visions of Committed Voters: Fantasy Theme Analysis of a Large Sample Survey'. **Critical Studies in Mass Communication** 1, pp. 287-310.
Breger, L. & McGaugh, J.L. (1969). 'A Critique and Reformulation of Learning Theory Approaches to Psychotherapy and Neurosis'. **Psychological Bulletin**, 69, pp. 642-645.
Bremer, G.J. (1980). **Over klagen, in het bijzonder het klagen bij de dokter.** Alphen aan de Rijn.
Brown, G. & Yule, G. (1983). **Discourse Analysis.** Cambridge.
Brown, P. & Levinson, S. (1978). 'Universals in Language Usage: Politeness Phenomena'. In: E. Goody (ed.) **Questions and Politeness: Strategies in Social Interaction.** Cambridge, 1978.
Burger, H. (1984). **Sprache der Massenmedien.** Berlin/New York.

Campbell, K.K. (...). 'Criticism: Ephemeral and Enduring'. **Speech Teacher** 23, pp. 13-24.
Campbell, K.K. & Jamieson, K.H. (eds.) (1977). **Form and Genre. Shaping Rhetorical Action.** Leesburg Pike.
Candlin, C.N. (1983a). The Language of Unequal Encounters: Discoursal Features in a Police-Witness Interview. (mimeo)

Paper delivered at the Hatfield Polytechnic Conference on Discourse Structure. 1983.

Candlin, C.N. (1983b). Beyond Description to Explanation in Cross-Cultural Discourse. (mimeo) Paper delivered at the East-West Center, Honolulu Conference on English as an International Language: Discourse Patterns across Cultures. 1983.

Candlin, C.N., Bruton, C.J. & Leather, J.H. (1976a). 'Doctors in Casualty: Applying Communicative Competence to Components of Specialist Course Design' IRAL, 14, (3), pp. 245-272.

Candlin, C.N., Bruton, C.J. & Leather, J.H. (1976b). 'Doctor Speech Functions in Casualty Consultations: some Quantified Characteristics of Discourse in a Regulated Setting'. In: G. Nickel (ed.) **Proceedings of the III AILA World Congress**. Stuttgart, 1975.

Candlin, C.N. et al. (1978). **Doctor-Patient Communication Skills Vols I and II**. Graves Medical Audio-Visual Library, Chelmsford England (published version of C.N. Candlin, C.J. Bruton & J.H. Leather (1975) **Doctor-Patient Communication Skills: Working-Papers I-IV**. Department of Linguistics & Modern English Language, University of Lancaster, Lancaster. (mimeo).

Candlin, C.N. et al. (1981). 'Designing Modular Materials for Communicative Language Skills'. In: In Selinker, E. Tarone & V. Hanzeli (eds.) **English for Academic and Technical Purposes: Studies in Honor of Louis Trimble**. Newbury House, Rowley, Massachusetts.

Candlin, C.N., Coleman, H. & Burton, J. (1980). **Dentist-Patient Communication** (Report plus Appendix). General Dentist Council & University of Lancaster. Lancaster England.

Candlin, C.N., Coleman, H. & Burton, J. (1983). 'Dentist-Patient Communication Communicating Complaint'. In: N. Wolfson & E. Judd (eds.) **Sociolinguistics and Second Language Acquisition**. Newbury House, Rowley, Massachusets.

Candlin, C.N. & Lotfipour, K. (1983). 'Processes of Discourse'. **Journal of Applied Language Study** I, (2).

Carpenter, M.D. (1976). 'Sensitivity to Syntactic Structure: Good versus Poor Premorb Schizophrenics'. **Journal of Abnormal Psychology** 85, (1), pp. 41-50.

Chaffee, S. (1978). 'Presidential Debates- Are They Helpful to Voters?. **Communication Monographs** 45, pp. 330-346.

Chaika, E. (1974). 'A Linguist Looks at Schizophrenic Language'. **Brain and Language** 1, pp. 257-76.

Chapman, L.J., Chapman, J. & Miller, G. (1964). 'A Theory of Verbal Behaviour in Schizophrenia'. In: B.A. Maher (ed.) **Progress in Experimental Personality Research, Vol I.** New York, 1964.

Chapman, L.J. Chapman, J. & Daut, R.L. (1985). 'Schizophrenic Inability to Disattend from Strong Aspects of Meaning'. **Journal of Abnormal Psychology** 85, pp. 35-40.

Chase, S. (1938). **The Tyranny of Words.** New York.

Churchill, L. (1978). **Questioning Strategies in Sociolinguistics.** Rowley, Massachusetts.

Cicourel, A.V. (1972). 'Basic and Normative Rules in the Nego tiation of Status and Role'. In: D. Sudnow (ed.) **Studies in Social Interaction.** New York/London, 1972.

Cicourel, A.V. (1980). 'Three Models of Discourse Analysis; the Role of Social Structures'. **Discourse Processes** 3, pp. 101-132.

Cicourel, A.V. (1982). 'Language and Belief in a Medical Setting'. In: H. Byrnes (ed.) **Georgetown University Round Table on Languages and Linguistics 1982.** Washington D.C.

Cicourel, A.V. (1983). 'Language and the Structure of Belief in Medical Communication'. In: S. Fisher & A.D. Todd (eds.) **The Social Organization of Doctor-Patient Communication.** Washington, 1983, pp. 221-241.

Clarke, D. (1975). 'The Use and Recognition of Sequential Structure in Dialoque'. **British Journal of Social and Clinical Psychology** 14, pp. 333-339.

Clausewitz, F. (1970). 'Lehre vom Gebrauche der Gefechte zum Zwecke des Krieges'. In: E. Obermann (ed.) **Verteidigung. Ein Handbuch.** Stuttgart, 1970.

Cole, P. & Morgan, J.L. (eds.) **Syntax and Semantics 3: Speech Acts.** New York.

Conrad, P. & Kern, R. (eds.) 1981. **The Sociology of Health and Illness: Critical Perspectives.** New York.

Conte, R. (1981). 'Aspects of Interaction in a Medical Interview'. **Journal of Pragmatics** 5, pp. 113-144.

Corea, G. (1977). **The Hidden Malpractice: How American Medicine Treats Women as Patients and Professionals.** New York.

Corsaro, W.A. (1981). 'Communicative Processes in Studies of Social Organization: Sociological Approaches to Discourse Analysis'. **Text** I, (1), pp. 5-63.

Corsaro, W.A. (1982). 'Something Old and Something New: The Importance of Prior Ethnography in the Collection and Analysis of Audiovisual Data'. **Sociological Methods and**

Research, Vol. II, (2), pp. 145-166.
Cragan, J.f. & Shields, D.C. (1981). **Applied Communication Research: A Dramatistic Approach.** Prospect Heights, Illinois.
Croce, B. (1978). **Aesthetic. As Science of Expression and General Linguistic.** Transl. by D. Ainslie. Boston.

Davis, K. (1984). Problem (Re)formulation in Psychotherapy. Rotterdam, **Konteksten 4**.
Deeds, S. (1973). **A Guidebook for Family Planning Education.** DHEW Publication (HSA) 74-16002 US Department of Health, Education & Welfare, Public Health Service, HSA Bureau of Community Health Services. Rockville, Maryland.
Devoge, J.T. & Beck, S. (1978). 'The Therapist-Client Relationship in Behaviour Therapy'. In: M. Hersen, R.M. Eisler & P.M. Miller (eds.) **Progress in Behaviour Modification 6.** New York.
Dewey, J. (1934). **Art as Experience.** New York.
Dijk, T. van (1977). 'Context and Cognition: Knowledge Frames and speech Act Comprehension'. **Journal of Pragmatics** 1, pp. 211-232.
Dijk, T. van (1981). 'Review of R.O. Freedle (ed.) (1979) 'New Directions in Discourse Processing'. **Journal of Linguistics** 17, pp. 140-148.
Dreifus, C. (ed.) (1977). **Seizing Our Bodies.** New York.
Dreitzel, H.P. (ed.) (1977). **Recent sociology II.** New York/London.
Dubber, C. & Weijdema, W. (1980). 'Funkties van herhaling in verbale interactie'. In: A Foolen et al. (eds.) **Conversatieanalyse.** Groningen, 1980, pp. 224-241.
Dubos, R. (1959). **Mirage of Health.** New York.

Ecker, H.P. et al. (1977). **Textform Interview.** Düsseldorf.
Edelman, M. (1977). **Political Language: Words that Succeed and Policies that Fail.** New York.
Eemeren, F.H. van & Grootendorst, R. (1984). **Speech Acts in Argumentative Discussions. A Theoretical Model for the Analysis of Discussions Directed towards Solving Conflicts of Opinion.** Dordrecht/Cinnaminson.
Eemeren, F.H. van, Grootendorst, R. & Kruiger, T. (1984). **The Study of Argumentation.** New York.
Ehlich, K. & Rehbein, J. (eds.) (1983). **Kommunikation in Schule und Hochschule.** Tübingen.
Ehrenreich, B. & Ehrenreich, J. (1970). **The American Health**

Empire. New York.
Ehrenreich, B. & English, D. (1978). For Her Own Good. New York.

Fairclouth, N. (to appear). 'Critical and Descriptive Goals in Discourse Analysis'. Journal of Pragmatics.
Fehlenberg, D. (1983a). 'Die empirische Analyse der Visitenkommunikation: Institutionskritik und Ansätze für eine reflektierte Veränderung institutioneller Praxis'. Osnabrücker Beiträge zur Sprachtheorie 24, pp. 29-56.
Fehlenberg, D. (1983b). Doctor-Patient Interaction During Daily Ward Rounds: The Traditional Setting and Exploration of the Psychomatic Approach. (mimeo). Linguistic Workshop 'Medical Communication'. Tilburg.
Fehlenberg, D. & Köhle, K. (1984). 'Das ärztliche Gespräch während der klinischen Visite und in der Sprechstunde'. Internist 25, pp. 682-693.
Ferrel, W.A. & Salerno, N.A. (1973). Strategies in Prose. (3rd edition) New York.
Fiedler, P.A. (1976). Teilstandisierte vs. verhaltensanalytische Gruppentherapie'. Mitteilungen der DGVT 8, pp. 161-173.
Fisher, S. (1982). 'The Decision-Making Context: How Doctor and Patient Communicate'. In: R.J. Di Pietro (ed.) Linguistics and the Professions. New Jersey.
Fisher, S. (1982). Doctor-Patient Communication; A Social and Micro-Political Performance. (mimeo). Paper presented at the International sociological association meetings, Mexico City, 1982.
Fisher, S. (1983). 'Doctor Talk/Patient Talk: How Treatment Decisions are Negotiated in Doctor/Patient Communication'. In: S. Fisher & A. Todd (eds.) The Social Organization of Doctor-Patient Communication. Washington, (to appear).
Fisher, S. (1984). 'Was Ärzte sagen- was Patientinnen sagen: Die Mikropolitik des Entscheidungsprozesses im medizinischen Gespräch'. In: S. Trömel-Plötz (ed.) Gewalt durch Sprache. die Vergewaltigung von Frauen in Gesprächen. Frankfurt aM.
Fisher, S. (1984). 'Institutional authority and the Structure of Discourse'. Discourse Processes 7, pp. 201-224.
Foets, M. & Peeters, R. (1982). 'De sociologische belangstelling voor ziekten en gezondheid'. In: Y. Nuyens (ed.) Sociologie en Gezondheidszorg. Antwerpen, 1982, Vol. I, pp. 47-65.

Foolen, A. Hardeveld, J. & Springorum, D. (eds.) (1980) **Conversatie-analyse.** Groningen.

Fotion, N. (1979). 'Speech Activity and Language Use'. **Philosophia** 8, (4), pp. 616-638.

Fowler, R. et al. (1979). **Language and control.** London.

Franke, W. (1985). 'Taxonomie der Dialogtypen'. In: W. Kurschner (ed.) **Sprachtheorie, Pragmatik, Interdisziplinares. Akten des 19. Linguistischen Kolloquiums, Vechta 1984.** Tübingen.

Frankel, R.M. 81984). 'From Sentence to Sequence: Understanding the Medical Encounter through Microinteractional Analysis'. **Discourse Processes** 7, pp. 135-170.

Freidson, E. (1962). 'Dilemmas in the doctor-patient relationship'. In: A. Rose (ed.) **Human Behaviour and Social Processes.** London, 1962.

Freidson, E. (1970). **Profession of Medicine.** New York.

Friedrichs, J. (1976). 'Journalistische Praxis: Das Interview'. **Fernsehen und Bildung** 10, pp. 169-197.

Fromkin, V.A. (1975). A Linguist Looks at 'A linguist Looks at Schizophrenic Language'. **Brain and Language** 2, pp. 498-503.

Fumaroli, M. (1984). **L'âge de l'éloquence. Rhétorique et "res literaria" de la Rénaissance au seuil de l'époque classique.** (4th edition) Paris.

Geest, T. van der (1978). **Entwicklung der Kommunikation.** Bochum.

Geest, T. van der (1982). Therapist-Client and Doctor-Patient Conversation. (mimeo). Paper presented to the International sociological association meetings. Mexico City, 1982.

Geest, T. van der (1983). 'Adaptie in arts-patient communicatie; enkele methodologische kanttekeningen bij een onderzoeksopzet'. **Tabu,** 1983, pp. 71-98.

Geest, T. van der (1985a) 'Leiderschapsstijlen: autoriteit en afstand als kenmerkende dimensies voor het taalgegebruik'. In: W.K.B. Koning (ed.) **Taalbeheersing in theorie en praktijk.** Dordrecht, 1985.

Geest, T. van der (1985b).**Interactie, onderwijsorganisatie en taalvaardigheid.** (SLO). Enschede.

Geest, T. van der & Fehlenberg, D. (eds.) (1982). **Kommunikationsanalysen in der Verhaltenstherapie.** Bochum.

Geldrop, G. van, Hoekman, K. & Krol, L. (1978). **Medisch probleemoplossen.** Amsterdam.

Gerver, D. (1967). 'Linguistic Rules and the Perception and Recall of Speech by Schizophrenic Patients'. **British Journal of Social Clinical Psychology** 6, pp. 204-211.

Gevers, Th., Kapsenberg, I. & Straatman, W. (1980). **Het professionele tweegesprek**. Lisse.

Gibbard, G.S., Hartman, J.J. & Mann, R.D. (eds.) (1974). **Analysis of Groups**. San Francisco.

Giles, H. & St. Clair, R. (eds.) (1979). **Language and Social Psychology**. London.

Goffman, E. (1961). 'The Medical Model and Mental Hospitalization; Some Notes on the Vicissitudes of the Tinkering Trades'. In: E. Goffman. **Asylums**. Harmondsworth, pp. 281-336.

Goffman, E. (1967). 'On Face-Work'. In: E. Goffman. **Interactional Ritual. Essays on Face-to-Face Behavior**. New York, 1967, pp. 5-46.

Goffman, E. (1971). **Relations in Public: Microstudies of the Public Order**. New York.

Goffman, E. (1974). **Frame analysis. An Essay on the Organization of Experience**. New York.

Goodwin, C. (1984). 'Prefaces to Assessments'. Contribution to the 'International and Multidisciplinary Conference on Interaction and Language Use'. **British Sociological Association of Language Study Group**. Plymouth.

Goody, E. (ed.) (1978). **Questions and Politeness. Strategies in Social Interaction**. Cambridge.

Gordon, L. (1974). **Woman's Body, Woman's Right: A Social History of Birth Control in America**. New York.

Gottman, J.M. (1979). **Marital Interaction**. New York.

Green, A. (1977). 'Atome de parenté et relations oedipiennes'. In: C. Lévi-Strauss. **L'Identité, Séminaire interdisciplinaire dirigé par C. Lévi-Strauss au College de France 1974-1975**. Paris.

Green, J.L. & Wallat, C. (eds.) (1981). **Ethnography and Language in Educational Settings**. Norwood, New Jersey.

Grice, H.P. (1975). 'Logic and Conversation'. In: P. Cole & J.L. Morgan (eds.) **Syntax and Semantics 3: Speech Acts**. New York, pp. 41-58.

Gück, J., Matt, E. & Weingarten, E. (1983). 'Zur interaktiven Ausgestaltung der Arzt-Patient-Beziehung in der Visite'. In: U. Gerhardt et al. (eds) **Jahrbuch Medizinische Soziologie 3**. Frankfurt, 1983.

Gumperz, J.J. (1982a). **Discourse Strategies**. Cambridge.

Gumperz, J.J. (ed.) (1982b). **Language and Social Identity**.

Cambridge.

Haberland, H. & Mey, J.L. (1981). 'Wording and Warding: The Pragmatics of Therapeutical Conversation'. **Journal of Pragmatics** 5, pp. 103-111.
Habermas, J. (1971). 'Vorbereitende Bemerkungen zu einer Theorie der kommunikativen Kompetenz'. In: J. Habermas & N. Luhmann. **Theorie der Gesellschaft oder Sozialtechnologie- was leistet die Systemforschung?** Frankfurt a.M.
Habermas, J. (1972). 'Towards a Theory of Communicative Competence'. In: H.P. Dreitzel (ed.) **Recent Sociology II**. New York/London.
Habermas, J. (1973). **Kultur und Kritik**. Frankfurt.
Habermas, J. (1981). **Theorie des kommunikativen Handelns**. Frankfurt a.M.
Halder, P. (1977). **Verhaltenstherapie und Patientenerwartung**. Bern
Hale Ho'ola Hou: **Kalihi-Palama Health Clinic Annual Report** 1983.
Halloran, M. (1977). 'Doing Public Business in Public'. In: Campbell et al. (eds.) **Form and Genre. Shaping Rhetorical Action**. Leesburg Pike, 1977.
Hammersley, M. (1977). 'School Learning: The Cultural Resources Required by Pupils to answer a Teacher's Question' In: P. Woods & M. Hammersley (eds.) **School Experiences**. Croome Helm, 1977.
Hang, H.-G.(1976). **Die Fragesignale in der gesprochenen deutsche Standardsprache**. Göppingen.
Harari, J.V. (ed.) (1980). **Textual Strategies. Perspectives in Post-Structuralist Criticism**. London.
Harris, S. (1984). 'Questions as a Mode of Control in Magistrates Courts'. In: H. Coleman (ed.) **Language and Work**. In: **International Journal of the Sociology of Language**. (to appear).
Haselkorn, F. (1968). **Family Planning: The Role of Social Work**. Adelphi University School of Social Work. Adelphi.
Hauser, S.T. (1981). 'Physician-Patient Relationships'. In: E. Mishler, et al. (eds.) **Social Contexts of Health, Illness, and Patient Care**. London.
Hayakawa, S.I. (1972). **Language in Thought and Action**. New York.
Heath, S.B. (1979). 'The Context of Professional Languages: An Historical Overview'. In: J.A. Alatis & G.R. Tucker (eds.) **Georgetown university Round Table on Languages and**

Linguistics 1979. Washington D.C.

Henley, N. (1977). **Body Politics: Power, Sex and Nonverbal Communication.** New Jersey.

Heritage, J.C. & Watson, D.R. (1979). 'Formulations as Every Objects'. In: G. Psathas (ed.) **Everyday language. Studies in Ethnomethodology.** Irvington, 1979.

Heritage, J.C. (1984). 'A Change of State Token and Aspects of its Sequential Placement'. In: J.M. Atkinson & J.C. Heritage (eds.) **Structures of Social Action.** Cambridge, 1984.

Heritage, J. (1984). **Garfinkel and Ethnomethodology.** Cambridge.

Hoermann, H. (1976). 'The concept of Sense Constancy', in: **Lingua** 39. pp. 269-280.

Hoffman, L. (1980). 'Zur Pragmatik von Erzählformen vor Gericht'. In: K. Ehlich (ed.) **Erzählen im Alltag.** Frankfurt aM.

Hoffmann, R.R. (1982). **Politische Fernsehinterviews.** Tübingen.

Holdcroft, D. (1979). 'Speech Acts and Conversation'. **Philosophical Quarterly** 29 (115), pp. 125-141.

Houtkoop-Steenstra, J.P. (1980). '**"Je hebt wel gelijk, maar ..." Enige pragmatische aspecten van concessief-adversatieve "wel"-"maar"-constructies**'. Publikaties van het Instituut voor Algemene Taalwetenschap 28. University of Amsterdam. Amsterdam.

Houtkoop-Steenstra, J.P. (1981). 'Taalgebruik en konversationele strategieën'. In: **Kongresbundel Zomeruniversiteit Vrouwenstudies.** Amsterdam, 1981.

Houtkoop-Steenstra, J.P. (1985). 'Kan een verzoek met "Ja" worden geaccepteerd?'. **Tijdschrift voor Taal- en Tekstwetenschap** 5 (1), pp. 23-41.

Hudson, K. (1978). **The Language of Modern Politics.** London.

Hymes, D. (1967). On Communicative Competence. (mimeo) Paper delivered at the Yale Linguistics Club.

Hymes, D. (1972). 'Models of the Interaction of Language and Social Life'. In: J. Gumperz & D. Hymes (eds.) **Directions in Sociolinguistics.** New York, 1972, pp. 35-71.

Hymes, D. (1979). 'The Scope of Sociolinguistics'. In: Hymes, D. **Foundation in Sociolinguistics. An Ethnographic Approach.** London, 1977, pp. 193-209.

Jaffe, J. (1964). 'Verbal Behaviour Analysis'. In: D. Rioch & F. Weinstein (eds.) **Disorders of Communication** 42.

Jankowski, P et al. (eds.) (1976). **Klientzentrierte Gesprächspsychotherapie.** Göttingen.
Jefferson, G. (1983). 'On the Interactional Unpackaging of a "Gloss"'. **Tilburg Papers in Language and Literature 29.**
Jefferson, G. ( ). "At First I thought": A Normalizing Device for Extraordinary Events. (unpubl.).
Jefferson, G. & Lee, J.R.E. (1981). 'The Rejection of Advice: Managing the Problematic Convergence of a 'Troubles Telling' and a 'Service Encounter''. **Journal of Pragmatics** 5, pp. 399-422.

Kennedy, A.K. (1983). **Dramatic Dialogue. The Duologue of Personal Encounter.** Cambridge.
Kessel, W. van (1976). 'Der Psychotherapeutische Prozess'. In: P. Jankowski et al. (eds.) Klientenzentrierte Gesprächspsychotherapie. Göttingen, 1976.
Kinneavy, J.L. (1971). **A. Theory of Discourse. The Aims of Discourse.** Englewood Cliffs, New Jersey.
Klamer, E. (1978). **Paragraph Tense: a Basic Rhetoric.** New York.
Knapp, M.L. (1978). **Social Intercourse. From Greeting to Goodbye.** Boston.
Knoke, D. & Burke, P.J. (1980). **Log-Linear Models.** Beverly Hills.
Knorr-Centina, K. & Cicourel, A.V. (1981). **Advances in Social Theory and Methodology: Toward an Integration of Micro- and Macro-Sociologies.** Boston.
Koning, W.K.B. (ed.) (1985). **Taalbeheersing in theorie en praktijk.** Dordrecht.
Kress, G. & Hodge, R. (1981). **Language as Ideology.** London.
Kress, G. & Trew, A. (1978). 'Ideological Transformation of Discourse; or How the Sunday Times Got Its Message Across'. **Journal of Pragmatics** 2, pp. 311-329.
Krol, L.J. (1979). 'Ongerustheid en causa ignota'. **Nederlands Tijdschrift voor Geneeskunde** 123, (21), pp. 865-868.
Kropf, D. (1976). **Grundprobleme der Gesprächspsychotherapie.** Göttingen/Toronto.
Kurschner, W. (ed.) (1985). **Sprachtheorie, Pragmatik, Interdisziplinares. Akten des 19. Linguistischen Kolloquiums, Vechta 1984.** Tübingen.

Labov, T. (1980). The Communication of Morality: Cooperation and Commitment in a Food Coperative. Columbia,(unpublished).

Labov, T. (1983). Moral Language: A Sociological Analysis of Cooperation and Commitment. (mimeo). Paper given at Japanese Assoc. of College English Teachers. Hachioji, Japan.

Labov, W. (1972). Sociolinguistic Patterns. Philadelphia.

Labov, W. (1972). 'The Transformation of Experience in Narrative Syntax'. In: W. Labov. Language in the Inner City. Studies in the Black English Vernacular. Oxford, 1972.

Labov, W. (1972). Language in the Inner City. Studies in the Black English Vernacular. Oxford.

Labov, W. (1975). 'Empirical foundations of Linguistic Theory', in: R. Austerlitz (ed.). The Scope of American Linguistics. The First Golden Anniversary of the Linguistic Society of America. Lisse. pp. 77-133.

Labov, W. (unp.) Intensity. Georgetown Monographs on Languages and Linguistics. Washington D.C. (to appear).

Labov, W. & Fanshel, D. (1977). Therapeutic Discourse: Psychotherapy as Conversation. New York.

Lakoff, R.T. (1982). 'Persuasive Discourse and Ordinary Conversation, With Examples From Advertising'. In: D. Tannen (ed.) Analyzing Discourse: Text and Talk. Washington, D.C., 1982, pp. 25-42.

Leech, G.N. (1977). 'Language and Tact'. Linguistic Agency University of Trier. (mimeo). Series A Paper 46, 1977.

Leech, G.N. (1983). Principles of Pragmatics. London/New York.

Lefcourt, H.M. (1976). Locus of Control. Current Trends in Theory and Research. New York.

Lennard, H. & Bernstein, A. (1960). The Anatomy of Psychotherapy. New York.

Levelt, W.J.M. & Flores d'Arcais, G.B. (eds.) (1978). Studies in the Perception of Language. Chichester, Sussex.

Levinson, S.C. (1979). 'Activity Types and Language'. Linguistics 17, pp. 365-399.

Levinson, S.C. (1983). Pragmatics. Cambridge.

Lévi-Strauss, C. (1958). 'Analyse structural en linguistique et en anthropologie (I)'. In: C. Lévi-Strauss. Anthropologie structurale (I). Paris, pp. 37-62.

Lint, P. van (1973). 'Wat mot die goser van me'. Levende Talen 297, pp. 178-191.

Lint, P. van, Hoek, K.W. van de & Kagie, R. (1977). Ja kijk, mag ik dit zeggen. Opmerkingen over de verbale strategieën van een ministerpresident en zijn ondervragers in elf televisie-interviews van januari tot maart 1976. Groningen.

Lint, P. van, Hoek, K.W. van de & Kagie, R. (1980). **Vormen van taalverkeer. Een elementaire inleiding in de leer van de verstandhoudingsmiddelen.** De mondelinge vormen. Groningen.
Lint, P. van, Hoek, K.W. van de & Pauw, I. (1981). **Iedereen kijkt mee, hopen we ... De eerste vijf maanden van het kabinet-Van Agt/Wiegel retorisch weerspiegeld in 21 TV-gesprekken.** Twee dln. Groningen.
Lint, P. van (1981). 'Taalexpressie als Taalvaardigheid II. Over de speelse vormen van Taalverkeer, vooral de Voorlezing en de Voordracht'. In: M.F. Steehouder & C.J.M. Janssen (eds.) **Taalbeheersing 1981: Lezingen op het VIOT-taalbeheersingscongres** (...). Enschede 1981. pp. 33-40.
Lint, P. van, Hoek, K.W. van de & Pauw, I. (1984). 'Aspekten van taalexpressie'. In: Lint, P. van, Hoek, K.W. van de & Pauw, I. **Taalexpressie als taalvaardigheid. Reader voor taalexpressie** (**onderbouw**). Groningen (unpublished).
Lint, P. van (1985). 'Retorische Kritiek en Politieke Retorica. Socioretorische aspekten van politieke retorica, in het bijzonder in de ethermedia'. **Massacommunicatie** 13, (2), pp. 54-70.
Lucas, J.L. (1983). The Therapeutic Interview: A Setting for Asymmetrical Discourse. (mimeo). Department of ESL, University of Hawaii at Manoa. Manoa.
Luker, K. (1975). **Taking Chances: Abortion and the Decision** Not to Contracept. Berkeley.
Lutz, R. (1978). **Das verhaltens-diagnostische Interview.** Stuttgart.
Lyons, W. (1980). **Emotion.** Cambridge.

Maher, B.A. (ed.) (1964). **Progress** in Experimental **Personality Research.** New York, 1964.
Mailer, N. (1960). **Advertisements for Myself.** New York.
Manisoff, M. (1970). **Family Planning Training for Social Service.** Planned Parenthood Federation of America Inc.
May, J. (1981). 'Practical Reasoning: Extracting Useful Information from Partial Informants'. **Journal of Pragmatics** 5, pp. 45-59.
McKnight, A. (1976). **Large-Group Conversation: Problems for Discourse Analysis.** MA Thesis (mimeo). Department of Linguistics and Modern English Language. University of Lancaster. Lancaster.
McLaughlin, M.L., Cody, M.J. & Rosenstein, N.E. (1983). 'Account Sequences in Conversations Between Strangers'.

Communication Monographs 50, pp. 102-125.

Meddens, H. & Sturm, A. (1977). 'De aanstaande verkiezingsstrijd, een interessant onderwerp voor moedertaalonderwijs'. **Moer** 2, pp. 4-14.

Mehan, H. (1979). **Learning Lessons.** Cambridge, Massachusets.

Meichenbaum, D. (1976). 'Cognitive Behaviour Modification'. In: J.T. Spence & R.C. Carson & J.W. Thibaut (eds.) **Behavioural Approaches to Therapy.** Morristown, New Jersey, 1976.

Merton, R. & Barber, E. (1963). 'Sociological Ambivalence'. In: E. Tirykian (ed.) **Sociological Theory.** Glencoe, 1963.

Minsky, M. (1975). 'A Framework for Representing Knowledge'. In: P.H. Winston (ed.) **The Psychology of Computer Vision.** New York, 1975.

Mishler, E.S. (1975). 'Studies in Dialogue and Discourse II. Types of Discourse Initiated by and Sustained Through Questioning'. **Journal of Psycholinguistic Research** 2, pp. 99-121.

Mishler, E.S. (1975). 'Studies in Dialoque and Discourse: An Exponential Law of Successive Questioning'. **Language in Society** 4, pp. 31-51.

Morgan, S. (1978). 'Sexuality After Hysterectomies and Castration'. **Women and Health** 3, pp. 5-10.

Morris, C. (1971) **Writings on the General Theory of Signs.** Den Haag.

Morris, R.J. & Suckerman, K.R. (1974). 'The Importance of the Therapeutic Relationship in Systematic Desensibilisation'. **Journal of Consulting and Clinical Psychology** 42, pp. 148-153.

Morris, R.J. & Suckerman, K.R. (1974). 'Therapist Warmth as a Factor in Automated Systematic Desensibilisation'. **Journal of Consulting and Clinical Psychology** 42, pp. 244-250.

Nothdurft, W. (1982). 'Zur Undurchlässigkeit von Krankenhausvisiten'. In: K. Köhle & H.-H. Raspe (eds.) **Das Gespräch während der ärztlichen Visite.** München.

Obermann, E. (ed.) (1970). **Verteidigung. Ein Handbuch.** Stuttgart.

Olmüller, W., Dolle, R. & Piepmeier, R. (1977). **Diskurs: Politik.** Paderborn.

Orwell, G. (1946). 'Politics and the English Language'. **Horizon** (april 1946).

Owen, M. (1983). **Apologies and Remedial Interchanges.**

Berlin.

Parsons, T. (1951). The Social System. New York.
Pateman, T. (1975). Language, Truth and Politics. Devon.
Pateman, T. (1980). Language, Truth and Politics. Sussex.
Pauw, I. (1984). Indelen en onderverdelen. Een retorisch onderzoek naar opvattingen over en kenmerken van Taalexpressie. Groningen (unpublished).
Persoon, J.M.G. (1975). Veranderingen in de patient-huisarts relatie. Nijmegen.
Persoon, J.M.G. (1978). 'Arts-patient relaties'. In: C.W. Aakster & G. Kuiper (eds.) Leerboek Medische Sociologie. Sociale wetenschappen toegepast in de gezondheidszorg. Groningen, 1978, pp. 228-236.
Piët, S. (1980). Een vraag en een weet. Gereedschap voor het vraaggesprek. Baarn.
Pomerantz, A. (1984). 'Agreeing and Disagreeing with Assessments: Some Features of Preferred/Dispreferred Turn Shapes'. In: J.M. Atkinson & J.C. Heritage (eds.) Structures of Social Action. Cambridge, 1984.
Popper, K. (1974). Objective Knowledge. Oxford.
Popper, K. & Eccles, J.C. (1977). The Self and Its Brain. New York.
Portnoy, S. (1973). 'A Comparison of Oral and Written Verbal Behaviour'. In: K. Salzinger & R.S. Feldman (eds.) Studies in Verbal Behaviour: An Empirical Approach. New York, 1973.
Prather, J. & Fidell, L. (1975). 'Sex Differences in the Content and Style of Medical Advertisements'. Social Science and Medicine 9, pp. 23-26.
Psathas, G. (ed.) (1979). Everyday Language: Studies in Ethnomethodology. New York.

Quintillianus, M.F. (1968). Institutio Oratoria. With an English Translation by H.E. Butler. London.

Read, H. (1956). Education Through Art. London.
Rehbein, J. (1977). Komplexes Handeln. Elemente zur Handlungstheorie der Sprache. Stuttgart.
Reiser, D.E. & Rosen, D.H. (eds.) (1984). Medicine as a Human Experience. Baltimore.
Riesbeck, C. & Schank, R. (1978). 'Comprehension by Computer: Expectation-Based Analysis of Sentences in Context' In: W. Levelt & G.B. Flores d'Arcais (eds.) Studies in the

Perception of Language. Chichester, Sussex.
Rioch, D. & Weinstein, F. (eds.) (1964). **Disorders of Communication.**
Rochester, S.R., Martin, J.R. & Thurston, S. (1977). 'Thought-Process Disorder in Schizophrenia: The Listener's Task'. **Brain and Language 4**, pp. 95-113.
Rochester, S.R. & Martin, J.R. (1979). **Crazy Talk, a Study of the Discourse of Schizophrenic Speakers.** New York.
Rogers, C. (1951). **Client-centered therapy.** London.
Ross, W.D. (1968). **Foundations of Ethics.** Oxford.
Rumelhart, D. & Ortony, A. (1977). 'The Representation of Knowledge in Memory'. In: R. Anderson et al. (eds.) **Schooling and the Acquisition of Knowledge.** Hillsdale, New Jersey,
Rutter, D.R. (1979). 'The Reconstruction of Schizophrenic Speech'. **British Journal of Psychology 134**, pp. 356-360.
Ruzek, S.B. (1978). **The Women's Health Movement.** New York.
Ryan, E. & Giles, H. (eds.) (1982) **Attitudes towards Language Variation: Social and Applied Contexts.** London.

Sacks, H. (1973). On the Preference for Agreement and Contiguity in Sequences in Conversation. (unpublished).
Sacks, H. **Unpublished Lecture Notes.**
1967, Fall, lecture 13.
1968, May 29. 1967, Fall, Lecture 13.
1970, Spring, lecture 5.
1970, Winter, lecture 2.
Salzinger, K. et al. (1970). 'The Immediacy Hypothesis and Response-Produced Stimuli in Schizophrenic Speech'. **Journal of Abnormal Psychology 76**, pp. 258-264.
Salzinger, K. & Feldman, R.S. (eds.) (1973). **Studies in Verbal Behaviour: An Empirical Approach.** New York.
Schank, R. & Abelson, R. (1977). **Scripts, Plans, Goals and Understanding: An Inquiry into Human Knowledge Structures.** Hillsdale, New Jersey.
Schegloff, M. (1972). 'Notes on a Conversational Practice: Formulating Place'. In: D. Sudnow (ed.) **Studies in Social Interaction.** New York/London, 1972.
Schouten, J.A.M. (1982). **Anamnese en advies : nieuwe richtlijnen voor de informatie-uitwisseling tussen arts en patient.** Alphen aan de Rijn.
Schulte, D. (1974). Ein Schema für Diagnose und Therapieplanung in der Verhaltenstherapie. In: D. Schulte (ed.) **Diagnostik in der Verhaltenstherapie.** München, 1974.

Schwitalla, J. (1979). **Dialogsteuerung in Interviews.** München.

Schwitalla, J. (1979b). 'Nonresponsive Antworten'. **Deutsche Sprache** 7, pp. 193-211.

Scully, D. (1980). **Men Who Control Women's Health.** Boston.

Scully, D. & Bart, P. (1973). 'A Funny Thing Happened on the Way to the Orifice: Women in Gynecological Textbooks'. **American Journal of Sociology** 78, pp. 1045-1050.

Seaman, B. & Seaman, G. (1977). **Women and the Crisis in Sex Hormones.** New York.

Searle, J. (1969). **Speech Acts.** Cambridge.

Searle, J. (1975). 'Indirect Speech Acts'. In: P. Cole & J.L. Morgan (eds.) **Syntax and Semantics 3: Speech Acts.** New York.

Searle, J.R. (1976). 'A Classification of Illocutionary Acts'. **Language in Society** 5, pp. 1-23.

Sexton, M. (1976). **Acceptance, Defiance and Backing Down in a Psychiatric Interview.** MA paper, Department of Linguistics & Modern English Language. University of Lancaster. Lancaster, (unpublished).

Siegrist, J. (ed.) (1978). **Arbeit und Interaktion im Krankenhaus.** Stuttgart.

Silverman, D. (1981). 'The Child as a Social Object: Down's Syndrome Children in a Paediatric Cardiology Clinic'. **Sociology of Health and Illness** 3, (3), pp. 254-274.

Sloan, D. et al. (1981). 'Risk of Myocardinal Infarction in Relation to Current and Discontinued Use of Oral Contraceptives'. **The New England Journal of Medicine** 302.

Smith, M.J. (1982). **Persuasion and Human Action.** Belmont, California.

Spence, J.T., Carson, R.C. & Thibaut, J.W. (eds.) (1976). **Behavioural Approaches to Therapy.** Morristown, New Jersey.

Sperber, H. (1955). 'Expressive Aspects of Political Language'. In: H. Werner & B. Kaplan (eds.) **On Expressive Language. Papers presented at the Clark University Conference** on Expressive Language Behavior. Worcester, Massachusetts.

Springorum, Th. P.A.F. (1982). **Dialoogstructuur. Een onderzoek naar structuuraspecten van directiefdialogen.** Nijmegen.

Stappers, J.G. (1983). 'Mass Communication as Public Communication'. **The Journal of Communication** 33, (3), pp. 141-145.

Stevens, R. (1971). **American Medicine and the Public Inte-**

rest. New Haven.

Streeck, J. (1980). 'Speech Acts in Interaction: A Critique of Searle'. **Discourse Processes** 3, pp. 133-154.

Strong, P.M. (1979). **The Ceremonial Order of the Clinic**. London.

Stubbs, M. (1973). **Discourse Analysis**. Oxford.

Sudnow, D. (ed.) (1972). **Studies in Social Interaction**. New York.

Tannen, D. (ed.) (1982). **Analyzing Discourse: Text and Talk**. Washington D.C.

Tannen, D. & Wallat, C. (1982). Interactive Frames and Knowledge Structure Schemas in Interaction: Examples from a Pediatric Examination. (mimeo). Paper prepared for US-France Joint Seminar on Natural Language Comprehension. St. Paul les Durances France.

Taylor, P.W. (1975). **Normative Discourse**. Westport, Connecticut.

Terasaki, A.K. (1976). 'Pre-Announcement Sequences in Conversation'. **Social Sciences Working Paper 99**.

Thomas, J. (1983b). 'Cross-Cultural Pragmatic Failure'. In: **Applied Linguistics** 4, (2), pp. 91-112.

Thomas, J. (1983c). 'Cross-Cultural Discourse as Unequal Encounter'. (mimeo). Department of Linguistics and Modern English Language: University of Lancaster. Lancaster.

Todd, A.D. (1982). The Medicalization of Reproduction: Scientific Medicine and the Diseasing of Healthy Women. San Diego, (unpublished).

Todd, A.D. (1982). Doctor-patient Discourse in the Prescription of Contraception to Women. (mimeo). Paper presented to the International sociological association meetings. Mexico City, 1982.

Todd, A.D. (1983a). 'A Diagnosis of Doctor-Patient Discourse in the Prescription of Contraception'. In: S. Fisher & A.D. Todd. (eds.) **The Social Organization of Doctor-Patient Communication**. Washington-D.C.

Todd, A.D. (1983b). 'Women's Bodies as Diseased and Deviant: Historical and Contemporary Issues'. In: S. Spitzer & R. Simon (eds.) **Research in Law Deviance and Social Control**. JAI-Press.

Todd, A.D. (1984). 'The Prescription of Contraception: Negotiations between Doctors and Patients'. **Discourse Processes** 7, pp. 171-200.

Touw-Otten, F. & Verbeek-Heida, P. (1980). 'Hulpzoekend en

ziektegedrag'. In: C.W. Aakster& G. Kuiper (eds.) **Leerboek Medische Sociologie. Sociale wetenschappen toegepast in de gezondheidszorg.** Groningen, 1978, pp. 237-247.

Turner, R. (1972). 'Some Formal Properties of Therapy Talk'. In: D. Sudnow (ed.) **Studies in Social Interaction.** New York.

Vanoye, F. (1973). **Expression, Communication.** Paris.

Wagner, K.R. (1978) **Sprechplanung. Empirie, Theorie und Didaktik der Sprecherstrategieen.** Frankfurt.

Waitzkin, H. & Stoekle, J.D. (1976). 'Information Control and the Micropolitics of Health Care: Summary of an Ongoing Research Subject'. **Social Science and Medicine** 10, pp. 263-276.

Waitzkin, H.B. & Waterman, B. (1974). **The Exploitation of Illness in Capitalist Society.** Indianapolis.

Wells, G. (ed.) (1981). **Learning through Interaction.** Cambridge.

Weiss, E. & English, O.S. (1944). **Psychomatic Medicine. The Clinical Application of Psycho-Pathology to General Medical Problems.** Philadelphia.

Werlich, E. (1975). **Typologie der Texte. Entwurf eines textlinguistischen Modells zur Grundlegung einer Textgrammatik.** Heidelberg.

Werner, H. & Kaplan, B. (eds.) (1955). **On Expressive Language. Papers presented at the Clark University Conference on Expressive Language Behaviour.** Worcester, Massachusetts.

Wertz, R.W. & Wertz, D.C. (1981). 'Notes on the Decline of Midwives and the Rise of Medical Obstetricans'. In: P. Conrad & R. Kern (eds.) **The Sociology of Health and Illness.** New York.

West, C. (1982). 'When the Doctor is a Lady: Power, Status and Gender in Physician-Patients Conversations'. In: A. Stromberg (ed.) **Women, Health and Medicine.** Palo Alto.

West, C. (1983). 'Ask Me No Questions ... An Analysis of Queries and Replies in Physician-Patient Dialogue'. In: S. Fisher & A. Todd (eds.) **The Social Organization of Doctor-Patient Communication.** Washington, D.C.

West, C. (1984). 'Medical Misfires: Mishearings, Misgivings, and Misunderstandings in Physician-Patient Dialogues'. **Discourse Analysis** 7, pp. 107-113.

White, G.M. & Robillard, A.B. (1982). Doctor Talk and Hawaiian "Talk Story". (mimeo). Paper presented to the International sociological association meetings. Mexico City, 1982.

Winkler, A.C. & McCuen, J.R. (1978). **Rhetoric made Plain.** New York.

Winston, P.H. (ed.) (1975). **The Psychology of Computer Vision.** New York.

Wodak, R. & Craen. P. van de (eds.) (1985) **Highways and Byways in Communication Disorders.** Clevedon, Avon.

Woods, P. & Hammersley, M. (eds.) (1977). **School Experiences.** London.

Wykes, T. (1980). 'Editorial, Language and Schizophrenia'. **Psychological Medicine 10**, pp. 403-406.

Yates, S. et al. (eds.) (1982). **A Manual of Cross Cultural Training.** **National Centre for Industrial Language Training.** Southall UK.

Zappen, M. (1980). Carl Rogers and Political Rhetoric. **Pre/Text 1**, (1-2), pp. 95-115.

Zee, H. van der (1979). **Het vraaggesprek als instrument bij praktijkonderzoek. Leren door te vragen: hoe doe je dat?** Meppel.

Contributors

M.Bax
Nederlands Instituut, Rijksuniversiteit Groningen
Grote Kruisstraat 2-1
9712 TS Groningen, The Netherlands

J.Berenst
Nederlands Instituut, Rijksuniversiteit Groningen
Grote Kruisstraat 2-1
9712 TS Groningen, The Netherlands

A. van Berkel
Nederlands Instituut, Rijksuniversiteit Groningen
Grote Kruisstraat 2-1
9712 TS Groningen, The Netherlands

D. van Bijsterveld
Psychiatrisch Ziekenhuis Endegeest, A-gebouw
Endegeesterstraatweg 5
2342 AJ Oegstgeest, The Netherlands

E.G.Bormann
Department of Speech Communication, University of Minnesota
317 Folwell Hall
9 Pleasant St. S.E.
Minneapolis, Minnesota 55455, U.S.A.

C.N.Candlin
Department of Linguistics and Modern English Language,
University of Lancaster
Bailrigg, Lancaster
England LA14YT

F. van Eemeren
Instituut voor Neerlandistiek, Universiteit van Amsterdam
Spuistraat 134
1012 VB Amsterdam, The Netherlands

T.Ensink
Nederlands Instituut, Rijksuniversiteit Groningen
Grote Kruisstraat 2-1
9712 TS Groningen, The Netherlands

H.Ettema
Instituut voor Klinische Psychologie, Rijksuniversiteit Groningen
Turfsingel 46
9712 KR Groningen

A.J.van Essen
Instituut voor Toegepaste Taalkunde, Rijksuniversiteit Groningen
Grote Kruisstraat 2-1
9712 TS Groningen

M.Fahrenfort
Faculteit der Geneeskunde, Vrije Universiteit Amsterdam
Vakgroep Gedragswetenschappen
Postbus 7161
1007 MC Amsterdam, The Netherlands

D.Fehlenberg
Sonderforschungsbereich 129, Universität Ulm
Am Hochsträss 8
D-7900 Ulm, West-Germany

S.Fisher
Wesleyan University
Department of Sociology
Middletown, Connecticut 06457, U.S.A.

D.Franck
Instituut voor Algemene Literatuurwetenschap, Universiteit van Amsterdam
Spuistraat 210
1012 VT Amsterdam, The Netherlands

T.van der Geest
Nederlands Instituut, Rijksuniversiteit Groningen
Grote Kruisstraat 2-1
9712 TS Groningen, The Netherlands

R.Grootendorst
Instituut voor Neerlandistiek, Universiteit van Amsterdam
Spuistraat 134
1012 VB Amsterdam, The Netherlands

P.ten Have
Sociologisch Instituut, Universiteit van Amsterdam
Oude Hoogstraat 24
1012 CE Amsterdam, The Netherlands

H.Houtkoop-Steenstra
Subfaculteit Letteren i.o., Katholieke Hogeschool Tilburg
Postbus 90153
5000 LE Tilburg, The Netherlands

W. and T. Labov
University of Pennsylvania
Department of Linguistics
Room 619 Williams Hall CU
Philadelphia 19104, U.S.A.

P. van Lint
Nederlands Instituut, Rijksuniversiteit Groningen
Grote Kruisstraat 2-1
9712 TS Groningen, The Netherlands

J. Lucas
University of Hawaii at Manoa
Hawaii, U.S.A.

J. Schwitalla
Institut für Deutsche Sprache, Sitz Mannheim
Postfach 5409
D 6800 Mannheim 1, West-Germany

Th. Springorum
Instituut Nederlands, Katholieke Universiteit Nijmegen
Erasmusplein 1
6525 HT Nijmegen, The Netherlands

J.G.Stappers
Instituut voor Massacommunicatie, Katholieke Universiteit Nijmegen
Postbus 9108
6500 HK Nijmegen, The Netherlands

A. D. Todd
Suffolk University
Boston, MA, U.S.A.